# Sustainable Diets.

How can huge populations be fed healthily, equitably and affordably while maintaining the ecosystems on which life depends? The evidence of diet's impact on public health and the environment has grown in recent decades, yet changing food supply, consumer habits and economic aspirations proves hard.

This book explores what is meant by sustainable diets and why this has to be the goal for the Anthropocene, the current era in which human activities are driving the mismatch of humans and the planet. Food production and consumption are key drivers of transitions already underway, yet policy makers hesitate to reshape public eating habits and tackle the unsustainability of the global food system.

The authors propose a multi-criteria approach to sustainable diets, giving equal weight to nutrition and public health, the environment, socio-cultural issues, food quality, economics and governance. This six-pronged approach to sustainable diets brings order and rationality to what either is seen as too complex to handle or is addressed simplistically and ineffectually. The book provides a major overview of this vibrant issue of interdisciplinary and public interest. It outlines the reasons for concern and how actors throughout the food system (governments, producers, civil society and consumers) must engage with (un)sustainable diets.

**Pamela Mason** took her first degree in pharmacy and then studied nutrition, gaining an MSc and a PhD in nutrition from King's College London, UK. She has an MSc in food policy from City University of London, UK. She is a registered public health nutritionist with the UK Association for Nutrition. She works with local food networks in Monmouthshire, South Wales.

**Tim Lang** is Professor of Food Policy at the Centre for Food Policy, City University of London, UK. He founded the Centre for Food Policy in 1994 and was Director until 2016. He is co-author of *Food Wars* (2015), *The Unmanageable Consumer* (2015), *Ecological Public Health* (2012) and *Food Policy* (2009). He is policy co-lead on the EAT-Lancet Commission on Healthy Diets from Sustainable Food Systems (2016–17).

# Sustainable Diets

## How Ecological Nutrition Can Transform Consumption and the Food System

# Pamela Mason and Tim Lang

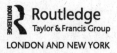

Routledge
Taylor & Francis Group
LONDON AND NEW YORK

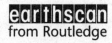

earthscan
from Routledge

First published 2017
by Routledge
2 Park Square, Milton Park, Abingdon, Oxon OX14 4RN

and by Routledge
711 Third Avenue, New York, NY 10017

*Routledge is an imprint of the Taylor & Francis Group, an informa business*

© 2017 Pamela Mason and Tim Lang

*British Library Cataloguing-in-Publication Data*
A catalogue record for this book is available from the British Library

*Library of Congress Cataloging-in-Publication Data*
A catalog record for this book has been requested

ISBN: 978-0-415-74470-6 (hbk)
ISBN: 978-0-415-74472-0 (pbk)
ISBN: 978-1-315-80293-0 (ebk)

Typeset in Goudy
by Swales & Willis Ltd, Exeter, Devon, UK

# Contents

# Figures

# Tables

# Acknowledgements

No book is ever written by the author(s) alone. When writing one draws on hundreds, often thousands, of other people directly and indirectly. This book is no exception. We have tried to cite people and organisations wherever possible. But some people have been directly helpful to us, as we wrote, answering queries, providing quick summaries, pointing us to data or papers, and simply providing encouragement! Others have simply been inspiration. We thank all the following for their varied input to our thinking over the years this book has been germinating: Mark Ainsbury, Tony Allan, Thomas Allen, Annie Anderson, Marta Antonelli, David Baldock, David Barling, Mike Barry, Mark Barthel, Tim Benton, Laura Blake, Rosie Boycott, João Breda, Francesco Branca, Chris Brown, Gianluca Brunori, Barbara Burlingame, Geoffrey Cannon, Martin Caraher, Annika Carlsson-Kanyama, Mike Childs, Kate Clancy, Charlie Clutterbuck, Bruce Cogill, Sandro Dernini, Sue Dibb, Jane Dixon, Corné van Dooren, Liz Dowler, Marielle Dubbeling, Gareth Edwards-Jones (RIP), Florence Egal, Sara Eppel, Jessica Fanzo, Kate Flanagan, Carl Folke, Harriet Friedmann, Émile Frison, Anthony Froggatt, Yiannis Gabriel, Tara Garnett, Joan Dye Gussow, Michael Hamm, Peter Harper, Corinna Hawkes, Michael Heasman, Colin Hines, Arjen Hoekstra, Ingrid Hoffmann, John Ingram, Michael Jacobson, Phil James, Jørgen Jensen, Tim Johns, Andy Jones, Hugh Joseph, Ingrid Keller, Unni Kjaernes, Niels Heine Kristensen, Geoff Lawrence, Mark Lawrence, Claus Leitzmann, Jennie MacDiarmid, Jim Mann, Terry Marsden, Phil McMichael, Tony McMichael (RIP), John Middleton, Erik Millstone, Carlos Monteiro, Kevin Morgan, Donal Murphy-Bokern, Miriam Nelson, Marion Nestle, Danielle Nierenberg, Kaare Norum, Clare Oxborrow, Carlo Petrini, Michael Pollan, Barry Popkin, Jonathan Porritt, John Roy Porter, Jules Pretty, Geof Rayner, Shivani Reddy, Lucia Reisch, Pete Ritchie, Johan Rockström, Luca Ruini, Sergio Schneider, Olivier De Schutter, Barb Seed, Lindy Sharpe, Vaclav Smil, Pete Smith, Roberta Soninno, Gunhild Stordalen, Tristram Stuart, Geoff Tansey, Ann Thrupp, Bill Vorley, Mark Wahlquvist, James Walton, Alan Warde, Steve Wiggins, Walter Willett, Duncan Williamson and Jon Woolven. We have also received great inspiration from the wonderful work since 2006 by Tara Garnett and the Food Climate Research Network, and more recently the EAT-Lancet Commission (2016–17) and the Stockholm Resilience Centre. We are also grateful for the support and input from colleagues at City, University of London's Centre for Food Policy and the Food Research Collaboration, the inter-University UK collaboration with civil society: Mary Atkinson, Victoria Schoen, Nadia Barbu, Talvinder Sehmbi, and the researchers and colleagues who contribute to that. We thank too all the wonderfully active and questioning researchers who are at or pass through or taught at the Centre for Food Policy. Our thanks too to the many people engaged with sustainable diets in civil society, public health and environmental movements around the world, such as Consumers International, Chatham House, the Sustainable Consumption Institute, and the UK's Sustain and Eating Better. We also salute all those engaged in this agenda from whom we have learned, in Sweden, Australia, France, Germany, the Netherlands, the UK and USA. Any failings in the text or analysis are ours not theirs.

We have also been served well by the team at Routledge – Tim Hardwick, Ashley Wright and all the Swales & Willis infrastructure crew who get scripts to book form. We are grateful not least for their patience, civility, humour and professionalism.

Finally, we want to thank Ambrose Mason and Liz Castledine (the latter also for her watercolours for the cover). They have been wonderful in their support and encouragement, almost beyond belief.

We started this book in a United Kingdom but completed it when the UK had narrowly and fractiously voted to leave the European Union, from which huge amounts of its food came. And then President Trump was elected in the USA. Such shifts are reminders of how food systems are part of the wider political economy. The necessity for the transition to sustainable diets is unlikely to fade, however. We therefore sign this from our particular British regions, just in case the political fragmentation continues. Whether it does or does not (we hope the latter), the issue of sustainable diets will demand attention. We are heartened that so many scientists, academics, analysts and food campaigners now know this, although politicians lag somewhat. That the scale of the task is immense must not deter us, nor deflect our resolve to help societies to face what needs to be faced.

Pamela Mason, Usk, Monmouthshire, Wales
Tim Lang, London, England
January 2017

# Acronyms and abbreviations

| | |
|---|---|
| ADD | average Danish diet |
| AHEI | Alternative Healthy Eating Index |
| AI | adequate intake |
| AMR | antimicrobial resistance |
| AOC | *Appellation d'Origine Controlée* (French designation) |
| APEC | Asia-Pacific Economic Corporation |
| ASEAN | Association of South East Asian Nations |
| BII | Biodiversity Intactness Index |
| BMI | body mass index |
| bn | billion |
| BOP | back of pack (labelling) |
| BSE | bovine spongiform encephalopathy |
| BSI | British Standards Institute (linked to ISO) |
| BST | bovine somatotrophin |
| CAFO | Concentrated Animal Feeding Operations |
| CAP | Common Agricultural Policy |
| CBD | Convention on Biological Diversity |
| CCC | Committee on Climate Change |
| CDC | Centers for Disease Control and Prevention (USA) |
| CGIAR | Consultative Group on International Agricultural Research |
| CHD | coronary heart disease |
| CIHEAM | Centre international de hautes études agronomiques méditerranéennes |
| CINE | Centre for Indigenous Peoples' Nutrition and Environment |
| CIWF | Compassion in World Farming |
| CO$_2$e | carbon dioxide (CO$_2$) equivalent |
| Codex | Codex Alimentarius Commission (joint WHO/FAO body) |
| COROS | Common Objectives and Requirements of Organic Standards |
| CPI | Consumer Price Index |
| CSIRO | Commonwealth and Scientific Research Organisation |
| CVD | cardiovascular disease |
| DASH | Dietary Approaches to Stop Hypertension diet |
| DDS | Dietary Diversity Score |

| | |
|---|---|
| Defra | Department for Environment, Food and Rural Affairs (UK) |
| DFID | Department for International Development |
| DGA | Dietary Guidelines for Americans |
| DRV | dietary reference value |
| EAR | estimated average requirement |
| EFCOVAL | European Food Consumption Validation Project |
| EFSA | European Food Safety Authority |
| EIPRO | Environmental Impact of PROducts |
| EPIC | European Prospective Investigation into Cancer and Nutrition |
| ERS | Economic Research Service of the USDA |
| ETI | Ethical Trade Initiative |
| EU | European Union |
| EUFIC | European Food Information Council |
| FAO | Food and Agriculture Organization (of the UN) |
| FAWC | Farm Animal Welfare Council (UK) |
| FBDG | food-based dietary guidelines |
| FCA | full cost accounting (an approach to cost externalised impacts) |
| FCRN | Food Climate Research Network |
| FDA | Food and Drug Administration (USA) |
| FIES | Food Insecurity Experience Scale (of the UN) |
| FP | front of pack (labelling) |
| FPPP | Food Purchasing Power Parity |
| FSA | Food Standards Agency (UK) |
| FUSIONS | Food Use for Social Innovation by Optimising Waste Prevention Strategies |
| GAP | good agricultural practice |
| GATT | General Agreement on Tariffs and Trade |
| GDA | Guideline Daily Amounts |
| GDP | gross domestic product |
| GEF | Global Environment Facility |
| GHG | greenhouse gases |
| GHGEs | greenhouse gas emissions |
| GIS | geographical information system |
| GLOBIO | Global Methodology for Mapping Human Impacts on the Biosphere |
| GM | genetic modification |
| GMO | genetically modified organism |
| GNP | gross national product |
| HACCP | Hazards Analysis Critical Control Point |
| HANCI | Hunger and Nutrition Commitment Index |
| HDI | Healthy Diet Indicator |
| HDDS | Household Dietary Diversity Score |
| HDL | high-density lipoprotein |
| HEI | Healthy Eating Index |

| | |
|---|---|
| HIV/AIDS | human immunodeficiency virus infection and acquired immune deficiency syndrome |
| IACFO | International Association of Consumer Food Organizations |
| ICN | International Conference on Nutrition (1992) |
| ICN2 | International Conference on Nutrition (2014) |
| IFAD | International Fund for Agriculture |
| IFOAM | International Federation of Organic Agriculture Movements |
| IFPRI | International Food Policy Research Institute |
| IGD | Institute of Grocery Distribution |
| ILO | International Labour Organization |
| IMF | International Monetary Fund |
| IPCC | Intergovernmental Panel on Climate Change (UN advisors) |
| IPES-Food | International Panel of Experts on Sustainable Food Systems |
| ISO | International Standards Organisation |
| kcal | kilocalorie (nutritional energy) |
| kg | kilo (weight) |
| LCA | life-cycle analysis |
| LDL | low-density lipoprotein |
| LEAF | Linking Environment and Farming (an assurance scheme) |
| LIDNS | Low Income Diet and Nutrition Survey (UK) |
| LPI | Living Planet Index |
| MDI | Marine Depletion Index |
| MPI | multidimensional poverty index |
| MRSA | methicillin-resistant staphylococcus aureus |
| MSA | Mean Species Abundance |
| mt | metric tonne |
| MTI | Marine Trophic Index |
| NAFTA | North American Free Trade Agreement |
| NCD | non-communicable disease |
| NDNS | National Diet and Nutrition Survey (UK) |
| NEF | New Economics Foundation |
| NGO | non-governmental organisation |
| NHANES | National Health and Nutrition Examination Survey (of the USA) |
| NHNS | National Health and Nutrition Survey (Japan) |
| NIOSH | National Institute for Occupational Safety and Health |
| NND | new Nordic diet |
| NNR | Nordic Nutritional Recommendations |
| ODI | Overseas Development Institute |
| OECD | Organisation for Economic Co-operation and Development |
| OIE | World Organisation for Animal Health (*Office International des Épizooties*) |
| ONS | Office for National Statistics (of the UK) |
| PANDiet | an index of probability of adequate nutrient intake (24 nutrients) |

| | |
|---|---|
| PAS | Publically Available Standard (of the BSI) |
| PBL | Netherlands Environmental Assessment Agency |
| PCB | polychlorinated biphenyl (a chlorine compound) |
| PDO | Protected Designation of Origin |
| PGI | Protected Geographical Indication |
| POPs | persistent organic pollutants |
| PPP | public–private partnership |
| QALY | quality adjusted life year |
| RCT | randomised controlled trial |
| RDA | recommended dietary allowance |
| RN | reactive nitrogen |
| RSPCA | Royal Society for the Prevention of Cruelty to Animals |
| RUAF | Resource Centres on Urban Agriculture and Food Security |
| RUMA | Responsible Use of Medicines in Agriculture Alliance |
| SCC | somatic cell count |
| SDC | Sustainable Development Commission |
| SDG | Sustainable Development Goals (of the UN) |
| SETAC | Society of Environmental Toxicology and Chemistry |
| SHDB | Social Hotspots Database |
| SNAP | US Supplemental Nutrition Assistance Programme |
| TCDD | 2,3,7,8-Tetrachlorodibenzodioxin |
| TRA | Theory of Reasoned Action |
| trn | trillion |
| TTIP | Transatlantic Trade and Investment Partnership |
| UK | United Kingdom |
| UN | United Nations |
| UNCTAD | United Nations Conference on Trade and Development |
| UNEP | United Nations Environment Programme |
| UNEP-WCMC | World Conservation Monitoring Centre |
| UNESCO | United Nations Educational, Scientific and Cultural Organization |
| UNICEF | United Nations Children's Fund |
| US | United States (of America) |
| USA | United States of America |
| USD | US dollars |
| USDA | United States Department of Agriculture |
| WBCSD | World Business Council for Sustainable Development |
| WCRF | World Cancer Research Fund |
| WHO | World Health Organization (of the United Nations) |
| WRAP | Waste Resources Action Programme (UK) |
| WRI | World Resources Institute |
| WTO | World Trade Organization |
| WWF | World Wide Fund for Nature |

# Introduction
## What's the problem?

### Contents

## Introduction

Our motive for writing this book was to map and broaden discussion about the issue of sustainable diets. This has been one of those issues which simmer on the policy back-burner and are tussled over by cognoscenti but don't exactly hit the headlines. It's been around for decades, quietly gathering interest, but has still not received sufficient high-level, let alone mass, attention. Yet what could be more important than the nature, quality and sufficiency of diet for the planet?

For years there has been growing disquiet about the sustainability of food systems as they are over-reliant on oil, wasteful and polluting the environment, but it took the rapid growth of obesity to grab attention in the 2000s. A tension surfaced between health focus and environmental concerns. Alongside these, the long-standing question about how to feed the world's population raised murkier questions about population and global inequalities. This complex mix of food-related problems seemed to make politicians nervous.

Then, seemingly overnight, when oil prices doubled in 2007–8 and raised food prices, the issue of diet momentarily had some traction among leaders of the developed world. They were shocked that their interests, their food prices and their voters might be affected. But these concerns were mostly then channelled into production rather than consumption considerations – given a strong steer by agricultural-oriented scientists understandably frustrated at being marginalised for decades. Just produce more food to get things back on track, they urged.

The debate then became centred on the food quantities needed in the future to feed growing populations rather than what the optimum diets should be to improve health and well-being in the first place. It was assumed that consumption looks after itself. Of course, one needs to consider food production and the viability of supply chains, but surely these ought to be shaped by the goal of producing a good diet? Could one say what a good diet is for the twenty-first century? Dietary guidelines for human health have been developed worldwide for many years at the national level, and with a degree of consensus, but attention on what a sustainable diet looks like is newer, although the question has been asked.[1]

The good news given in this book is that there are today even more data, evidence and ideas than there were when the rich world momentarily nervously caught its breath. Indeed, there is ample work on which to draw. This book tries to do justice to that body of knowledge. There was and still is strong evidence about current distortions in consumption and their effects on health, ecosystems and food cultures. And there are rich ideas on what a sustainable diet means.

Our motives for the book are a mix of the personal, professional and public. We have each been intrigued by the need to clarify how food and sustainability and health are addressed for decades. In different ways we have been involved in the growing interest in sustainable diets across the sciences, from nutrition to the social sciences. But the issue of sustainability of diet is not a private matter. If you, the reader, or we, the writers, ate a low carbon diet tomorrow and for the rest of our lives, it makes little difference unless such changes occur at the population level. Sustainability is partly personal but, most importantly, it is also public and planetary-wide. We are not alone in our interest in the public implications of deciding what type of diet is appropriate, in what proportions of different foods and how much to eat. Indeed, one of the pleasures of writing this book has been the opportunity to acknowledge the great work of hundreds of scientists, academics and policy analysts who have come to see this issue of the sustainability of diets as one of the key issues for our times. Dietary sustainability depends on understanding how to feed huge populations equitably, healthily and in ways that maintain the ecosystems on which humanity depends. This book grapples with the immensity of this challenge for the twenty-first century.

Food and diet are increasingly linked to tough challenges: under-nutrition alongside malnutrition and obesity; safety alongside nutrition concerns; climate change alongside water scarcity, soil erosion and biodiversity loss; food waste alongside global poverty. Many rural livelihoods worldwide depend on the food system yet increasing numbers of food producers are threatened from loss of land, changes in weather and poor remuneration. In the wake of welfare cuts, food banks have become among the fastest growing charities in rich countries. All these issues are reflective of a food system that is against many indicators unsustainable.

Though there is increasing scientific and academic agreement on these sustainability challenges for the food system, responses to date have been inadequate to meet the scale of the challenge. We think that there are several reasons for this. First, changes in consumer behaviour and food consumption will be needed, with the need to shift the dietary balance to one with a higher proportion of plant foods relative to animal foods, challenging the right of the consumer to choose and raising questions about concepts of progress and food as we have known them since the middle of the twentieth century. Given food's huge challenges, can we really eat what we like? Is choice the pre-eminent principle which politicians and industry say it is?

Second, achieving a coherent set of messages to policy makers and the public has not been helped by different perspectives and interests being voiced by diverse disciplines and stakeholders. It would help, we argue in this book, if there was an attempt to chart common ground. We try to do just that. The involvement of nutrition scientists in sustainable diets is essential but we particularly salute those who are engaging with environmental impacts. Most interest has been shown in the impact of diet on energy and greenhouse gases,[2] and in the synergies between a healthy diet and an environmentally friendly diet.[1, 3] Engagement of nutrition with other aspects of sustainable diet such as social and economic impacts has been more limited. Nutrition science in recent decades has been dominated by an intellectual focus on the nutritional content of food at the expense of how and why the food arrived on the consumer's plate. Some in the health sciences, too, see sustainable diet as a potential deviation from the non-communicable diseases (NCDs) such as obesity, cardiovascular disease, diabetes and cancers. But a good diet, of course, requires these diseases to be tackled just as much as food safety. Also, how can we separate diet from the troubling evidence about antimicrobial resistance from profligate and routine use of antibiotics on livestock as well as humans? This surely makes the case for a rethink of the connection between consumption and production, and the role of agricultural and veterinary sciences and their professions. Engineering is another source of knowledge competing for attention, which ought to be encouraged to sing from a new sustainable diet 'hymn sheet'. It brings vital involvement in resource management and technological solutions. The social sciences, meanwhile, are concerned about human behaviour and how social mores and cultural norms shape what people like to eat. The economists, too, can bring important insights into the limitations of monetary analysis in tackling human welfare. These different perspectives collectively could sing more in harmony. Too often in the past there has been policy cacophony, discordant voices vying for influence, each arguing that their research questions, their use and their interpretations are the right ones. This simply means that the 'solutions' proposed talk at cross purposes, and justify policy makers and the public retreating to the status quo. Business-as-usual wins.

Third, part of the reason for trying to chart a potential common ground on sustainable diets is to push governments and any social forces with leverage to make stronger commitments on sustainable diet. Some sort of guidance on sustainable dietary choices for consumers has come in recent years from governmental organisations in Germany,[4] Sweden,[5] France[6] and the Netherlands,[7, 8] but these initiatives lost momentum following the advent of the Eurozone fiscal crisis. Also, as we show later in the book (Chapter 8), the rational appeal of sustainable diets does not mean they are received positively.

Let us give an example from our own country, the UK. In 2008–9, the UK's Sustainable Development Commission (SDC), on which one of us (TL) was a commissioner, published a review of academic research and expert reports, concluding that there was sufficient coherence to guide the formulation of sustainable dietary guidelines, with benefits for UK consumers from eating a more plant-based diet and eating less overall.[9] However, this expert body was closed down in 2011 by the 2010–15 UK Coalition Government. The baton passed to civil society in the UK and it was WWF, a conservation organisation, which commissioned research on healthy and environmentally sustainable diets from the Rowett Institute of Nutrition and Health at Aberdeen University, published as the pioneering Livewell report.[10] Then the UK's lead food ministry again picked up the baton, but only temporarily. The Defra Green Project's Sustainable Consumption working groups endorsed the need for sustainable diet and sketched draft principles for healthy, sustainable diets.[11] After that for some years, there was silence, and then on March 17, 2016 Public Health England altered the Eatwell plate to advise UK consumers to 'eat less red and processed meat' (www.gov.uk/government/publications/the-eatwell-guide). This little tale illustrates much about sustainable diets: a mix of crabby, reluctant progress, steps forward and backwards, some triumphs, lots of hard work but not big enough a shift. Yet!

Some people argue that issues of diet should be left to market forces. There already is interest in sustainable diets from some quarters of industry.[12, 13, 14] Industry research groups study how industry can meet nutrition and sustainability objectives.[15] But can individual companies resolve world food systems problems? Although we think that industry has a key role to play, there is a need for independent modelling of sustainable diets to create the vision, provide policy coherence and focus the political will.

Despite these huge challenges and complexities, we are hopeful that transition to sustainable diets can take place. Dietary change is not new. Big changes in diet took place in the twentieth century, partly in response to industrialisation. But there is now need for leadership, a unified vision and policy coherence on food consumption. Rayner and Lang's 'ecological public health' approach provides one such framework. This views health as a function of ecological relationships, a web of connections between humans, planet and society.[16] The perspective taken on sustainable diets in the book is informed by that. Progress is dependent on how political processes manage four domains of existence: the material (the environment), the physiological (biological processes), the social (human interaction) and the cognitive or life-world (cognition and culture).

The ecological public health perspective does not see these dimensions as separate, but as strands which should be integrated, woven and bound together to create the framework for a diet that is green, healthy and fair for the long term. This approach helps break down barriers between nutrition and environment, food safety and plentiful food supply, quantity and quality, production and consumption. A good food system is seen as one that creates the conditions to meet all these goals and one that does not prioritise short-term gains over long-term losses. In reality, the current food system is doing the opposite. It mines resources and fails to protect the means for future generations to eat well. Ecological public health could, in our view, be an intellectual framework for sustainable diets, but there are other perspectives available too, and we do our best to cover those wherever appropriate. The book is amply referenced to enable readers to pursue these other lines of thought. And each chapter begins with a core argument short summary.

## Outline of the book

Chapter 1 introduces the terrain and key ideas explored in this book. It outlines what is meant by the notions of sustainable diets and sustainability. We introduce the need to pose questions about what is a good diet and a good food system.. We dissect the terms 'sustainability' and 'sustainable diet'. We introduce the framework employed to structure the book. It builds on work begun by the UK Sustainable Development Commission in 2009.[9] This proposed six core headings or clusters for food and sustainability: environment (from climate change to biodiversity and soil); health (nutrition, food safety, access and availability); social values (culture, animal welfare); quality (taste, authenticity); economy (affordability, labour, prices); and governance (systems of decision-making). These are summarised.

Chapter 2 presents a review of existing metrics and methods such as life-cycle analysis, the measurement of carbon, water and nitrogen footprints, and various existing dietary health measures. It recognises that there will not be movement on sustainable diets unless there is good measurement to help target-setting and audits.

Chapters 3–8 then evaluate the impact of diet on the six headings we use to operationalise what is meant by 'sustainable' in sustainable diets. These six headings are fundamental to how we have addressed the complexities in the body of knowledge, and are how the book is structured. They are: health and nutrition (Chapter 3); environment (Chapter 4); social values (Chapter 5); quality (Chapter 6); economy (Chapter 7); and governance (Chapter 8). Chapters 3–8 follow a broadly similar format: posing the problems, while providing a review of the evidence and weaving in any solutions or policy responses, while taking a critical stance on how adequate these are.

Chapter 9 summarises the case made in Chapters 1–8 for conceptualising sustainable diets. It reviews definitions of a sustainable diet and evaluates formulations developed to date by governments, business and civil society. The chapter also explores whether the pursuit of sustainable dietary guidelines can fit the UN's Sustainable Development Goals in what we call an $SDG^2$ strategy – sustainable diet guidelines to deliver sustainable development goals.

# References

1  Harland J, Buttriss J, Gibson S. Achieving Eatwell plate recommendations: is this a route to improving both sustainability and healthy eating? *Nutrition Bulletin*, 2012; 37(4): 324–43

2  Macdiarmid JI, Kyle J, Horgan GW, *et al*. Sustainable diets for the future: can we contribute to reducing greenhouse gas emissions by eating a healthy diet? *The American Journal of Clinical Nutrition*, 2012; 96(3): 632–9

3  Macdiarmid JI. Is a healthy diet an environmentally sustainable diet? *Proceedings of the Nutrition Society*, 2013; 1(1): 1–8

4  German Council for Sustainable Development. *The Sustainable Shopping Basket: a Guide to Better Shopping* (3rd Ed.). Berlin: German Council for Sustainable Development, 2008

5  National Food Administration Sweden's Environmental Protection Agency. *Environmentally Effective Food Choices: Proposal Notified to the EU*, 15 May. Stockholm: National Food Administration and Swedish Environmental Protection Agency, 2009

6  Agence de l'Environnement et de la Maîtrise de l'Energie (France). *Espace Ecocitoyens: Alimentation; 2012*. Available at: www.ecocitoyens.ademe.fr/mes-achats/bienacheter/alimentation (accessed October 6, 2012), 2012

7  Minister of Agriculture, Nature and Food Quality. *The Policy Document on Sustainable Food: Towards Sustainable Production and Consumption of Food*. Den Hag: Ministry of Agriculture, Nature and Food Quality, 2008

8  Health Council of the Netherlands. *Guidelines for a Healthy Diet: the Ecological Perspective*. The Hague: Health Council of the Netherlands, 2011

9  Reddy S, Lang T, Dibb S. *Setting the Table: Advice to Government on Priority Elements of Sustainable Diets*. London: Sustainable Development Commission. Available at: www.sd-commission.org.uk/publications.php?id=1033 (accessed October 18, 2013), 2009

10  WWF-UK in collaboration with the Rowett Research Institute of Nutrition and Health University of Aberdeen. *Livewell: a Balance of Healthy and Sustainable Food Choices*. Available at: http://assets.wwf.org.uk/downloads/livewell_report_jan11.pdf (accessed August 6, 2016), 2011

11  Defra. *Sustainable Consumption Report: Follow-Up to the Green Food Project*, July. Available at: https://www.gov.uk/government/publications/sustainable-consumption-report-follow-up-to-the-green-food-project (accessed October 19, 2013), 2013

12  Barilla Center for Food and Nutrition. *2011 Double Pyramid: Healthy Food for People, Sustainable for the Planet*. Available at: www.barillacfn.com/uploads/file/99.en_PositionPaper-BarillaCFN_DP.pdf 2011 (accessed August 6, 2016)

13  Unilever. *Sustainable Living Plan 2010*. London: Unilever PLC. Available at: www.sustainable-living.unilever.com/the-plan/ (accessed October 7, 2013), 2010

14  Pepsico. *Performance with Purpose*. Available at: www.pepsico.co.uk/purpose (accessed October 12, 2013), 2010

15  Institute of Grocery Distribution (IGD). *Sustainable Diets*. Available at: www.igd.com/sustainablediets (accessed October 12, 2013), 2013

16  Lang T, Rayner G. Ecological public health: the 21st century's big idea? An essay by Tim Lang and Geof Rayner. *BMJ*, 2012; 345

# Chapter 1

# Sustainable diets
## Welcome to the arguments

## Contents

## Core arguments

This chapter introduces the terrain and key ideas explored in this book. It outlines what is meant by the notions of sustainable diets and sustainability, and describes the practical and conceptual problems of sustainability and food. We introduce some key debates and problems. Not everyone favours exploration of sustainable diets. Some question whether it matters, others whether sustainable diets are possible, and there are serious discussions about how and whether human health and environmental health conflict or coincide. The chapter sets out the framework for the book. It summarises the conventional approach to sustainability as being about three overlapping concerns – environment, society and economy. Instead, we propose that food requires a more subtle and complex combination of factors, arguing that sustainable food and diets can usefully be viewed under six broad headings: quality, health, environment, social values, economy and governance. These headings form the structure for this book and, after a look at indicators, are addressed in turn in Chapters 3–8.

## Sustainable diets: both a practical and conceptual problem?

This is a book about sustainable diets or sustainable eating. This simple two-word phrase – sustainable diet – has become associated with a variety of meanings. The word 'sustainability' is tricky enough. It means different things to different people. It entered everyday and policy language in the 1980s to provide a different set of criteria by which human activity could be judged, and mainly to try to achieve a better alignment of environmental, economic and societal goals. In common parlance the word came to refer to living in a manner that is environmentally benign. The meaning narrowed in common usage to refer to the capacity of the environment (or what is often now referred to as 'ecosystems') to maintain humanity. Yet the wider meaning remains crucial. Even if people want to use the word 'sustainable' only to mean the environmental, they have also to consider how other factors impinge on the environment. In practice sustainability can be highly contested, as this book shows. Sustainability in food and diets can be interpreted in either a soft or hard way. One could choose a meal, for example, and claim that this or that feature is environmentally sound or that it is slightly healthier than normal (implying some sacrifice on what would be ideal or normal). Or, on the other hand, one could be rigorous and only eat a total diet across a month or year measured as being low fat, low sugar, low salt, low carbon, low impact everything. The soft version implies minor choice change. The harder version could be made to sound like a culinary hair shirt. Yet both versions could lay claim to being sustainable. Also, both versions have to draw upon other factors than the environment such as culture, cost, values, production, social norms and more. This book explores what is entailed if whole societies really want to eat more sustainably.

What about the 'diet' word? And food? While people mostly think they know what is meant by food or diets, these too can mean different things. Food is nutrients and is essential for the maintenance of human life, but humans are not the only species that eat. Food sits in a web of relationships both human and non-human: plants, climate, animals, insects – the web of life in a Darwinian sense. Diet and food also have cultural meanings. What people eat varies by social class, ethnicity, culture, income, history, aspiration and occasion. Feast-day diets are exceptional. But what if any society starts to eat feast-day diets everyday? This change of dietary pattern is precisely what happened in the twentieth century in the rich world, and it has spread around the world rapidly with economic development in the twenty-first century. This dietary shift or nutrition transition, as it is called, has got to the point where the rich world eats as though there are multiple planets, and yet its diet is seen as optimal – feast-day food on most days.

The word 'diet' is not just a matter of the food. Like the environment, the word 'diet' carries baggage and its reality is shaped by socio-cultural pressure such as human preferences, availability, normality, cost, moral values. What you like to eat might not be what others like and vice versa. Diets are more complex than the simplicity of the word implies. The word refers to the total intake of foods across a period of time. It is more than a meal; it's a sequence and even a lifetime of meals, a total dietary intake and pattern. In that respect, diet is about normality, habits, acculturation, what people eat conventionally across a year or their full lifespan. Seen in that way, as social scientists and nutritionists all agree, trying to capture what a diet is at the population level requires considerable tracking of data. A snapshot of one meal or one day may not convey the longer term shifts in dietary patterns. That is why longitudinal studies are so interesting and important for policy makers.

What happens if these two deceptively simple terms – sustainable + diet – are put together as 'sustainable diet'? The complexities multiply. If scientists want to measure the sustainability of diet in the USA or Europe, can they use the same indicators as in Africa, India or China? Also, is a sustainable diet the same in the USA or Europe as in Africa, India or China? Doesn't what people eat make a difference to any evaluation? And what about cultural, economic or terrain differences? We should note, too, that sometimes the phrase is used in the singular 'sustainable diet', sometimes in the plural 'sustainable diets'; in this book we use both.

The term is often used to refer to both health and environment, and to encapsulate the multiple goals of eating well for human health, in a manner that causes least environmental damage or, at best, even promotes environmental resilience, and that meets other socio-economic and cultural goals. But what does health imply and what is environmental resilience? As we show in these pages, the exploration of how food links human health with environment raises complex challenges for terminology and theory, for practicality and policy, for production and consumption, for people and the planet. Health and well-being are not just purely physiological or contextual matters. They are social, cultural, economic and policy constructs. Sustainable diet is a broad, perhaps even loose, term that signifies all this. That is why this book argues that, if the term is to be retained, consumers, producers and policy makers all need to recognise that it is more than just health + environment. As we argue in the following chapters, even if one does seek only to focus on health and environment, other values and considerations creep in. One cannot understand 'the environment' without bringing in the economy, culture and more. It is arbitrary and narrow, moreover, to restrict 'health' to the purely physiological because, for example, bodily functions are framed by social location, life chances, culture and history.

Before you, the reader, cast the book aside, thinking that this is a study in philosophy or epistemology (the theory of knowledge), and that the clarification of sustainable diets is impossible, let us assure you that the purpose of the book is to unpick some of the complexity and looseness to get at the practical matters that need to be addressed. We do this throughout, but especially in the final chapters. We also propose a simple but pragmatic template for 'sustainability', which enables you – whether your interest is the pursuit of better eating or better policy or supply – to think practically about how to reduce impact and improve prospects. The six headings we use to investigate sustainable diets are a useful heuristic for everyday life. A sustainable diet is one that optimises good sound food quality, health, environment, socio-cultural values, economy and governance.

On these fronts the evidence from science is becoming overwhelming and clear. The good news is that the academics are offering some broad pointers as to what a sustainable diet is and must be. The bad news is that this poses some tricky problems for policy makers and some food industries, particularly associated with meat and dairy and highly processed foods. It also poses a challenge to consumers who are highly divided globally and over- and mal-consuming in the West while under-consuming in low-income countries. Food culture is awry. Consumers eat only partially aware of the consequences. The strength of evidence on all this is why academics are becoming firmer in their advice. There is agreement within the natural and social sciences concerned with food that the twenty-first-century food system is in a troubled state, and that the consequences of not changing course are serious. What humanity eats has major impacts on public health, the economy, the environment and the future. The economic model of farm and food develop-ment pursued over the last half century might foster aspirations to eat like a North American or European but, if this continues, the implications will be even more devastating for biodiversity, climate change, land use, food availability, public health, and much more. The prognoses are troubling and can no longer be ignored.

Far from being banished as a problem area, as the post-Second World War food policy planners hoped, food has returned as a major worry in the twenty-first century. Yet the twentieth century seemed such a success; never was the growth of food production more successful and the capacity to feed more mouths more enthusiastically pursued. Defeat was being snatched from the jaws of victory. The massive outpouring of food sought by policy makers for centuries – and delivered by policy makers, scientists and farmers from the mid-twentieth century – had created a new mass era of diet-related non-communicable disease: heart diseases, strokes, obesity, diabetes, etc. These are now collectively the major cause of pre-mature death globally. Also, coinciding with this self-inflicted policy wound, was mounting evidence that food was a major – and in some measures the major – factor in environmental degradation. Prime, ancient biodiverse forests, for instance, were being bulldozed in the last and present centuries to produce hundreds of thousands of hectares of soya to feed to pigs or, elsewhere, massive plantations of palm for palm oil – all for unnecessarily highly processed foods, often high in salt, sugar and fats.

As such evidence emerged, it was relayed and played out in public forums and the world's media, championed by civil society and science. The twentieth-century success now needed to be re-evaluated. Thus the simple questions that drive this book surfaced: what is a good diet? What should people eat? Indeed, is it possible to eat well for both environmental and bodily health? Can this be done in a culturally acceptable manner? If so, does this mean eating sparsely? Is it afford-able by all? Must fun and social pleasure be sacrificed on the altar of environmental resilience? Does a sustainable diet mean eating minimally? These are real questions with which growing numbers of scientists and policy analysts began to engage in the new millennium. But change is still elusive or not at sufficient scale. One theme of the book, therefore, is to explore what stops the transition to sustainable diets.

Before we expand on this problem, let us be clear that such complexity is not wholly new for the world of food. Food has been both a problem and a pleasure for humans since time immemorial. What has changed recently is the form this combination takes, the reasons for change, the urgency of the evidence, and the stubbornness of current drivers and dynamics going in contrary directions. That's why the term 'sustainable diet' began to take on a totemic value. It stood for a different path for progress. Instead of waste, excess, feast-day food every day, eating beyond planetary or health welfare and policy advice, could a different approach to population health and well-being be charted? Could this link human and planetary health? These questions are real daily challenges and also of fundamental importance at a population level. They can be immensely threatening to some sectoral interests with power in and influence over food systems and food policy. The sustainability or unsustainability of diets has implications that go to the heart of the definition of progress, development and the celebration of consumer choice. That is why we end the book addressing whether and how broad advice can be given at both population and individual levels.

Food is necessary for life. It motivates action. It gives meaning. It is both work and rest. It is the largest source of labour on the planet: 1.5 billion people are involved in primary growing or rearing of food. Their efforts and struggles to produce food for humanity is a theme throughout history. This history is peppered with both success and failure, sometimes at the same time in the same place. At one moment in history there are famines dislocating lives and causing premature death; the next moment, there is abundance and an era in which food can become a matter for art, leisure and display. Some people are fed while, alongside them, others experience malnutrition to the point of premature death. Some over-consume, while others under- or mal-consume.

If the picture of food today, as in the past, is full of paradoxes and contradictions, should people be surprised that sustainable diets is an issue of some complexity and some contestation? No. This is a normal situation for food policy matters. Indeed, the social history of food is one of constant change, variability and disruptions. Since modern humans emerged from their ancestral past around 400,000 years ago, food has been characterised by fluctuations of availability. Settled agriculture is estimated to have begun around 10,000 or 12,000 years ago and, as knowledge and techniques grew, the long struggle of humans to push back the effects of seasons, events, climate changes, wars and biological processes has been waged. Technical innovation replaced the Darwinian process of slow evolution. Humans had already discovered they could breed plants and animals, both of which were transported around the world in new trading routes and with migration (people take their seeds, not just goods, if they can). Civilisation generated scientific understanding. Societies borrowed, stole and bought foodways from each other.

In this sense, the modern problem of sustainable diets is a new phase in the long challenge of living within environmental circumstances, eating from what is available or can be made available. And yet, to take an overview of the academic literature in the 1990s and 2000s (up to the commodity price crisis of

2007–8), one could be forgiven for thinking that sustainable diets was a problem of minor significance, an issue of fringe importance. We profoundly disagree with that view. There is clear evidence of the need for diets and the food system to be calibrated to enable humans to live within environmental limits. This is not just a technical challenge but a cultural one. Societies have to meet multiple objectives – health, environment, social acceptability, pleasure, affordability, etc. – in different ways appropriate to their location and circumstance. One reason sustainable diets is such an important issue is that it punctures the twentieth-century myth – perhaps even a norm – that humans can eat what they like, when, and as much as they like with no consequences to anyone else except perhaps the individual consumer.

In truth, this is nonsense, a fantasy, and this book tries to summarise why diet and food are now such problems for public health, the environment, society, policy and the economy, and, historically, on such an unprecedented scale. The world's population has more overweight people from access to too much food than people thin from hunger. The pursuit, invention, marketing and sales of energy-dense processed foods now contributes to a distorted food system. Critics argue that the meat and dairy industries, for example, have turned domestic farm animals into short-life machines that are helped through life by antibiotics; semi-captive existences that emulate Thomas Hobbes' dictum about the lives of the British in 1651 – 'nasty, brutish and short'.[1] Food's role in environmental degradation is also, sadly, beyond dispute. The food system is implicated in climate change, water misuse and scarcity, loss of biodiversity, land use, soil erosion and waste. Yet more people eat, we stress again, in unprecedented numbers, and eat well, if by that is meant greater life expectancy, but rampant life inequalities are also being exacerbated by uneven access, poor availability and income disparities. Food is also hard work, often in poor conditions and out of sight. Hundreds of millions of people globally are badly paid or not paid at all for their food labour.

Governance is a problem for sustainable diets. By 'governance', we mean not just who takes decisions, but the processes, tone and style whereby frameworks of thinking and policy are set. Food is a matter of trust relationships not just control. Although the case for change is strong, there is reluctance by decision-makers to begin the processes of change. Why is this? And isn't the wide gap between evidence, policy and behaviour a recipe for trouble? If 'normality' is dislocated later, won't people later ask their leaders: why didn't you act? You knew but did nothing! To be fair to the politicians, they also were under pressure to deliver ever cheaper food. But herein lies a tricky political problem: modern economics downplays the true and full costs of food. Food may be cheap in a supermarket, but other bills are paid elsewhere; the full health, environmental and social costs are not included. Cheap food isn't cheap; extra costs lie elsewhere.

This, dear reader, is the sober critique of what civilisation has delivered to you in the name of food progress. It is not insurmountable, but there are tricky challenges. One is choice. Can people really eat what they like? Everyone likes to think so but the sustainable diet debate suggests that there are limits to how far this is true. That is why we share in this book the broad line that eating less (for the West) actually means eating differently and better.

## Sustainable diet as code for better consumption

Where has this discussion gone so far? In one sentence: sustainable diet is code for better consumption. The notion of sustainable diet proposes that a good diet for the twenty-first century is one that is health-enhancing, has a low environmental impact, is culturally appropriate and economically viable. Using a variety of indicators – land use, biodiversity loss, water use, climate change gas emissions, health, economic costs, etc. – this book summarises trends in world diet, showing that they are not in a sustainable direction. Why is this? Broadly, the position is that, for the last half century, a process of major change has occurred in what is produced, sold and consumed. This is all framed by a marketisation of the food system, encouraged by a consumerist ethic in which choice is god; this marks the triumph of neoliberal thinking.[2, 3] In this neoliberal world, a good food system has been characterised by the pursuit of surplus (beyond mere sufficiency), expanded choice (as individual rights), lower prices (via efficiency from mass production) and free flow of foods and goods (through market economics). This has been a remarkably influential policy package in the twentieth century. But now, data suggest that consumption patterns are in some respects out of sync with reality, having disproportionate impacts on biodiversity, health, culture, land use, water and other resources.[4] That is why there is now a need to reconfigure what is meant by a good diet for the twenty-first century.[5–13]

From the 1970s to today evidence mounted about modern food systems' impact on the environment, public health and social justice.[4, 14] This evidence did not just suddenly emerge. It came from observing the effects of decades of food systems change in farming through to consumer service industries. These changes were broadly popular; they lowered prices and increased the range of foods available. Industrialised agriculture – which has been estimated to feed about 30% of the world's population while most is 'hand to mouth' small-scale production[15] – has been hugely successful in facilitating vast quantities of highly processed foods and the emergence of mass-scale food retailers and food service companies. But this apparent success is now tarnished. Mass commodity production has led to a model of eating associated with 'Western' or affluent lifestyles. The world, not just an elite few nations, is going through the 'nutrition transition'.[16, 17] This refers to the process in which populations change from simpler diets, initially to a better range (because they can afford it), but then to mass consumption of foods high in fats, sugars and salt (because they are ubiquitous and cheap). This new abundance of pre-processed foods has reshaped culinary traditions in older rich societies and is in the process of doing the same in newly affluent middle income societies today. The result is a world with vastly more people overweight and obese (1.5 billion) than hungry (0.9 billion), and a mismatch of people, physiology, health and food economy that has created new complex forms of inequality and distortion, a toxic mix of over-, mal- and under-consumption. It is for this complex world that the term 'sustainable diet' is now also a code for change. Evidence for doing so comes from diverse starting points in science – health, climate change, land use, nutrient flows, water availability, and so on.[18] The debate about sustainable diet is thus part of a wider one on rethinking consumption. All of us must keep asking: what is a good diet and how can we get it in an era where we know eco-systems, human health and food production capacity are linked?[19, 20]

## The intellectual case for sustainable diets

The term 'sustainable diet' is usually traced back to papers by two US academics, Joan Dye Gussow and Kate Clancy of Columbia and Syracuse Universities who, in 1986, argued that nutrition education was too narrow and should engage with this wider discourse and outline new dietary guidelines.[21–23] The intellectual roots are in fact much older, arguably coalescing in the 1970s food policy reawakening that followed the first oil crisis, the early environmental movement, famines in the Sudan, Biafra and Bangladesh, with a sprinkling of input from the Western counter-cultural pursuit of simpler lives and anti-consumerism.[24] And the roots go even deeper, back into the Malthusian problem of food supplies within a finite world.[25] The span of thought, therefore, ranges from Malthusian demography and political economy to modern concerns about 'living within planetary limits', sustainable development and the oil-based approach to the food economy – all of which are discussed in later pages. This rich and wide range of sources impelled sustainable diets into serious policy discussion in the 2000s.[6, 13, 26–29] By 2010 the Food and Agriculture Organization (FAO) and Bioversity International (part of the UN-affiliated CGIAR, an agricultural research consortium) hosted a large scientific conference in Rome, which formulated the much-cited definition:

> Sustainable Diets are those diets with low environmental impacts which contribute to food and nutrition security and to healthy life for present and future generations. Sustainable diets are protective and respectful of biodiversity and ecosystems, culturally acceptable, accessible, economically fair and affordable; nutritionally adequate, safe and healthy; while optimizing natural and human resources.[10]

This definition, the production process of which was co-chaired at the FAO Rome headquarters by one of us (TL), implies a better alignment of consumption with eco-systems.[30] Who could be against that? In fact it coincided with a period of the gradual reassertion of business-as-usual food policies, after a few years of crisis thinking that had followed the 2007–8 commodity price spike. Developed economies had been destabilised by rocketing oil and food prices, so policy makers began to consider longer term analyses.[31] The data on food's high carbon, water, land use and biodiversity impact persuaded the G8, for example, that their food systems (not just Africa's or Asia's) faced considerable tensions.[32, 33] Models like that in Figure 1.1 began to surface. But this broader thinking faded and, by 2010–11, G8 had 'bought' the case that more food needed to be produced without troubling their consumers. Their macro-economic priorities were to rebuild consumer confidence while bailing out the financial system and cutting back the state to pay for it. Their policy focus was to reassert productionism. They ignored the academic analyses that power over land use and food now no longer resides with agriculture itself but with traders, processors, food service and retailers off the land. Productionism narrows the policy focus to farming when the modern food system is more than that. In the USA, the US Department of Agriculture estimates that farming only receives 17.2 cents of every dollar consumers spend on food.[34] In the UK, to give another rich society example, farming has just 4.6% of the value-added as food travels through a food chain on which the ultimate consumers (eaters) spent £201 billion in 2015, while caterers and retailers took 13% and 14% added-value respectively.[35] The latter sectors dwarf farming in employment too. In 2015, UK agriculture employed 476,000 people, compared with food manufacturing's 433,000 but retailing's 1,157,000 and catering's 1,658,000.

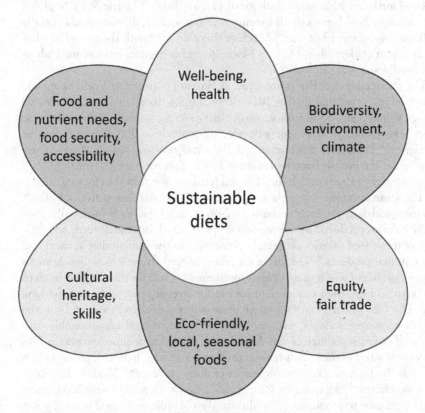

*Figure 1.1* The FAO-Bioversity International model of sustainable diets at the centre of multi-criteria sustainable food systems

Source: FAO and Biodiversity International, 2012.

The farm-oriented politicians also ignored the health toll from current dietary patterns as part of the picture. According to the World Health Organization (WHO), worldwide obesity has nearly doubled since 1980.[36] By 2008, more than 1.4 billion adults, 20 years old and above (35% of the world's population), were overweight. Of these, over 200 million men and nearly 300 million women were obese (11% of the world's population). Sixty-five per cent of the world's population live in countries where being overweight and obesity kills more people than being underweight. More than 40 million children under the age of five were overweight in 2011. Health problems from over-, under- and mal-consumption and non-communicable diseases now co-exist even in low-income countries.[37] Rates of death due to non-communicable diseases in sub-Saharan Africa, for instance, are predicted to rise 17% in the next decade.[38] The most recent global burden of disease review (an approach pioneered by WHO with the World Bank) summarised the effect of mal- and over-consumption as resulting in over 18 million deaths annually caused by different diet-related factors: high blood pressure (9.4 million), high body mass index (3.4 million), high fasting blood glucose (3.4 million) and high total cholesterol (2.0 million).[39] In the WHO's global assessment of health risks in all income levels of society, diet featured centrally in 10 out of the top 19 factors.[40] Much of this coincides with the spread of what the Brazilian epidemiologist Carlos Monteiro and colleagues have termed 'ultra-processed' foods and drinks.[41, 42]

The financial cost of this is immense. A Harvard University/World Economic Forum review estimated that in 2010–30 NCDs, i.e. those significantly affected by diet, would cost US$30 trillion, equivalent to 48% of global GDP in 2010, the effect being greater in low-income developing countries, a dire drag on economic 'efficiency'.[43] Alongside this human toll, the environmental impact of agriculture is immense. It currently contributes around 14% of greenhouse gas emissions.[44] Of these, animals are responsible for 31% and fertilisers for 38%.[45] In Europe, food is the European consumer's biggest source of greenhouse gas emissions (GHGEs),[46] and meat and dairy products account for 24% of their GHGEs.[46, 47] Globally, 36% of the calories produced by the world's crops are used for animal feed, and only 12% of those feed calories ultimately contribute to the human diet as meat and other animal products.[48] This drive for grains to feed animals as well as humans plays a significant role in destroying ecosystems.[49] It is little wonder that modern food systems have their immense impact in biodiversity loss, water use and land use.[4] The UN Millennium Ecosystem Assessment calculated that, of 24 of the world's ecosystem services, five are being degraded or used unsustainably, and that food is a major source of this degradation. Global agriculture consumes 70% of all fresh water extracted for human use[50] and intensive livestock production is probably the largest sector-specific source of water pollution.[44] Modern diets consume significant 'hidden' water; for instance, one Dutch study found 200 litres of water were used to produce a 200 millilitre glass of milk, and 2,400 litres of water to produce a 150-gram hamburger.[51] In the twentieth century as a whole, an estimated 75% of the genetic diversity of domestic agricultural crops inherited from the nineteenth century was lost.[52] At the same time there has been increasing concentration on particular crops.[53] By the end of the twentieth century, 12 plant species accounted for 75% of global food supply, and only 15 mammal and bird species accounted for 90% of animal agriculture.[54, 55] While nutrition guidelines worldwide encourage the consumption of fish and fish oil, FAO calculates that over half (52%) of global wild fish stocks are already 'fully exploited'.[56]

Overviews of data such as these have led more scientists to appeal for policy change, arguing that too many planetary boundaries have already been exceeded and others, such as the rate of biodiversity loss, the nitrogen cycle and climate change, are approaching those points.[57, 58] Meanwhile, never has so much food been produced in all human history, only to deliver unprecedented food waste. Two hundred and twenty million tonnes a year globally is wasted, equivalent to the total food production of sub-Saharan Africa.[59] In low-income countries, food waste occurs near the farm while consumers waste very little. In high-income countries, by contrast, consumers waste up to a third of what they buy.[59] In the European Union (EU), 89 million tonnes of food waste are generated each year, with a monetary value of about £950 (US$1,500) per tonne per household.[60] The EU rate of waste is growing such that, if not checked, it will be 126 million tonnes by 2020. Across the world, growing populations and changing dietary demands that follow from rising incomes in developing countries mean competing demands on land use for housing, fuel, food, water, wood and amenity everywhere.

The United Nations Environment Programme (UNEP) estimates that, even if more land is made available for food growing, only 0.2 hectares (1,970 m²) of crop-able land per person will be available by 2030.[61] Such figures have fuelled the intense debate about rising meat and dairy consumption, in particular, and about the inefficiency of feeding animals approximately half of all cereals grown globally.[62–64] The FAO took a major role in this with its 2007 Livestock's Long Shadow report showing animal husbandry's considerable environmental impact.[62] A 2013 report then proposed that, if all livestock management were to be as efficient as the best, those impacts could come down significantly.[65] But then it conceded that, if global consumption of meat and dairy continues to rise, all those efficiency gains would be neutralised. In short, whether policy makers like it or not, we have to talk about consumption. Burying our heads in the sand about sustainable diets is folly.

## Reactions to the case for sustainable diets

How have policy makers responded to the issue of sustainable diet? In Chapter 8 we set out the diversity of reactions from across the sectors in more depth, but meanwhile here we sketch eight different policy positions on sustainable diets. We give these now, to keep in mind as the book unfolds. They are the politics, as it were, of sustainable diets. Within organisations and sectors, there may be differences as to which is right, or to be supported.

One position questions whether the issue of sustainable diets can or should be tackled at all. Some say it is too complex. Others are frankly in denial. Climate change deniers see no problem in food's GHGEs; any blips are epi-phenomena or bias. The science is wrong, they say. Others downplay the rise of non-communicable diseases as consumers' self-inflicted harm, or not the responsibility of the state anyway. Still others argue that, even if there is a problem, the cost of tackling this all is simply too great, and that events must follow their course.[66] Others that this is nobody's interest but the consumer's. This category is the Old Guard in policy circles; fractious but influential (particularly since Mr Trump's election); unhappy even to consider the issue. Smoother adherents might smile sweetly, say soothing words, but walk away. Others might be overtly hostile. Collectively, it has the upper hand on the noisy rhetoric score.

A second position sees this all as a technical problem, one that can be addressed by technical solutions. The future lies with functional foods, nanotechnology, developing insects as a source of human food, the application of biotechnology or automation, or new controlled diets and agri-technology. It anticipates a big opportunity for business through technical fixes that basically leave the current business model intact.

The third says this is interesting but not the priority for food policy makers whose main task should be preventing and resolving hunger. This position sees sustainable diets as a deviation from the true moral path of twentieth-century food policy: to feed the poor. The worry is that sustainable diets might be a fig leaf for rich society protectionism. Here we are spreading Western diets and choice to the world, and suddenly this new elite view emerges which says 'don't eat as we have done'. The motives here are honourable; the objective of development is to feed the hungry and to do this with urgency, whether by raising incomes or applying technical fixes. This is a policy insider's position. They do not necessarily oppose the juxtaposition of health and environment as a food policy. It's just that there are other priorities.

The fourth position takes a different tack. This puts responsibility onto consumers, by promising (if not fully providing) tools for change. Leave it to consumers. If diets are unsustainable, consumers need to be made responsible for changing them. Put the details on food labels. There's no need for regulation; only use soft policy measures such as information. In 2007, for instance, the Carbon Trust, a UK government body set up to champion carbon reduction, experimented with giant snack manufacturers Walkers (part of Pepsico) and put a carbon label onto some products; others followed. The scheme met fierce criticism and Tesco, for one, withdrew in 2012.[67] Attention was by then focusing on helping companies to improve monitoring and carbon reduction across key products.[68-70] The carbon labelling experience is interesting. On the one hand it showed the limitations of labelling; no significant consumer behaviour change followed and the British continued to munch crisps (chips). On the other hand, it persuaded companies to audit their own carbon footprints more rigorously. But could a label really resolve sustainability? Only if it was huge and complex. And wouldn't a label require an auditing scheme, probably national or even international, something like the Nordic keyhole scheme, a national logo to signify sustainability? But this misses the point of sustainable diets which is not so much about individual products as the impact of the whole diet. Moreover, if there were to be labels for all the issues requiring consumer action, all foods would have to be packaged to carry the labels which would drown consumers in information overload. This would almost certainly meet opposition from sensitive brand owners, let alone not meeting the need to cut packaging waste. On the other hand, big investment in informatics would fuel this booming tech sector, and shopping would become nirvana for app-fiends.

The fifth response is for producers to act below the consumer radar and to choice-edit. 'Choice-editing' alters choice without giving the consumer the option to reverse how the choice is structured other than to purchase elsewhere.[71] This is change led by food companies; the restriction of choice without admitting it. It is what is currently adopted by those companies and advisors who are concerned about aspects of sustainability. Leave it to us; we'll sort out decarbonisation. One study of choice-editing in fish concluded that it is unlikely to be used when a company sees no added brand value from doing so.[72] The method most used in choice-editing is reformulation, changing the recipe, tweaking ingredients. This is corporate responsibility as change by stealth, not tackling consumer consciousness or choice reduction. It can be effective, but it does not rein in consumption. People can continue to eat more of a 'sustainable' product and their diets continue to be unsustainable.

The sixth response is to focus on one issue or 'magic bullet'. This is a reductionist approach which has, in part, been encouraged by some arguments within the sustainable diet discourse. Forget the complexity of sustainable diets, let's just focus on 'big hits'. Two hotspots have dominated attention: meat and dairy, and food waste. There is a strong case for rich societies to reduce their meat and dairy consumption,[73] which meets fierce farmer and meat trade opposition. Food waste, however, has wider apparent appeal.[60, 74, 75, 76] Who can be against waste reduction? In fact, there are important tensions about why there is waste and how to tackle it. Some waste campaigners see waste as systemic and as a case where rich consumers need to eat differently.[75] Others see it as an opportunity for engineering and managerial interventions to create new standards of technical efficiency.[77] Others see waste merely as an opportunity to generate biogas and to recycle.[78] The analysis varies, although the term 'waste' is common. In fact, it is all of these, and more. Estimates that reducing consumer food waste could save $300 billion yearly by 2030 add policy interest.[79]

The seventh policy position is an appeal not to dilute the health message with environmental concerns and to remain focused on health because that yields what's needed. This is a subtle position. It does not downplay the environment; rather it suggests that, broadly, if consumers in the developed world were to follow dominant health advice, their diet's environmental impact would fall, certainly with regard to greenhouse gases.[29, 80] One recent UK study shows that, if consumers followed WHO nutrition advice, their dietary greenhouse gas emissions would fall by 17%.[9] The implication is that there is no need to create specific sustainable dietary advice. To fuse dietary health and environmental advice into sustainable dietary guidelines (as Gussow and Clancy first suggested) is messy and a deviation. The problem with this policy position is that it misses the significance of culture and the importance of appealing to consumers to change their consumption norms. This is despite the fact that the nutrition transition is precisely what has fuelled the diet-related burden of ill-health: eating all day, switching from water or infusions to sugary soft drinks, eating snacks not meals, being bombarded by advertising messages, and so on. This is a policy position primarily directed at rich societies but may be of less relevance in low- or middle-income countries or, in richer countries, for low-income consumers.

An eighth position is to take sustainable diets seriously, to model them, to explore how the pursuit of sustainable diet is a useful policy goal for consumers, to see them as a vehicle that sends different signals back down the food supply chain and make it fit for the twenty-first century.[8, 28, 29, 81, 82] It accepts that markets are a matter of both production and consumption. It implies a redesign of food systems, land use and production, but debates how extensive this needs to be. This position too meets resistance (see Chapter 8). In 2015, for example, the US Government received formal advice, after a two-year process, to integrate health and environmental criteria into the new 2015 Dietary Guidelines for Americans.[83] This is the formal dietary advice which, in theory, should shape the US food system. The meat and farming industries were unhappy. The US Secretary of Agriculture poured scorn on the scientific advice, saying even his young grandson didn't need such advice. But then something surprising happened, an outpouring of public support for the advice to be both health and environmentally based. The formal consultation process was extended to 75 days,[84] with sceptics thinking this was to allow industry opponents to get more critical comments on to the record. If so, it backfired; 29,976 comments were logged, with a huge number favouring the linking of environment and human health. The comments make fascinating reading and show the value of 'open government'.[85] But still the integrated sustainable dietary advice was rejected by the US Secretaries of State for Agriculture and Health – and this was under President Obama. If ever proof was needed that sustainable diets can be politically charged, this was it (see Chapter 8 for other examples).

## The framework used in this book: six key headings

The notion of sustainability is often associated with the 1987 report of the World Commission on Environment and Development, usually known as the Brundtland report. This was chaired by Norway's first woman Prime Minister, Dr Gro Harlan Brundtland, later the Director General of the World Health Organization. The Brundtland report suggested the new policy framework for development should give equal and overlapping emphasis to the environment, society and economy. A focus on any one of these was not enough; none on its own would deliver security to future generations. Hence the report's much-cited definition:[86]

> Sustainable development is development that meets the needs of the present without compromising the ability of future generations to meet their own needs. It contains within it two key concepts:

the concept of needs, in particular the essential needs of the world's poor, to which overriding priority should be given; and

the idea of limitations imposed by the state of technology and social organization on the environment's ability to meet present and future needs.

(*Our Common Future: Report of the World Commission on Environment and Development*, page 43)

Admirable and influential though it is and was, the Brundtland triple focus does not quite fit the complexity that we have already shown is raised by the challenge of sustainability in either diets or the wider food system. Health is missing or not emphasised sufficiently, also true for important cultural dynamics such as quality, taste and social life. Can all these be covered under the heading of 'society'? Perhaps, but not with adequate detail, fit for policy implementation.

*Table 1.1* Sustainability as a complex set of 'omni-standards' or 'poly-values'

| Quality | Social values |
| --- | --- |
| Taste | Pleasure |
| Seasonality | Identity |
| Cosmetic | Religion |
| Fresh (where appropriate) | Animal welfare |
| Authenticity | Equality and justice |
| | Cultural appropriateness |
| | Skills (food citizenship) |

| Environment | Health |
| --- | --- |
| Climate change | Safety |
| Energy use | Nutrition |
| Water | Equal access |
| Land use | Availability |
| Soil | Social determinants of health, e.g. |
| Biodiversity | affordability |
| Waste reduction and circularity | Information and education |
| | Protection from marketing |

| Economy | Governance |
| --- | --- |
| Food security and resilience | Science and technology evidence base |
| Affordability (price) | Transparency |
| Efficiency | Democratic accountability |
| True competition | Ethical values (fairness) |
| Fair return to primary producers | International aid and development |
| Jobs and decent working | Trust |
| conditions | |
| Fully internalised costs | |
| Circular economy (full recycling) | |

Source: modified from SDC, 2011.[87]

To fill this gap and make a more realistic policy framework, tailored and appropriate for the challenge of food and sustainability, the UK's Sustainable Development Commission in 2011 proposed a six-point approach for policy makers, supply chains and consumers (see Table 1.1). This offered a more complex approach to food sustainability, which it termed an omni-standards or poly-values approach.

This six-heading framework is what we have used to structure this book. We think it is useful and provides sensible policy-relevant categories through which to view and address sustainable diets. Although the rest of the book provides much evidence (and references) for why these issues matter, in the following paragraphs we provide an introduction to what Table 1.1 means and why the issues itemised there are of significance for the subject of this book.

The issue of quality (top left in Table 1.1) is of fundamental importance in food and is addressed in Chapter 6. Food businesses battle over quality; they are often criticised for altering what consumers think of as quality – cosmetic or 'mouthfeel' appeal taking priority over nutritional quality or long-term impacts. For consumers, however, the notion of quality is paramount. People might differ in what they think quality is and how they interpret it but, whatever someone's culture, she or he will always prefer something tasty, something they like, something they judge to have the right characteristics. Quality is also about the eye; what the food looks like or how it smells can help or hinder sales. Seasonality is listed under quality because a food in season tastes better and is likely to be lower in embedded carbon than if it was long distance and trucked, shipped or flown.[88] If people want foods out of season – strawberries in mid-winter, for example – these will be lower in carbon if trucked from where they are still being grown in more benign climates. Local is not necessarily always the lowest in carbon. Nevertheless, when the Swedish Government's National Food Administration and Environmental Protection Agency produced their combined advice in 2008, they strongly recommended seasonality as a consumer principle.[89] We include freshness, not because it can always be delivered (particularly in countries with short growing seasons), but again because fresh foods often taste better. What can be better than a blackberry picked from a hedgerow or a wild bit of a park? Also, authenticity is included under quality, not as some elite notion but because, whatever their diets, people always want something they judge to be 'real'.

Chapter 5 addresses the importance of social values (top right in Table 1.1) in shaping food systems and what individual consumers eat. Consumers everywhere see food as pleasure, whether they are people suffering acute hunger or people who rarely think of food because it is so plentiful. Food and pleasure (and pain) are linked in ways that have fascinated social scientists. So is the fact that food expresses identity. The diet people eat indicates who they are, their aspirations, class, ethnicity and background. Food also raises opportunities for people to express values beyond themselves. Religious beliefs shape taste and frame what one thinks of as culturally appropriate. Hindus don't eat cow meat. Muslims only eat meat killed according to halal rules. Jews don't eat pork. Vegetarians, of course, make a conscious decision not to eat meat of any kind; some eat dairy products while vegans do not. Social values are invoked to give equal or even higher priority to animal welfare. Eating is an act that can either meet or flout principles of social justice and these vary according to your moral compass. It is also a matter of skills. What skills are needed for sustainable diets? Science to ensure standards, of course, but also domestic skills such as cooking. How food is cooked and where this is done (at home or in the factory) can shape its environmental and nutrient intake. A mass factory-cooked food is likely to be more energy efficient in its mode of cooking but might raise questions about control. This illustrates the problem of 'trade-offs' raised later.

The environment is, of course, of significance in any discussion of sustainable diet and food (see Chapter 4). Even recently, one could encounter people working in public health who saw the 'environment' as important but not their core responsibility. Such thinking has become less tenable with mounting evidence on climate change. In this book we range widely across environmental matters: climate change (it determines what grows), energy use (food is embedded energy and one of the major energy users on the planet), water (food is the single greatest water use on the planet), land use (where the vast majority of food is grown), the seas (fish are harvested; the seas are part of the planet's complex eco-system), soil (its status affects nutrient uptake in plants); biodiversity (food production is one of the greatest drivers of biodiversity destruction); and waste. This latter issue cuts across the whole book. One of the key rationales for the mid-twentieth-century revolution in food production, distribution and marketing – in which so much was altered about how food was grown, processed, sold and consumed – was that modernity would reduce waste. Pioneers of this revolution in food systems argued rightly that previous generations had been blighted by waste – bad storage and transportation. Technology would resolve and prevent this, they argued. Yet, by the early twenty-first century, evidence had emerged about vast and continuing waste. Consumers in rich countries like the USA and UK wasted up to a third or more of the food they purchased. In poorer societies food is more likely to be wasted near production; consumers see food as too important and expensive to waste.[59]

The relevance of health and nutrition for this book is self-evident and is covered in Chapter 3. It warrants its separate category in Table 1.1 because the main thinkers on sustainability have tended to see health as an outcome of other leading factors, rather than of primary importance in itself. In food, this is impossible to justify. There is little point in food unless it maintains and enhances public and intergenerational health and well-being. Nutrition is important but so too is safety. In low-income countries unsafe food and water are key determinants of infant mortality. Poor sanitation can retain and recycle pools of infection. Social factors also determine diet and health. Indeed, an entire school of thinking about public health analyses the 'social determinants' of health. Equality of access to food is one such determinant – one of the Five As: access, availability, affordability, attitudes and advertising. Unless people have access to food, its protective capacities are denied to them. Availability depends on food production and distribution systems.

So too does information and education. To economists these are prerequisites for the effective working of markets; efficiencies depend on consumers having access to knowledge about foods. But, in the real world, a vast flow of information is in the form of marketing and advertising. An issue raised by sustainable diets is where and how to revalidate information flows. How can consumers be better educated and be protected from misleading or distorting advertising?

The importance of economics in sustainability was always clear in Brundtland and is addressed in Chapter 7. The word 'economics' comes from the Greek *oikos* meaning 'house' and *nomos* meaning 'custom' or 'law'. Economics thus came to mean the 'rules of the house'. It had a domestic connotation. Early writers, indeed the eighteenth-century architects of what is meant by economics today, tended to see economics as a moral and political pursuit; the 'rules' of living are malleable; they represent political choices. However, economics, as a twentieth-century discipline, has become something different, trying to sever the political dimension and claiming value-neutrality. In this book we take the broader older view of economics. We look at food not just through the lens of cost, money and financial transactions, important though these are. We are interested in how food availability and some of the social values raised earlier are translated into financial and management systems. Thus our attention in the book is on matters such as food security and resilience, prices (whether they reflect the true and full costs), what is meant by efficiency and where the money goes in food systems. This last point is intriguing in that, throughout the twentieth century, the length of food supply chains grew. More and more people work in the food system off rather than on the land. Farming and growing may remain the world's largest employers by far but most money (profit and value-added) flows off the land. That is why the issue of true prices is such a hot issue for sustainable diets. Do food prices reflect the real cost of production and consumption? The evidence suggests they do not. So what is a fair return to each sector of the supply chain? This is clearly a political (and moral) question. Cheap food is not cheap if it's high in salt, sugar and fat and adds to the burden of non-communicable disease. Economists call this the externalisation of costs. Cheap food has costs dumped on society elsewhere – as healthcare costs, or environmental pollution or societal dislocation with its on-costs. Yet mass-produced, mass-marketed foods are frequently produced in conditions conventional economists think are efficient: factories churning out products in great quantities, thus lowering the price of each unit of food. In this situation, moral and political questions to consider about food economics include not just fair returns to primary producers (they grow the food, after all), but what are good jobs and decent working conditions. Food economics might be altered by attempting to combat waste, not just by preventing it and getting consumers to eat what they buy, but to recycle food 'waste' back into the nutrient cycle as part of what is called the 'circular economy'. A transition to sustainable diets could imply a wholesale economic restructuring, not least for the treatment of sewage (the final point of linear food supply chains) and the need to ensure that human waste (faeces and urine), rich in nutrients, can be safely returned to the soil to nurture future food growth.

All the above five headings bring us towards the sixth sector of the analytic framework used in this book: food governance (see Chapter 8). The word here, note, is not 'government' but 'governance'. This word is used to mean more than what government does, often taken to be making decisions and managing the strategic direction of society. Governance means something broader: how decisions are made, by whom, with what effect. It recognises that a range of actors apart from government is involved. It denotes style and process as well as substance. Under food governance we include the evidence base for decision-making. How good is the evidence? From which sciences? What technological and engineering assumptions are made? Is the governance 'transparent', namely open and clear and intelligible? Are the means of decision-making democratically accountable? When decisions are made, are there procedures to review, audit, recall and upgrade them? These questions are part of our framework because studies and experience have shown that food is a trust relationship. People buy and consume food in good faith. If the food looks OK, they'll eat it. But what if there are hidden bacteria and unknown effects? Food adulteration scandals throughout the ages show that people are furious if this happens. Questions raised about quality and adulteration in rich societies from the 1970s on, for instance, led to a powerful set of ethical questions, not least over animal welfare. Indeed, the ethics of food are now a key driver of the debate about sustainable food systems and of sustainable diets. Moral and ethical questions are raised by how people eat. If we eat a diet high in embedded carbon and water (i.e. much has been used to get the food to us), how does this affect others who eat less well? Our diets become international developmental issues. They are planetary and population issues, not just personal matters.

To conclude, this chapter has introduced the notion of sustainable diets. It has introduced the conceptual framework used in the book, the six headings summarised just above here. It has shown that sustainability, diet and food systems raise many questions, explored in more depth in the following chapters. The next turns to the issue of methods: how, why and when can the (un)sustainability of diets be measured? And do we need better indicators?

## References

1 Hobbes T, MacPherson Ce. *Leviathan*. London: Penguin Classics, 1981 [1651]
2 McMichael P. *The Global Restructuring of Agro-food Systems*. Ithaca; London: Cornell University Press, 1994
3 Goodman D, Watts MJ (Eds). *Globalising Food: Agrarian Questions and Global Restructuring*. London: Routledge, 1997
4 UNEP, Nellemann C, MacDevette M, *et al*. *The Environmental Food Crisis: The Environment's Role in Averting Future Food Crises. A UNEP Rapid Response Assessment*. Arendal, Norway: United Nations Environment Programme/GRID-Arendal, 2009
5 Garnett T. Food sustainability: problems, perspectives and solutions. *Proceedings of the Nutrition Society*, 2013; 72(1): 29–39

6  Garnett T. *What Is a Sustainable Diet? A Discussion Paper*. Oxford: Food & Climate Research Network, Oxford Martin School, University of Oxford, 2014: 31

7  Lang T, Barling D. Food security and food sustainability: reformulating the debate. *The Geographical Journal*, 2012; 178(4): 313–26

8  Carlsson-Kanyama A, Gonzalez AD. Potential contributions of food consumption patterns to climate change. *The American Journal of Clinical Nutrition*, 2009; 89 (Supplement): 1S–6S

9  Green R, Milner J, Dangour AD, *et al*. The potential to reduce greenhouse gas emissions in the UK through healthy and realistic dietary change. *Climatic Change*, 2015; 129(1–2): 253–65

10  Burlingame B, Dernini S (Eds). *Sustainable Diets and Biodiversity: Directions and Solutions for Policy, Research and Action*. Proceedings of the International Scientific Symposium 'Biodiversity and Sustainable Diets United against Hunger', 3–5 November 2010, FAO Headquarters, Rome. Rome: FAO and Bioversity International, 2012

11  Fanzo J, Cogill B, Mattei F. *Metrics of Sustainable Diets and Food Systems*. Rome: Bioversity International (CGIAR), 2012

12  Macdiarmid JI, Kyle J, Horgan GW, *et al*. Sustainable diets for the future: can we contribute to reducing greenhouse gas emissions by eating a healthy diet? *The American Journal of Clinical Nutrition*, 2012; 96(3): 632–9

13  van Dooren C, Marinussen M, Blonk H, *et al*. Exploring dietary guidelines based on ecological and nutritional values: a comparison of six dietary patterns. *Food Policy*, 2014; 44: 36–46

14  WHO. *World Health Report 2002: Reducing Risks, Promoting Healthy Life*. Geneva: World Health Organization, 2002

15  ETC. *Who Will Feed Us? Questions for the Food and Climate Crisis*. Ottawa: ETC Group, 2009: 31

16  Popkin B. *The World Is Fat: the Fads, Trends, Policies and Products That Are Fattening the Human Race*. New York: Avery/Penguin, 2009

17  Popkin BM. An overview on the nutrition transition and its health implications: the Bellagio meeting. *Public Health Nutrition*, 2002; 5(1A): 93–103

18  Millward DJ, Garnett T. Food and the planet: nutritional dilemmas of greenhouse gas emission reductions through reduced intakes of meat and dairy foods. *Proceedings of the Nutrition Society*, 2009; 69: 1–16

19  McMichael AJ. *Human Frontiers, Environment and Disease*. Cambridge: Cambridge University Press, 2001

20  Smith P. Delivering food security without increasing pressure on land. *Global Food Security*, 2, 2012

21  Gussow JD. Mediterranean diets: are they environmentally responsible? *American Journal of Clinical Nutrition*, 1995; 61(6 Suppl): 1383S–89S

22  Gussow JD, Clancy KL. Dietary guidelines for sustainability. *Journal of Nutrition Education*, 1986; 18(1): 1–5

23  Herrin M, Gussow JD. Designing a sustainable regional diet. *Journal of Nutrition Education*, 1989; 21(6): 270–5

24  Lang T, Barling D, Caraher M. *Food Policy: Integrating Health, Environment and Society*. Oxford: Oxford University Press, 2009

25  Malthus TR. *An Essay on the Principle of Population, as it affects the future improvement of society with remarks on the speculations of Mr. Godwin, M. Condorcet and other writers*. London: Printed for J. Johnson, 1798

26 Macdiarmid J. Is a healthy diet an environmentally sustainable diet? *Proceedings of the Nutrition Society*, 2012; 72(1): 13–20

27 Lang T, Barling D. Nutrition and sustainability: an emerging food policy discourse. *Proceedings of the Nutrition Society*, 2013; 72(1): 1–12

28 Carlsson-Kanyama A. Climate change and dietary choices: how can emissions of greenhouse gases from food consumption be reduced? *Food Policy*, 1998; 23(3/4): 277–93

29 Carlsson-Kanyama A, Ekström MP, Shanahan H. Food and life cycle energy inputs: consequences of diet and ways to increase efficiency. *Ecological Economics*, 2003; 44 (2–3): 293–307

30 FAO. *Final Document – International Scientific Symposium: Biodiversity and Sustainable Diets: 3–5 November 2010 – Definition of Sustainable Diets*. Rome: Food and Agriculture Organization. Available at: www.fao.org/ag/humannutrition/23781-0e8d8dc364ee46 865d5841c48976e9980.pdf (accessed February 12, 2016), 2010

31 OECD. *Agricultural Policies in OECD Countries: Monitoring and Evaluation*. Paris: Organisation for Economic Co-operation and Development, 2009

32 G8. *G8 Leaders Statement on Global Food Security*. Available at: www.whitehouse.gov/news/releases/2008/07/20080708-6.html (accessed February 12, 2016), 2008

33 G8. *'L'Aquila' Joint Statement on Global Food Security, L'Aquila Food Security Initiative (AFSI), 10 July 2009*. Rome: G8 Leaders. Available at: www.g8italia2009.it/G8_Allegato/LAquila_Joint_Statement_on_Global_Food_Security%5B1%5D,0.pdf (accessed February 12, 2016), 2009

34 USDA ERS. *Food Dollar* series. Washington, DC: United States Department of Agriculture Economic Research Services. Available at: www.ers.usda.gov/data-products/food-dollar-series/documentation.aspx (accessed February 12, 2016), 2015

35 Defra. *Agriculture in the UK 2015*. London: Department for Environment, Food and Rural Affairs, 2016

36 WHO. *Obesity and Overweight: Factsheet 311*. Geneva: World Health Organization, 2013

37 WHO. *Global Status Report on Noncommunicable Diseases, 2010*. Geneva: World Health Organization. Available at: www.who.int/nmh/publications/ncd_report2010/en/ (accessed April 15, 2016), 2011

38 Scott A, Ejikeme CS, Clottey EN, *et al.* Obesity in sub-Saharan Africa: development of an ecological theoretical framework. *Health Promotion International*, 2013; 28(1): 4–16

39 Moodie R, Stuckler D, Monteiro C, *et al.* Profits and pandemics: prevention of harmful effects of tobacco, alcohol, and ultra-processed food and drink industries. *The Lancet*, 2013; 381(9867): 670–9

40 WHO. *Global Health Risks: Mortality and Burden of Disease Attributable to Selected Major Risks*. Geneva: World Health Organization, 2009

41 Monteiro CA. Nutrition and health: the issue is not food, not nutrients, so much as processing. *Public Health Nutrition*, 2009; 12(5): 729–31

42 Monteiro CA, Levy RB, Claro RM, *et al.* Increasing consumption of ultra-processed foods and likely impact on human health: evidence from Brazil. *Public Health Nutrition*, 2011; 14(1): 5–13

43 Bloom DE, Cafiero ET, Jané-Llopis E, *et al.* *The Global Economic Burden of Noncommunicable Diseases*. Geneva: World Economic Forum and Harvard School of Public Health, 2011

44 UN. *World Economic and Social Survey 2011: The Great Green Technological Transformation*. New York: United Nations Department of Economic and Social

Affairs. Available at: www.un.org/en/development/desa/policy/wess/wess_current/ 2011wess.pdf (accessed April 15, 2016), 2011

45  Stern N. *The Stern Review of The Economics of Climate Change: Final Report*. London: HM Treasury, 2006

46  Tukker A, Huppes G, Guinée J, *et al*. *Environmental Impact of Products (EIPRO): Analysis of the Life Cycle Environmental Impacts Related to the Final Consumption of the EU-25. EUR 22284 EN*. Brussels: European Commission Joint Research Centre, 2006

47  Tukker A, Bausch-Goldbohm S, Verheijden M, *et al*. *Environmental Impacts of Diet Changes in the EU*. Seville: European Commission Joint Research Centre Institute for Prospective Technological Studies, 2009

48  Cassidy ES, West PC, Gerber JS, *et al*. Redefining agricultural yields: from tonnes to people nourished per hectare. *Environmental Research Letters*, 2013; 8: 034015

49  Millennium Ecosystem Assessment. *Ecosystems and Human Well-Being: Synthesis*. Washington, DC: Island Press, 2005

50  WWF. *Thirsty Crops: Our Food and Clothes: Eating Up Nature and Wearing Out the Environment?* Zeist (NL): WWF, 2006

51  Chapagain AK, Hoekstra AY. *Water Footprints of Nations, vols. 1 and 2*. UNESCO-IHE Value of Water Research Report Series No 16. Paris: UNESCO, 2006

52  FAO. *Dimensions of Need: An Atlas of Food and Agriculture*. Rome: Food and Agriculture Organization, 1995

53  Khoury CK, Bjorkman AD, Dempewolf H, *et al*. Increasing homogeneity in global food supplies and the implications for food security. *Proceedings of the National Academies of Science*, 2014; 111(1): 4001–6

54  FAO. *Women: Users, Preservers, and Managers of Agro-biodiversity*. Rome: Food and Agriculture Organization, 1998

55  FAO, Bioversity International. *Final Document: International Scientific Symposium: Biodiversity and Sustainable Diets – United against Hunger*. 3–5 November. Rome, Italy: Food and Agriculture Organization (FAO) Headquarters. Available at: www.eurofir.net/ sites/default/files/9th%20IFDC/FAO_Symposium_final_121110.pdf (accessed March 14, 2016), 2010.

56  FAO. *The State of World Fisheries and Aquaculture 2006*. Rome: Food and Agriculture Organization, 2007

57  Rockström J, Steffen W, Noone K, *et al*. Planetary boundaries: exploring the safe operating space for humanity. *Ecology and Society*, 2009; 14(2): 32. Available at: www. ecologyandsociety.org/vol14/iss2/art32/ (accessed March 20, 2011)

58  Rockström J, Steffen W, Noone K, *et al*. A safe operating space for humanity. *Nature*, 2009; 461(7263): 472–5

59  Gustavsson J, Cederberg C, Sonnesson U, *et al*. *Global Food Losses and Food Waste: Extent, Causes and Prevention*. Rome: Food and Agriculture Organization, 2011

60  House of Lords EU Committee. *Counting the Cost of Food Waste: EU Food Waste Prevention*. 10th Report of Session 2013–14. London: The Stationery Office, 2014

61  UNEP (Bringezu S, Pengue W, O'Brien M, Garcia F, Sims R, Howarth R, Kauppi L, Swilling M and Herrick J). *Assessing Global Land Use: Balancing Consumption With Sustainable Supply. A Report of the Working Group on Land and Soils of the International Resource Panel*. Nairobi: UN Environment Programme, 2014

62  Steinfeld H, Gerber P, Wassenaar T, *et al*. *Livestock's Long Shadow: Environmental Issues and Options*. Rome: Food and Agriculture Organization, 2006

63 UNCTAD. *Wake Up Before It Is Too Late: Trade and Environment Review 2013*. Geneva: UN Conference on Trade and Development, 2013: 341

64 Lymbery P, Oakeshott I. *Farmageddon: The True Cost of Cheap Meat*. London: Bloomsbury, 2014

65 Gerber PJ, Steinfeld H, Henderson B, *et al*. *Tackling Climate Change Through Livestock: A Global Assessment of Emissions and Mitigation Opportunities*. Rome: Food and Agriculture Organization, 2013

66 Dietz S, Stern N. Why economic analysis supports strong action on climate change: a response to the Stern Review's critics. *Review of Environmental Economics and Policy*, 2008; 2(1): 94–113

67 Quinn I. 'Frustrated' Tesco ditches eco-label. *The Grocer*. Available at: www.thegrocer. co.uk/channels/supermarkets/tesco/frustrated-tesco-ditches-eco-labels/225502.article (accessed February 18, 2016), 2012

68 Carbon Trust. *Carbon Trust Launches Carbon Reduction Label*. Press launch, 15 March. London: The Carbon Trust. Available at: www.carbontrust.co.uk/about/presscentre/ 160307_carbon_label.htm (accessed March 18, 2007), 2007

69 Carbon Trust. *Tesco and Carbon Trust Join Forces to Put Carbon Label on 20 Products*. London: Carbon Trust. Available at: www.carbontrust.co.uk/News/presscentre/29_04_ 08_Carbon_Label_Launch.htm (accessed June 3, 2008), 2008

70 Carbon Trust, Coca-Cola. *Personal Carbon Allowances White Paper: How to Help Consumer Make Informed Choices*. London: Carbon Trust Advisory and Coca-Cola plc, 2012

71 National Consumer Council, Sustainable Development Commission. *Looking Back Looking Forward: Lessons in Choice Editing for Sustainability: 19 Case Studies into Drivers and Barriers to Mainstreaming More Sustainable Products*. London: Sustainable Development Commission, 2006

72 Gunn M, Mont O. Choice editing as a retailers' tool for sustainable consumption. *International Journal of Retail & Distribution Management*, 2014; 42(6): 464–81

73 Audsley E, Brander M, Chatterton J, *et al*. *How Low Can We Go? An Assessment of Greenhouse Gas Emissions from the UK Food System and the Scope for Reduction by 2050*. Godalming, Surrey: FCRN and WWF, 2010

74 Lipinski B, Hanson C, Lomax J, *et al*. *Reducing Food Loss and Waste: Creating a Sustainable Food Future*. Washington, DC: World Resources Institute, 2013

75 Stuart T. *Waste: Uncovering the Global Food Scandal*. London: Penguin, 2009

76 European Commission DG Environment, AEA Energy & Environment, Umweltbundesamt. Preparatory Study on Food Waste across EU 27. Contract #: 07.03 07/2009/540024/SER/G4. Brussels: DG Environment. Directorate C Industry. Available at: http://ec.europa.eu/environment/eussd/pdf/bio_foodwaste_sum.pdf (accessed February 18, 2016), 2010

77 Institute of Mechanical Engineers. *Global Food: Waste Not Want Not*. London: Institute of Mechanical Engineers, 2013

78 Defra. *Reducing and Managing Waste: Anaerobic Digestion and Energy Recovery from Waste: Policy Statement*. London: Department for Environment, Food and Rural Affairs, 2013

79 Global Commission on Economy and Climate. *Final Report: Strategies to Achieve Economic and Environmental Gains by Reducing Food Waste*, report by WRAP for the Global Commission (New Climate Economy). Banbury, UK: WRAP and Global Commission on Economy and Climate, 2015

80  Sustainable Development Commission. *Setting the Table: Advice to Government on Priority Elements of Sustainable Diets*. London: Sustainable Development Commission, 2009

81  Smith P, Haberl H, Popp A, *et al.* How much land-based greenhouse gas mitigation can be achieved without compromising food security and environmental goals? *Global Change Biology*, 2013; 19(8): 2285–302

82  Blake L. *Zero Carbon Britain. People, Plate and Planet: The Impact of Dietary Choices on Health, Greenhouse Gas Emissions and Land Use*. Machynlleth: Centre for Alternative Technology, 2014

83  US Dietary Guidelines Advisory Committee. *Scientific Report of the 2015 Dietary Guidelines Advisory Committee to the Secretaries of the US Department of Health and Human Services and the US Department of Agriculture*. Washington, DC: US Department of Health & Human Services, 2015

84  Department of Health and Human Services. Solicitation of Written Comments on the Scientific Report of the 2015 Dietary Guidelines Advisory Committee; Extension of Comment Period. *Federal Register* 2015; 80(67): 18852

85  Department of Health and Human Services. Read Comments. Available at: http://health.gov/dietaryguidelines/dga2015/comments/readComments.aspx (accessed August 19, 2015). Washington, DC: Department of Health and Human Services, 2015

86  Brundtland GH. *Our Common Future: Report of the World Commission on Environment and Development (WCED)* chaired by Gro Harlem Brundtland. Oxford: Oxford University Press, 1987

87  Sustainable Development Commission. *Looking Forward, Looking Back: Sustainability and UK Food Policy 2000–2011*. Available at: www.sd-commission.org.uk/publications.php?id=1187 (accessed February 12, 2016). London: Sustainable Development Commission, 2011

88  Macdiarmid JI. Seasonality and dietary requirements: will eating seasonal food contribute to health and environmental sustainability? *Proceedings of the Nutrition Society* 2014; 73(3): 368–75

89  National Food Administration, Sweden's Environmental Protection Agency. *Environmentally Effective Food Choices: Proposal Notified to the EU*, 15 May. Stockholm: National Food Administration and Swedish Environmental Protection Agency, 2009

# Chapter 2

# Methodologies
Measuring what matters while not
drowning in complexity

## Contents

## Core arguments

Measurable, robust and verifiable indicators for sustainable diets are needed by policy makers, food companies, scientists and consumers themselves. There are and always will be gaps in understanding of what constitutes a sustainable diet for different populations and different contexts but this makes it all the more important to be able to measure progress over time. Measures and benchmarks are essential. Clarity is needed about how to assess what qualifies or quantifies a sustainable diet. This chapter identifies potential indicators for sustainable diets and methods to assess them with their associated advantages and disadvantages. It shows there are many methods already available, and a fast-growing body of knowledge, but they need to be pulled into a more coherent framework. The chapter reviews the range of methods and the many indicators available for public health and nutrition, environmental health, social and cultural considerations, food quality and economics. It concludes that, while some useful measures are available, additional indicators are always required. A number of major questions and themes are apparent in the development of appropriate methods and indicators: (a) is the best approach to generate multi-criteria and single composite indicators? (b) is a sustainable diet really just a healthy diet but produced from a sustainable food system? (c) does the sustainability of diets require qualitative data or will numerical quantitative approaches suffice? The chapter concludes that the issue of methods requires more attention but that the multi-criteria approach is probably the best route. It is why the book is structured around the SDC's six headings, summarised in Chapter 1.

## What is the point of indicators and measurement?

Methods and indicators are not the most immediately exciting of topics for ordinary consumers. Anyone beginning to be interested in sustainable diets might even be put off taking the issue seriously if discussion about methods became interminable. To debate such things might be loved by academics and scientists but can bore everyone else. So we begin this chapter by summarising why the matter of methods and indicators is actually both interesting and really important. We then sketch many types and methods.

Data matter. Indeed, we live in a society increasingly controlled by data. It's the era of Big Data – huge, unprecedented computer power enables consumers to be tracked. Every mood, every food choice can be filed and dissected to yield population patterns. Big food companies increasingly rely on Big Data. Knowledge is power. Vast research projects are now trying to build Big Data and then 'mine' it.[1-3] While companies collect consumer choice data to improve marketing and the sophistication of their methods for keeping food on the shelves, public agricultural and health scientists are actively exploring the ways in which they believe Big Data can help improve the lot of small farmers in Africa or knowledge sharing about health effects of diets.[3-6]

Consumers are on the data frontline in other respects, too. Apps are being offered to help them choose. Rightly so, as choice of foods and diets determines not just our own health and well-being but that of the planet and of our fellow human beings. So it is in consumers' own interest to know what is true and, just as importantly, what is not true about diet. They also need to know that sustainable diets is in the middle of this important battle over knowledge. Later chapters in this book document how issues that might appear to be common sense – looking after the environment or being civilised about how to eat – are in fact very sensitive. Releasing data can affect markets. So how the data are collected matters, which is why methods matter. Who collects information, how and for what reasons become really important elements of politics. This is why data collection is, today, cited in debates about civil liberties. The dystopias described by George Orwell or Aldous Huxley put the battles over information as both symbols and mechanisms of the new power. Also, data goes to the heart of what a modern democracy is. Freedom to speak, freedom to explore, freedom to choose . . . these are notions central to the long process of democratic expansion since the eighteenth century and to the Enlightenment itself, which promulgated knowledge from science. It matters, in short, who, how, when and where data are collected about food and eating, in general, and it certainly matters for sustainable diets.

The rest of the book gives ample information about why a growing body of evidence and opinion suggests that a good diet in the twenty-first century must be a sustainable diet. This chapter on methods and indicators is sited early in the book because we want to stress how important it is to be able to evaluate those deceptively simple words 'good' and 'sustainable'. There is no point a consumer plucking ideas out of thin air about what is sustainable. There are thousands of papers and years of thinking on which to draw that help sort the fads from the facts, the important from the unimportant, the big impact features from things that seem to matter but aren't actually that important.

Methods matter because they can be the gateway to creating, refining and using indicators of sustainable diets. While there has been an encouraging growth of good research into sustainable diets over the last 20 years, big questions and themes are yet to be addressed. One such question is whether sustainable diets inevitably require multiple indicators or whether it is possible that these could be fused into one. Is the dream to create one composite SustDietIndex? This becomes a debate between multi-criteria and single criteria measures.

Another theme is whether a sustainable diet is basically a healthy diet, with the 'sustainability' element simply being a matter of whether the means of production, distribution and consumption are sustainable. In short, is a sustainable diet simply a healthy one from a sustainable food supply chain? Or does a sustainable diet mean more than health? Different methods and indicators follow from each question.

Yet another question concerns whether the best methods for defining sustainability ought to be quantitative or whether there is a place for qualitative work? Philosophers, sociologists and even some psychologists might disagree that everything can be reduced to numbers. Food is a matter of values, ideas, concepts, they argue. A counter to this position is that researchers have already developed measures and indices on values; it is possible to quantify ethereal values, so why not do it for sustainable diets? The World Values Survey, for example, has plotted shifts in multiple values between and within countries over decades.[7]

The chapter therefore provides an overview of many different measures, indicators and methods, created by many organisations and researchers. In our view, what matters as we explore all this are the questions we have posed above: why measure? Who controls the data? What questions frame the methods and indicators? What use is made of them? How open are they?

With these philosophical questions in mind, we see the case for measurement and indicators as boiling down to the fact that they can:

- give precision to what is meant by 'good' and 'sustainable';
- help set clear goals and targets;
- measure progress towards definable goals and set key performance indicators;
- be of use to stakeholders in civil society, industry and government;
- aid decision-making processes;
- guide policy and programmes when data are incomplete;
- enable monitoring of outcomes and behaviour;
- help consumers choose wisely.

Measuring performance has become a widespread activity in modern societies and is the benchmark by which political and economic choices are regularly backed, audited and justified. Max Weber, the great German sociologist, argued that modern societies are characterised by the birth of bureaucracy as the triumph of the routinised, hierarchical, rational approach to social order.[8] The filing cabinet (it would now be the computer plus 'cloud') becomes the record and shows the pecking order of whose filing cabinet it is becomes the signifier of power. Data gives power, and societies seem to be moving towards ever more rationalised and bureaucratised forms. With such analyses in mind, to suggest that sustainable diets, too, should be measured and monitored raises supplementary but inextricably yoked questions: for whom and how and by whom? These questions are moral and political. But they go to the heart of the sustainable diet project. Could one imagine a society in which people were judged reprehensively if they did not eat sustainably? Possibly, in an Orwellian dystopian future. An argument in health insurance is that, if someone eats a poor diet, he or she ought perhaps to pay a higher insurance premium; poor diet is a self-administered added risk. Against that is the demographer's analysis that all populations will have a range of behaviours, so the best way to improve health is not to single out 'failing' individuals but to shift the fulcrum – or median – of the entire behaviour. This was the position articulated by Geoffrey Rose, the British epidemiologist.[9, 10] Since dietary choices are linked to socio-economic position and status, why get bogged down in whether 'choice' is really choice? Focus on shifting the entire population.

Such questions and arguments are reminders that numbers, methods and indicators are not value-neutral. It is quite easy to anticipate a benign use of measurement of sustainable diets too, to check up on availability, take-up, responsibilities, costs and impact. These would also be valuable for a more just and equitable society. Good methods and indicators, as we argued above, are a mechanism by which to hold society to account. They hold up a mirror. So it is important to ensure that the mirror is not distorting.

The debate about the limits of value-neutrality in science and measurement has been raging for decades in the philosophy of science. Although the 'use versus abuse' model of science and technology has been criticised, it keeps being resurrected. It posits that science and technology are value-neutral. A protein is a protein is a protein. A nutrient is a nutrient. What matters is whether knowledge is used, well used or abused. Facts are facts. In matters such as sustainable diets, however, what is being dealt with is not atomic matter on its own terms, or nutrients *qua* nutrients. The concern is about their flows, their impact, their relationship with other dimensions of existence. The chapters that follow adopt the position that has emerged from science policy analysts. This suggests that what matters is how problems are framed, and the social assumptions built into the pursuit of knowledge. Facts embed values and values shape what is sought as knowledge. Numbers and methods are essential, but care needs to be taken in decisions about which numbers and why. The value of this approach is amply demonstrated by noting how sensitive issues of nutrition labelling have been. Furious arguments within the food industry and governments have been waged over whether, when and how to display the nutritional content of food products.[11-13] Facts aren't just facts; it matters how they are generated and interpreted.

Assessing the performance of food systems and diets through the lens of sustainability is still a relatively new concern that requires careful analysis and reflection, both in terms of its scope and the issues to be assessed on the one hand, and the sustainability challenges targeted or the assessment methods used on the other. It is important to be clear about the objectives of an assessment as they will inform the methods used. Potential findings should also be considered at the start of the assessment process as findings support decision-making which could have unforeseen impacts.

Given that sustainable diets need to take account of the food and nutrition needs not only of the present but also of future generations, ideally no measure of sustainable diets should be restricted to the present time. Moreover, assessments should take account of the global scale, in that findings at a local level could drive decisions which, although appropriate for one place and time, might have an unforeseen global effect or an effect in another country or another part of the same country.

Inclusion of stakeholders in assessment approaches is increasingly considered normal; consultation processes can be long. Just as food and diet is conditioned by cultural, social, geographical and political environments, so assessments for sustainable diets would be deemed to be more robust if they were to have involved different stakeholders when developing the methodology and indicators.

In our view, no single indicator or method can hope to capture the complexity of food systems and diets in terms of their environmental, nutrition and health, social and economic aspects. This is the case for the multi-criteria approach, and is why we take as the starting point for this book the clusters or domains for sustainable diet identified in the Sustainable Development Commission (SDC) report that forms the framework for this book.[14]

The account above is a reminder that the methods and indicators used for sustainable diets are themselves a matter of considerable complexity. An element of pragmatism is inevitable. There is pressure for good methods and indicators because there are already strong reasons for dietary change. In everyday terms, the case for good methods and indicators can be summarised pithily. What is counted is what counts. If it cannot be measured, it cannot be monitored. Knowledge is power.

## Available indicators and measures of a sustainable diet

There are indicators and methods of measurement available for the domains of a sustainable diet identified in the SDC report. An 'indicator' is generally a quantitative measure that can be used to illustrate or communicate about complex phenomena such as, for instance, trends over time. Ideally, and to communicate effectively, indicators of sustainable diet should be:

- measurable and easy to apply;
- relevant to the objectives and attributes of interest;
- robust in terms of errors and be subject to minimal uncertainty;

- accepted by actors and stakeholders;
- credible for experts and interpretable without ambiguity;
- sensitive/responsive to changes over time in physical conditions;
- hierarchical (providing a clear overview, but amenable to expansion into detail or at finer scales);
- able to promote learning and provide effective feedback to decision-making.

Many agencies and organisations have developed sustainability indicators, but few are directly related to food and diet. The world's governments approved, for example, the 17 UN Sustainable Development Goals (SDGs) in 2015, which each have supplementary targets.[15] There are 169 targets. The Paris Climate Change accord, also struck in 2015, set out goals, but without tight targets or indicators.[16] At a regional level, the European Environment Agency, for example, employs indicators for air and ozone layer, biodiversity, climate, soil, water and energy. Other indicators apply specifically to waste, agriculture, fisheries and transport.[17] At a national level the UK Department for Environment, Food and Rural Affairs (Defra), as in many developed economies, has developed sustainable development indicators including those for greenhouse gas emissions, waste, resource use, obesity, infant health, fish stocks and the origin of food consumed in the UK.[18] In theory, these indicators should all stem from sound methods and be made up of indicators that make sense at all levels: global to local.

Measures provide data in support of indicators and ideally should be:

- valid and reliable (high quality);
- timely (indicating problems or progress while there is still time to act to prevent negative consequences);
- collected and reported regularly and consistently;
- publicly available;
- transparent and understandable.

The choice of an indicator or measure depends on the initial question to be answered, but also depends on the availability of data. Data are often inadequate and insufficiently adapted to the aim of assessing the sustainability of diet and food systems. This is notably the case with life-cycle analysis (LCA), which is a key procedure for product analysis but does not directly help for sustainable diets because it measures product life-cycles rather than population impacts of whole diets. Some data arise from public statistics generated internationally such as, for example, the FAO food balance sheets, or nationally such as, for example, the UK National Diet and Nutrition Survey. Such information is more complete for wealthy countries than low-income countries and there are insufficient data on food losses, wastage and waste management.

# Health indicators

Sustainable diets must protect and promote the health of populations by reducing the risk of diet-related disease and foodborne illness and by promoting food safety. A healthy, sustainable diet must also be accessible and available to everyone. Sustainability of diets can be assessed by public health indicators such as obesity, incidence of non-communicable disease (NCD) (for example, cardiovascular disease and diabetes); safety indicators such as pathogens, antibiotic and pesticide residues in food and prevalence of foodborne illness; nutrition indicators such as intakes of energy, macronutrients and micronutrients, healthy eating indicators, diet quality indicators, fruit and vegetable intake; indicators of access such as availability of food in retail outlets, community gardens and allotments.

## Public health indicators and measures

Key indicators of public health with a link to diet include:

- mortality and morbidity from diet-related NCDs (for example, cancer, CVD and diabetes);
- prevalence of obesity in children and adults;
- prevalence of hypertension;
- prevalence of anaemia in women of reproductive age;
- prevalence of anaemia in children under five years;
- prevalence of stunting in children under five years;
- prevalence of adults who are underweight;
- prevalence of vitamin A deficiency;
- prevalence of iodine deficiency.

The World Health Organization has proposed a set of ten global targets and indicators for reducing diet-related NCDs and their associated risk factors.[19]

Estimates of obesity and diet-related chronic diseases can be obtained from a number of global databases such as the WHO Global Infobase,[20] the World Obesity Federation's Obesity Data Portal[21] and the Global Health Data Exchange.[22] Several major national survey programmes include information about diet-related NCDs, including the US Centers for Disease Control and Prevention[23] and Public Health England, while the WHO has reported on links between NCDs and diet[24] and the World Cancer Research Fund (WCRF) on links between specific cancers and diet.[25] Other data sources for diet-related public health include the Demographic and Health Surveys,[26] the WHO STEPwise approach to Surveillance programme,[27] the Eurobarometer Surveys,[28] the UNICEF Multiple Indicator Cluster Surveys,[29] the WHO World Health Surveys,[30] the Survey of Healthy Ageing and Retirement in Europe,[31] the Eurodiet report[32] and the International Social Survey Programme.[33] National health ministry websites also have data from national health surveys and national longitudinal studies.

### Food safety indicators and measures

Food safety is an area of scientific inquiry concerned about the handling, preparation and storage of food in ways that prevent foodborne illness. This includes a number of routines between industry and the market and then between the market and the consumer. For industry, food safety considerations include the origins of food, including the practices relating to food labelling, food hygiene, food additives and pesticide residues, as well as policies on biotechnology and food guidelines for the management of governmental import and export inspection and certification systems for foods.

A key indicator for food safety is ISO 22000, a standard developed by the International Organization for Standardization (ISO) dealing with food safety. The ISO 22000 international standard specifies the requirements for a food safety management system that involves interactive communication, system management, prerequisite programs and Hazard Analysis and Critical Control Point (HACCP) principles. HACCP is a system – first developed to ensure perfect safety for the food of astronauts who could not get to a hospital from outer space – designed for food businesses to look at how they handle food and introduces procedures to make sure the food produced is safe to eat.[34] Risks could be reduced by focusing on the critical points in supply chains.

The Codex Alimentarius Commission, a joint body of the FAO and WHO, produces global positions and guidance on food safety.[35] Although the Codex recommendations are for voluntary application by its member states, in many cases Codex advice forms a basis for national legislation. Several regulatory agencies around the world, including the European Food Safety Authority (EFSA) and national agencies such as the US Food and Drug Administration (FDA) or the UK Food Standards Agency (FSA), are responsible for food safety and requirements for food safety standards. National authorities such as the UK FSA and the US Centers for Disease Control and Prevention (CDC) collect data on foodborne illness.

Monitoring of pesticide residues in food is also carried out by national authorities – in the Expert Committee on Pesticide Residues in Food and, in the USA, by the FDA. While Codex sets world standards, regional authorities such as the EFSA do it for intergovernmental collaborations. Standards are also in place for residues of veterinary medicines, including antibiotics, in food and are monitored at a national and regional level.

The Belgian Federal Agency for the Safety of the Food Chain has developed a tool to measure food safety throughout the entire food chain from farm to fork.[36] Known as the Food Safety Barometer, this tool covers the chemical, physical and microbiological hazards of food and consists of a basket of 30 food safety indicators covering the whole food chain for foods produced in Belgium and for food imports. Both products and processes are included in the basket of indicators. Indicators for products include the presence of chemical and biological hazards such as acrylamide, aflatoxins, dioxins, mercury, forbidden colourants, salmonella species and Escherichia coli, while indicators for processes include inspections and audits. The barometer also includes indicators for prevention in terms of self-checking, compulsory notification and traceability and recording of foodborne outbreaks (for example, salmonellosis and listeriosis). The relative importance for food safety of the 30 indicators has been weighted to define the food safety barometer, which is used to measure food safety in Belgium on an annual basis.

### Nutrition indicators and measures

Methods and indicators related specifically to nutrition can be divided into two main types:

- Those that compare consumption data with a dietary guideline (diet scores or indices). They construct indices on the quality and variety of the diet (for example, the Mediterranean or Nordic type diet, or the 'flexitarian' diet) or compliance with a national dietary guideline (for example, for fruit and vegetable consumption such as the UK's 5-a-day or the USA's 7-a-day or Greece's 9-a-day).
- Those based on measurement or observation of food and nutrition consumption (dietary consumption data). They construct indicators around intakes of macronutrients such as, for example, the percentage of daily energy intake from total fat, saturated fat, protein and carbohydrate including sugars. The prevalence of diets high in saturated fat and sugar is linked to cardiovascular disease and increased obesity risk and hence to diabetes.

Some 20 diet scores are in existence, many of which are derived from four main scores:

- *The Healthy Eating Index* (HEI). The Healthy Eating Index (HEI) is a measure of diet quality that assesses conformance to federal dietary guidance in the USA. It is used to monitor the quality of American diets; to examine relationships between diet and health-related outcomes and between diet cost and diet quality; to determine the effectiveness of nutrition intervention programmes; and to assess the quality of food assistance packages, menus and the US food supply. The HEI is a scoring metric that can be applied to any defined set of foods, such as previously collected dietary data, a defined menu or a market basket, to estimate a score. The most recent version, HEI-2010,[37] which assesses diet quality as specified by the 2010 Dietary Guidelines for Americans, is made up of 12 components. The total HEI-2010 score is the sum of the component scores and has a maximum of 100 points. The higher the score, the better the diet. However, these indices vary in their ability to predict the risk of chronic disease. The Alternative Healthy Eating Index (AHEI), which is based on foods and nutrients predictive of chronic disease, rather than the HEI which measures adherence to US dietary guidelines, is more strongly associated with chronic disease risk. [38, 39] Further improvements to these indices are warranted.[40, 41]

- *The Diet Quality Index.*[42] Dietary recommendations from the 1989 National Academy of Sciences publication *Diet and Health* have been stratified into three levels of intake for scoring. Individuals who meet a dietary goal are given a score of zero. Those who do not meet a goal but have a fair diet are given one point, and those who have a poor diet are given two points. These points are summed across eight diet variables to score the index from zero (excellent diet) to 16 (poor diet).
- *The Healthy Diet Indicator* (HDI).[43] The HDI is based on WHO guidelines for the prevention of chronic diseases. If a person's intake is within the recommended borders this variable is coded 1 and if the intake is outside these borders, it is coded 0. For example, a polyunsaturated fatty acid intake of 3–7% energy is coded as 1 and an intake below 3 or higher than 7 as 0. The HDI is calculated as the sum of 9 dichotomous variables (range 0–9).
- *The Mediterranean Diet Score.*[44] This score is based on eight component parts of the traditional diet in the Mediterranean region. Increase in the dietary score is associated with reduced mortality. Compared with other dietary patterns, higher adherence to the Mediterranean diet is associated with a favourable cardiometabolic, hepatic and renal risk profile.[45] The Mediterranean diet is also considered to be a sustainable dietary pattern with benefits for the environment and social justice.[46]

Dietary consumption data are essential to develop and evaluate policy measures for a healthier, safer and sustainable diet. However, finding out how much food people consume is not easy.

At the global level, data published by the FAO since the middle of the twentieth century have enabled assessments, by product and by country, of the levels and trends of food consumption patterns throughout the world. The FAO data, often referred to as FAO's food balance sheets, are based on estimates of production plus imports and minus exports of a country and enable an evaluation of national agricultural resources that, after the extraction of non-food uses (for example, seeds, animal feed, biofuels, etc.) and division by the number of inhabitants, leads to an assessment of average food availability per person. This availability is higher than the quantities actually ingested because it includes what has been lost after being made available to the consumer.

The US Department of Agriculture (USDA) Economic Research Service (ERS) also has a food availability (per capita) data system that, like the FAO balance sheets, provides proxies for actual consumption.[47] This includes food availability data, loss-adjusted food availability data and nutrient availability data.

In the UK, the Family Food survey looks specifically at the domestic or household aspect. It provides detailed statistics on food and drink purchases, expenditure and the derived nutrient content of those purchases from a large household survey covering the United Kingdom.[48] These data are used by Defra to compare household food purchases with the healthy eating recommendations of the Eatwell plate.[49]

Unfortunately, many users of these statistics fail to ascertain the actual meaning of the data and misleadingly refer to them as consumption data rather than food availability. The energy (calorie) content of national resources can clarify the pressures on these resources regarding the demand for food products and, notably, the land necessary within or outside the country to meet this demand.

More reliable information about actual food intake comes only from well-designed food surveys, and because prevailing habits and food preferences keep changing such investigations need to be periodically repeated in order to uncover consumption shifts. Conducting such dietary surveys is a costly endeavour because representative food consumption surveys must examine a sufficiently large number of households and should be conducted by well-trained personnel.

The US National Health and Nutrition Examination Survey (NHANES) began in 1971 and, repeated at regular intervals, obtains its dietary data on the basis of subjects providing a list of food eaten the previous day. This may be an expedient approach but its accuracy cannot equal that of a supervised survey that involves actual measurement of food consumed. Japan's National Health and Nutrition Survey (NHNS) is conducted by registered dietitians who weigh actual amounts of foods before and after preparation as well as food that is wasted and record the composition of food eaten outside of the home. Germany's National Nutrition Survey II, conducted between November 2005 and the end of 2006, two decades after the first such survey in West Germany, fell somewhere between the American and Japanese methods of estimating food intakes. Information on socio-demographic characteristics, state of health and eating habits were collected from interviews with 19,329 men and women aged between 14 and 80 years; 24-hour recall was used as the primary tool for determining food consumption, and a random selection of participants completed two four-day food weighing protocols that established exact amounts of individual consumption.[50] In France nutritional surveillance data were disparate before the year 2000 and were often limited to regions and research cohorts. The first French National Dietary Survey (INCA 1) was conducted in 1999, INCA 2 in 2006–7[51] and INCA 3 in 2013–14. Dietary intake data are collected by trained dietitians using three 24-hour recalls, including one on a weekend, randomly distributed over a two-week period. The UK National Diet and Nutrition Survey (NDNS), which was set up in 1992, surveyed the diets of pre-school children, young people and older people in the 1990s, with the most recent NDNS of adults aged 19 to 64 years carried out in 2000/1. More recently, the NDNS has operated as a rolling programme evaluating a wider range of ages each year but, instead of using weighed records of several days' duration, it now resorts to a less expensive method in the form of a four-day estimated food diary in order to reduce costs and the burden on participants.

Further information on the diverse methods used to collect dietary data in the European Union can be found in EFSA's food consumption database that covers 22 of the EU countries.[52] Survey methodologies range from recalling intake from the previous day (24-hour recall) to keeping a record of the consumption of food and drinks over several days (dietary record). The level of detail and the quality of the data collected is also uneven, affected by differences in the survey design, the tools used to collect and measure the data, the clustering of age groups, and food description and categorisation systems.

Given the disparity in methods used to collect dietary data, the European Food Consumption Validation (EFCOVAL) Project was established to develop and validate a standardised method for food consumption surveys, evaluating the intake of foods, nutrients and potentially hazardous chemicals in the European population. The conclusion from this project was that the repeated 24-hour dietary recall using EPIC-Soft (the software developed to conduct 24-hour dietary recalls (24-HDRs) in the European Prospective Investigation into Cancer and Nutrition (EPIC) Study) for standardisation, in combination with a food propensity questionnaire and modelling of usual intake, is a suitable method for pan-European surveillance of nutritional adequacy and food safety among healthy adults and maybe in children aged 7 years and older.[53, 54] The EU Menu Project aims to establish a European food consumption database of information gathered using harmonised methods and tools explained in EFSA guidance.[55]

## Indicators and measures of food access

There is no universally accepted definition of the term 'food access', but it has been described as 'the ability for all members of society to obtain sufficient food for healthy living and in particular whether people on low incomes can obtain enough nutritious food'.[56]

A range of social factors influence access to food, among which insufficient money is critical. However, other factors such as cooking skills, household facilities, lack of transport, neighbourhood crime, age and health can also have a significant influence on the ability of a person to access food and could therefore provide the basis of indicators.

Indicators that are currently available for measurement of food access include the Dietary Diversity Score (DDS) in urban areas, food retail provision (typically within 500 m to 2 km of where people live) and, in rural areas, access to land, water and agricultural inputs.

Household dietary diversity, which is the number of different food groups consumed over a given period, has been validated to be a useful proxy indicator for measuring household food access, particularly when resources for undertaking such measurement are scarce.[57] Measuring household dietary diversity is useful for the following reasons:

- A more diversified diet is an important outcome in and of itself.
- A more diversified diet is associated with a number of improved outcomes in areas such as birth weight, child anthropometric status and improved haemoglobin concentrations.

- A more diversified diet is highly correlated with such factors as energy and protein adequacy and household income. Even in very poor households, increased food expenditure resulting from additional income is associated with increased quantity and quality of the diet.

The WHO Household Dietary Diversity Score (HDDS) is a summing up (using the 24-hour recall method) of how many of the following food groups (cereals, fish and seafood, root and tubers, pulses/legumes/nuts, vegetables, milk and milk products, fruits, oil/fats, meat, poultry, offal, sugar/honey, eggs, miscellaneous) were consumed by members of the household during one day. Calculating the number of different food groups rather than the number of different foods consumed is a better indicator of dietary diversity and hence food access. Knowing that households consume, for example, an average of four different food groups implies that their diets offer some diversity in both macro- and micronutrients. This is a more meaningful indicator than knowing that households consume four different foods, which might all be cereals.

Retail provision of food in a locality typically involves food retail mapping or conducting a census of food outlets. This can be done by visiting shops and markets in a locality and drawing up a list, or consulting local databases and business directories or both. Geographical information system (GIS) software can be used to map food retail provision in relation to where people live, often including a pre-identified distance (typically, 500 m to 2 km) to reveal areas where food shops are lacking. Used alone, food retail mapping is suitable for examining the food retailing environment and it has been used to examine the distribution of food retail outlets and store types[58] as well as different types of food retailers (for example, bakers, butchers, fruit and vegetable sellers, convenience stores)[59] in deprived areas of Glasgow. Food retail mapping has been used in attempts to identify 'food deserts', particularly in the USA. However, it is an inadequate method for assessing the wider aspects of food access as it measures only distances to, and distribution of, shops and does not identify the range or price of the foods within the shops nor what people think about the choice and quality of food in the shops.

Other indicators of food access that could be considered include: the amount and placement of healthy food in retail outlets; the availability of community gardens and allotments and the number of people growing their own food; the proportion of farmland operated by small family farms and indigenous populations relative to contract-based and plantation-type farms; the availability of school lunches and breakfasts; or the scale of food assistance provided by the state such as the US Supplemental Nutrition Assistance Programme (SNAP) and food stamps, or the UK's Healthy Start. Charities are also providers such as through food banks or the UK's FareShare. Some of these programmes could only offer data too vague to be good indicators. For example, data on the amount and placement of healthy foods in retail outlets are proprietary, and 'healthy' does not have a standard definition in this context. The number of people growing their own food is increasing and data on allotments and community gardens are available at a local level, but the strength of these as indicators for health requires more research. Data on the use of both federal (for example, SNAP in the USA)[60] and charity food assistance (for example, Trussell Trust food banks in the UK)[61] are already available and can be used as a general indicator of compromised food access and the ability to access food with dignity. These offer useful snapshots but do not yet cover the range of what is needed to be solid national or local indicators.

Agricultural yields in terms of tonnes produced per area of land can be used as an indicator of food availability. However, one important US study proposed that a good indicator might be the number of people nourished per area of land.[62] Currently, 36% of the calories produced by the world's crops are being used for animal feed and only 12% of those feed calories ultimately contribute to the human diet (as meat and other animal products). Additionally, human-edible calories used for biofuel production increased fourfold between the years 2000 and 2010, from 1% to 4%, representing a net reduction of available food globally. Given the increasing and changing demand for food as a result of global population growth and changing dietary patterns, there are many calls to boost crop production. Making people nourished per hectare a key indicator rather than yield per hectare would allow even small shifts in the use of crops – whether for animals or direct for humans – to become a more subtle ecological public health indicator. Using land for growing food exclusively for direct human consumption could, in principle, increase available food calories by as much as 70%. This could feed an additional 4 billion people. This is far more than the projected 2–3 billion people arriving through population growth in coming decades.

### Advertising and information

On no issue is the power of knowledge and the importance of generating good data for sustainable diets (see beginning of this chapter) more sensitive than this. Advertising and other forms of communication in print, on radio and TV and on the internet have an impact on food choice, nutrition and health. The evidence is particularly strong for children and young people, shaping us when impressionable.[63, 64] Potential indicators of advertising related to nutrition might include the number of advertisements for products high in saturated fat, sugar and sodium or high in any of these, or the mix of items advertised, or the nutritional content of advertised products and the impact on food choices. The food industry is a major source of advertisements but is beginning to switch away from paid ads to soft media marketing methods, using the web and posting games and other means for blurring educational messages. There are too few public bodies monitoring this. The Australian organisation Adbusters is an exception.[65] Some research on types of advertisements show the collective messages mostly reinforce fatty, sugary, salty food product consumption.[66] Also, much of the advertising industry is self-regulating. But having some kind of indicator of commercial attempts to mould consumption in unsustainable ways would be useful.

## Environmental indicators in relation to diet

Environmental indicators include greenhouse gas (GHG) emissions, land use, water use, energy use, soil quality, soil erosion, disturbances in nitrogen and phosphate cycles and loss of biodiversity. In terms of food, these indicators are closely interrelated, mainly because the production and consumption of animal protein affects all of them and has a large environmental impact. The choice of environmental indicators may therefore make little difference at a global level, but can at a regional or local level.

Most research on the ecological effect of diets has been conducted with reference to only a small number of indicators, in particular GHG emissions, energy use, embedded or virtual water and land use. The effects on biodiversity have been studied mostly indirectly via the effects on land use with little research of the direct effects on biodiversity. Local indicators such as eutrophication and acidification have been studied principally in relation to the use of fertilisers, manure surpluses and crop protection chemicals, rather than in relation to diet.

Environmental indicators used include:

- life-cycle assessment (LCA)
- carbon footprint
- embedded energy
- input–output analysis
- ecological footprint
- food miles
- water footprint and virtual water
- biodiversity
- soil
- waste
- organic output or sales.

### Life-cycle assessment

The most frequently applied method for calculating environmental effects is the life-cycle assessment (LCA). Life-cycle assessment methodology and approaches are covered by international recognised standards, i.e. ISO 14040:2006.

In this method, an estimate is made of the effects on one or more environmental indicators over the whole, or a specific phase, of the life cycle of a specific product, such as a food, from production to processing, manufacturing, transport, consumption and finally disposal. This analytical method is often called cradle-to-grave, or farm-to-fork, field-to-fork or well-to-wheel depending on which product is being analysed and the measurement boundaries. Life-cycle assessment has been used to assess the environmental impact of single foods, most commonly through measurement of GHGs.[67, 68] Far fewer LCA studies have evaluated land use, water use and impacts on biodiversity. Life-cycle assessment studies evaluating single foods are of limited value for evaluating whole diets and their impact on populations. Single foods can be aggregated into meals and comparisons of different types of meals (for example, omnivorous, vegetarian, vegan) can provide illustrative conclusions to the environmental effects of food choices, but are not necessarily representative of whole diets.

### Carbon footprint

'Carbon footprint' is a term used to describe the amount of GHG emissions of a particular entity or activity. A Publically Available Specification (PAS 2050) was created by the British Standards Institute (BSI) in the early days of carbon auditing for the purposes of assessing product life-cycle GHG emissions and has been so useful that it is now internationally used as a benchmark.[69] Indirectly, carbon footprint also assesses the energy consumed by human activities. Frequently employed, it can be adapted to different scales, but usually remains limited to GHG emissions.

### Embedded energy

This is a method based on the principles of thermodynamics that takes account of the energy required to produce a product. In terms of food, embedded energy is derived from agriculture, transportation, processing, food sales, storage and preparation. A US study has evaluated the energy discarded in food waste using the concept of embedded energy.[70]

### Input–output analysis

Input–output analysis estimates the ecological influences of goods and services. The outcome is an estimate of the average ecological impact of a given product group. Many hybrid methods are in current use, in which outcomes of an input–output model are included in a life-cycle analysis. Input–output methodology can be used at global environmental scales but not at a detailed level.

The European Commission explored the environmental impact of products within the European Union (EIPRO – Environmental Impact of PROducts) using methods based on analysis of inputs and outputs, sector by sector. This study quantified the relationships between production and consumption systems in terms of purchases, sales, resource use, emissions and environmental impact. It highlighted the considerable environmental impact of food and drinks[71] and the environmental impacts of dietary change in the EU.[72, 73]

### Ecological footprint

The ecological footprint is an assessment of society's demand for resources and converts it into a measure of impact – hence the footprint metaphor. The ecological footprint is expressed in terms of global hectares, where a global hectare is a measure of productive area that is available to support society's demand. The area can be terrestrial or marine. Once the demand side has been estimated, it is possible to compare it to the supply side and to assess whether a society is using its resources in a sustainable manner. This method has been used to calculate, for example, the ecological footprint of food and drink in Cardiff, Wales and how food and drink consumption could be made more sustainable.[74]

The ecological footprint has several advantages: because it is an aggregate value it is fairly simple and clear, it is easy to understand and visualise and, therefore, it is a useful tool for policy and for educational purposes to convey a message about human ecosystems impact.[75] However, the ecological footprint is often criticised for not being refined enough when used at smaller scales and for hiding the complexity of the issue.[75, 76]

## Food miles

Transportation is one determinant of resource use in the consumption of food. The notion of food miles was coined in 1993 to highlight the distance that food products are transported from the producer to the final consumer.[77, 78] Even before mass use on the web, it went viral and the absurdities of lorries trucking back and forth was highlighted.[79] Countries whose food exports are associated with long-distance travel were alarmed that this measure might take hold.[80] However, the distance food travels is not necessarily an accurate measure of environmental impact or GHG.[81] For example, tomatoes grown outside in Spain and transported to the UK are associated with lower GHG emissions than tomatoes grown in heated greenhouses in the UK.[82] A US study found that most GHG emissions occur not in the travel but on or near the farm.[83]

In spite of these shortcomings, food miles has a useful role to play in communicating with consumers, and has highlighted some of the cultural downsides of the increase in food travelling long distances.[84] It questioned how 'efficient' food manufacturers are if they assemble ingredients from spread sources.[85] Also, it led to a new interest in the consequences (and absurdity) of flying foods around the world.[86] One study found that if a customer drives a round-trip distance of more than 6.7 km in order to purchase their organic vegetables, their carbon emissions are likely to be greater than the emissions from the system of cold storage, packing, transport to a regional hub and final transport to customer's doorstep used by large-scale vegetable box suppliers.[87] The food industry has even used it to redesign wasteful trucking systems. In the UK, for example, industry estimated that a quarter of all wagons on the UK roads were food and that half of them were empty, returning to factories or distribution hubs.[88] This led to projects by companies to share 'back-loading'. Food miles has spawned many offshoot measures from 'fair miles', a case defending the social values in food exports from small farmers in developing countries,[89] to 'needless miles' from a commercial report critically assessing a large food retailer,[90] and to 'misery miles' in relation to long-distance trucking of live animals across continents.[91]

## Water footprint and virtual water

Water footprint is a measure of water use, and can be calculated for individuals, businesses, cities and countries. Studies have used water footprint to measure the use of water in diets. It includes direct water use (for example, for drinking and cleaning) as well as indirect water (the water required to produce goods and services). This indirect water is described as 'virtual water'.[92] For example, the average UK household uses around 150 litres of water a day. However, if the embedded water used in the production of the goods people consume is also taken into account, daily water consumption per person in the UK is estimated to be 4,645 litres. The water embedded in food represents the majority, or 65%, of total water use in the UK.

The World Water Council has used the term virtual water to raise awareness of the difference in water consumption between a meat-rich diet (5,400 litres of virtual water a day) and a vegetarian diet (2,600 litres a day) among American consumers,[93] while an EU study showed that the water footprint of EU diets could be reduced by around a third by consuming either a healthy diet or a vegetarian diet rather than the current meat-based diet.[94]

Virtual water also links food with trade.[95] For example, it takes about 1,000 litres of water to produce a ton of grain. If the ton of grain is imported by a country short of fresh water or soil water, that country is spared the economic and political stress of mobilising 1,000 litres of water.[95] In the UK 62% of the water footprint is related to the consumption of imported products. The World Resources Institute measures and maps water risks in different countries of the world, including risks of flooding, droughts and access to water.[96]

## Biodiversity

Sustainable diets should be protective and respectful of biodiversity and ecosystems. Biodiversity, i.e. diversity of life on earth, is an important factor for sustainable diets in terms of improving nutrition and food security, but biodiversity is still incompletely understood. At its simplest, biodiversity can be measured as the number of species per hectare. However, there are several limitations associated with an emphasis on species. First, what constitutes a species is not often well defined. Second, simply counting the number of species in an ecosystem does not take into consideration how variable each species might be or its contribution to ecosystem properties.[97]

Indicators of terrestrial biodiversity include:

- *The Mean Species Abundance* (MSA). Mean Species Abundance has been developed by the GLOBIO consortium, which is a collaboration between the Netherlands Environmental Assessment Agency (PBL), UNEP

GRID-Arendal and UNEP-World Conservation Monitoring Centre (UNEP-WCMC).[98] Mean Species Abundance is an indicator of naturalness or biodiversity intactness. It is defined as the mean abundance of original species relative to their abundance in undisturbed ecosystems. An area with an MSA of 100% means a biodiversity that is similar to the natural situation. An MSA of 0% means a completely destructed ecosystem, with no original species remaining. Mean Species Abundance does not completely cover the complex biodiversity concept and can be considered a proxy for the Convention on Biological Diversity (CBD) indicator on trends in species abundance.[99]

- *The Biodiversity Integrity Index.*[100] This measures terrain diversity carrying capacity.
- *The Biodiversity Intactness Index* (BII).[101] The index links data on land use with expert assessments of how this impacts the population densities of well-understood taxonomic groups to estimate current population sizes relative to pre-modern times. The main difference between MSA and BII is that every hectare is given equal weight in MSA, whereas BII gives more weight to species-rich areas. It has been criticised for underestimating extents of land degradation.[102]
- *The Living Planet Index* (LPI).[103] The Living Planet Index was developed to measure the changing state of the world's biodiversity over time. It uses time-series data to calculate average rates of change in a large number of populations of terrestrial, freshwater and marine vertebrate species. The main difference between LPI and MSA is that MSA takes the pristine situation as a baseline, whereas LPI compares with the situation in 1970.

Biodiversity in relation to fish can be measured using:

- *The Marine Trophic Index* (MTI) (www.bipindicators.net/mti), which has been developed by the Sea Around Us project (www.seaaroundus.org) at the UBC Fisheries Centre in Canada (www.fisheries.ubc.ca) to investigate the impacts of fisheries on the world's marine ecosystems.[104] The MTI can be used to describe the complex interactions between fisheries and marine ecosystems and communicate a measure of species replacement indices by fisheries. The MTI is calculated from catch composition data collected by the FAO after being spatially allocated to exclusive economic zones of each country and large marine ecosystems or other relevant spatial ecosystem components. The concept and approach is now widely accepted.
- *The Marine Depletion Index* (MDI) which is defined as the weighted mean of the ratios of the biomass estimated for 2050 and that of 2004, per species.[105] It was adapted from the original depletion index described in 2007.[106]

A few studies have tried to introduce biodiversity in to the conceptual framework of LCA.[107–109] Swiss workers have proposed an assessment method for arable crops, grasslands and semi-natural areas in the LCA framework, which is only applicable in Switzerland,[110] while more recent work has more relevance at a global scale[109] although it is very preliminary. A Swedish case study used data on plant species' richness and the regeneration times of ecosystems derived from a literature review to assess the impact of conventional versus organic milk production on biodiversity and land use. Although organic milk production required about twice as much land as conventional milk production, it had lower direct land-use impacts on biodiversity.[111] Linking biodiversity, food and sustainable diets is a major research challenge.

## Soil

Soil is arguably the most precious resource human food systems have inherited. Any diet that does not protect the soil is of questionable sustainability. It is among the most important twenty-first-century challenges.[112] Soil provides many natural services for food to grow, such as nutrient availability, clean water and resistance to pests and diseases. It is teeming with life, yet can be destroyed by mistreatment and poor farming associated with excessive use of fertilisers and pesticides. Topsoil erodes when it loses its plant top cover and is blown by the wind (as happened in the USA in the 1930s Depression, leading President Roosevelt to sign his Statement on Soil in 1936 and John Steinbeck to write *The Grapes of Wrath*).[113, 114] Nutrient run-off to ground or surface water adds to problems. Maintenance of the organic matter content of the soil is therefore crucial as organic material strengthens the soil structure, feeds soil organisms, provides nutrients and contributes to the water-holding capacity of the soil. Organic matter is therefore an important indicator for soil quality. Another indicator that is more easily measured is pH (soil acidity). One of the greatest impacts on soil quality on a worldwide scale is water erosion so erosion potential is a third indicator for soil quality.

Methods for measuring these soil quality indicators are described by the Sustainable Agriculture Initiative, a coalition of big food companies, thus:[115]

- *Organic matter*: the indicator is the calculated organic matter content for the current farm situation (and future 30 years) expressed as a percentage of Soil Organic Matter in the top 30 cm of the soil.
- *Soil acidity*: the indicator is acidity in water expressed in pH.
- *Reduced erosion risk* (caused by wind and/or water) is expressed in a score between 0 and 14, determined by the natural situation of the field and erosion prevention measures by the farmer.

## Waste

An estimated one-third of all food produced for human consumption is lost or wasted.[116] Although reducing food waste to zero would be impossible, sustainable diets would generate as little waste as practicably possible. The economic costs of current food wastage are substantial and amount to about USD 1 trillion each year.[117] However, the hidden costs of food wastage extend much further. Food that is produced but never consumed still causes environmental impacts to the atmosphere, water, land and biodiversity. By contributing to environmental degradation and increasing the scarcity of natural resources, food wastage is associated with wider social costs that affect people's well-being and livelihoods.

Food waste is therefore an important indicator of economic, environmental and social costs. Quantifying the full costs of food wastage improves understanding of the global food system and enables action to address supply chain weaknesses and disruptions that are likely to threaten the viability of future food systems, food security and sustainable development.

The FAO has developed a full cost accounting (FCA) method that measures, and values in monetary terms, the externality costs associated with the environmental impacts of food wastage. The FCA framework incorporates several elements: a market-based valuation of the direct financial costs, a non-market valuation of lost ecosystems' goods and services and a well-being valuation to assess the social costs associated with natural resource degradation.

Using this FCA methodology, the FAO has made a preliminary estimate that, in addition to the USD 1 trillion of economic costs per year, environmental costs reach around USD 700 billion and social costs around USD 900 billion.[117] This is equivalent to USD 2.6 trillion annually, roughly equivalent to the gross domestic product (GDP) of France, or approximately twice the total annual food expenditure of the USA. Particularly salient environmental and social costs of food wastage according to this methodology include:

- Greenhouse gas emissions of 3.5 Gt $CO_2$e. Based on the social cost of carbon, these are estimated to cause USD 394 billion of damages per year.
- Increased water scarcity, particularly for dry regions and seasons. Globally, this is estimated to cost USD 164 billion per year.
- Soil erosion due to water is estimated to cost USD 35 billion per year through nutrient loss, lower yields, biological losses and off-site damages. The cost of wind erosion may be of a similar magnitude.
- Risks to biodiversity, including the impacts of pesticide use, nitrate and phosphorus eutrophication, pollinator losses and fisheries overexploitation, are estimated to cost USD 32 billion per year.
- Increased risk of conflict due to soil erosion, estimated to cost USD 396 billion per year.
- Loss of livelihoods due to soil erosion, estimated to cost USD 333 billion per year.
- Adverse health effects due to pesticide exposure, estimated to cost USD 153 billion per year.

In the UK, WRAP has estimated the quantity of food and drink wasted. There are three main estimates in this research: first, an estimate of the total amount of household food and drink waste in local authority collected waste streams; second, a waste compositional analysis estimated from approximately 1,800 households who gave their consent to be included, which gives detailed information on the types, 'avoidability' and state of food wasted; third, information on the types of food and drink wasted was recorded in diaries by 948 households. The diaries recorded, for each instance of waste, the amount of waste, the reason for disposal and which 'waste' stream was used. The research included waste streams that are hard to measure from compositional analysis (material poured down the kitchen sink or other inlets to the sewer, home composted or fed to animals).[118] The WRAP research also estimated the price of the avoidable food waste and the GHG and land use associated with the waste.

### Organic

Organic production respects natural systems and cycles and the use of internal inputs is preferred to that of external inputs. It is associated with maintenance of better biodiversity than non-organic production and hence can be considered to be a marker of environmental impact and hence of sustainable diet. However, for livestock production, evidence shows that, compared with non-organic production, organic production is associated with greater land use and increased GHG emissions on a weight for weight basis.

Organic certification is essentially the indicator for organic food and this generally involves a set of production standards for growing, storage, processing, packaging and shipping that include:

- avoidance of synthetic chemical inputs (for example, fertilisers, pesticides, antibiotics, food additives), genetically modified organisms, irradiation and the use of sewage sludge;
- use of farmland that has been free from prohibited chemical inputs for a number of years (often, three or more);
- for livestock, adhering to specific requirements for feed, housing and breeding;
- keeping detailed written production and sales records (audit trail);
- maintaining strict physical separation of organic products from non-certified products;
- undergoing periodic on-site inspections.

In some countries, certification is overseen by the government. The USA, EU, Canada and Japan have comprehensive organic legislation and commercial use of the term 'organic' is legally restricted. Certified organic producers are also subject to the same agricultural, food safety and other government regulations that apply to non-certified producers. Certified organic foods are not necessarily pesticide-free; certain pesticides are allowed. In countries without organic laws, government guidelines may or may not exist, while certification is handled by non-profit organisations and private companies.

Internationally, there is an aim to harmonise certification between countries to facilitate international trade. Equivalency negotiations are underway and some agreements are already in place. There are also international certification bodies, including members of the International Federation of Organic Agriculture Movements (IFOAM) working on harmonisation efforts. In 2011 IFOAM introduced a new program – the IFOAM Family of Standards – a set of standard requirements that functions as an international reference to assess the quality and equivalence of organic standards and regulations. It is known as the COROS (Common Objectives and Requirements of Organic Standards). The vision is that the Family of Standards will contain all organic standards and regulations equivalent to the COROS.

## Social values

The food system is a major driver of human and animal welfare. The social aspects of 'sustainability' have been under-researched but this is an area of evaluation and measurement in which there is an explosion of work, led by NGOs and the food industry.[119] A sustainable diet is one that is socially just and in which workers have safe, healthy, decent working conditions with appropriate application of labour laws and conventions, fair and living wages, absence of child labour, the right to strike and appropriate working contracts and hours of work. Food system workers should also have minimal exposure to pesticides and minimal risk for injury and accidents. Gender equity and indigenous rights and fair trade are also of increasing concern and public interest.

Measurement of both human and animal welfare issues is relatively new and is less straightforward than the measurement of health and environmental impacts. However, given the importance of measures to generate evidence for improving policy and social conditions in the food system, methodologies must be, and increasingly are, available. There are various certification bodies that have created standards for social values such as the Ethical Trade Initiative,[120] which are fairly widely used in the food system. These can be taken as proxy measures.

### Human welfare

Social indicators that can be considered include:

- the proportion of food system workers who have safe, healthy working conditions;
- the proportion of food system workers who have fair labour contracts and access to social welfare;
- the number of child workers in the food system;
- pesticide exposure is minimised;
- discrepancies between farm workers and other occupational groups in terms of cancer and neurological disorders;

- percentage of food system workers who belong to unions;
- the proportion of food system workers covered by fair and equitable immigration policy;
- the presence of policies that recognise workers' rights;
- the proportion of farmers who have fair access to credit and information;
- the percentage of fair trade labelled goods;
- small-scale producers are not disproportionately disadvantaged by regulations.

Human welfare issues are measured principally by a social impact assessment or a social life-cycle analysis (LCA), which may include both social indicators and some economic indicators such as worker wages. Social LCA methodology is discussed below (see page 62).

## Animal welfare

Animal welfare is an important feature of sustainable diets and is of considerable public interest, not only in Western societies but also worldwide. Animal welfare is strongly linked to animal health and is therefore of considerable interest to farmers as healthy animals require less medicine and are more productive.

The welfare of an animal includes its physical and mental state and, as such, good animal welfare implies both fitness and a sense of well-being. Indicators of animal welfare can be described in terms of the 'five freedoms', which are a compact of rights for animals under human control, including those intended for food or acting as working animals. The five freedoms were originally developed in 1965 from a UK Government investigation and subsequent report on livestock husbandry, led by Professor Roger Brambell, into the welfare of intensively farmed animals, partly in response to concerns raised in Ruth Harrison's 1964 book, *Animal Machines*.[121] The Brambell Report stated that animals should have the freedom to 'stand up, lie down, turn around, groom themselves and stretch their limbs'.[122] This short recommendation became known as Brambell's Five Freedoms. The five freedoms are used as the basis for the actions of professional groups, including vets, and have been adopted by representative groups internationally including the World Organization for Animal Health and the Royal Society for the Prevention of Cruelty to Animals (RSPCA).

These five freedoms form a framework for the analysis of basic welfare within any system, together with the steps and compromise necessary to safeguard and improve welfare within the proper constraints of an effective livestock industry. They are:

1  Freedom from hunger and thirst – achieved by ready access to fresh water and a diet to maintain full health and vigour.
2  Freedom from discomfort – by providing an appropriate environment including shelter and a comfortable resting area.

3   Freedom from pain, injury or disease – by prevention or rapid diagnosis and treatment.
4   Freedom to express normal behaviour – by providing sufficient space, proper facilities and company of the animal's own kind.
5   Freedom from fear and distress – by ensuring conditions and treatment that avoid mental suffering.

The Five Freedoms have been the cornerstone of much legislation and policy, and have been used widely in marketing and form the basis of welfare assessment. However, they focus on animal suffering and need. Some animal welfarists such as the US Humane Society and the UK Farm Animal Welfare Council (FAWC) suggest that the minimum animal welfare should be defined in terms of an animal's quality of life over its lifetime on the farm, during transport, at gatherings and at the abattoir, including the manner of its death. Essentially this proposal is that an animal's quality of life can be classified three ways: a life not worth living, a life worth living or a good life.[122] It led the European Commission to accept that animals are 'sentient beings'.[123, 124]

No single measure indicates the status of animal welfare. Factors that have an impact on animal welfare include both the resources available to the animal in its environment, for example space or bedding material, or the practices used to manage the animal on the farm, such as how and when the farmer feeds the animal or the procedures in place for weaning. These environmental factors offer only an indirect indication of animal welfare. A more complete indication of animal welfare can be obtained by the responses of the animal to factors in its environment – i.e. direct animal-based measures.

The rationale for this approach is that animal-based measures aim to directly determine the actual welfare status of the animal and therefore include both the effect of the environment as well as how the animal is managed. The industry-led Sustainable Agriculture Initiative expresses animal welfare according to 11 numerical scores across six indicators (see Table 2.1).[115]

The somatic cell count (SCC) is a main indicator of milk quality. The majority of somatic cells are leukocytes (white blood cells), which become present in increasing numbers in milk usually as an immune response to a mastitis-causing pathogen, and a small number of epithelial cells, which are milk-producing cells shed from the inside of the udder when an infection occurs.

The methodology is straightforward. In most cases the farmer's input data directly produce the indicator. This is the case with SCC, antibiotic use, longevity and fertility. The locomotion score and body condition score are standardised visual observations of the way animals walk and of their condition. In several countries farmers have this information by regular inspection of the animals and use these scores for their management. Some of these metrics are proxies for specific conditions, for example, SCC for mastitis prevalence. Other measures such as herd replacement rate are more general and reflect performance in a number of areas including fertility, genotype, animal management, nutrition and the impact

*Table 2.1* An example of indicators and metrics for animal welfare with a focus on dairy herds

| Indicator | Metric(s) |
| --- | --- |
| Somatic cell count (relevant to milk producing animals) | Number of cells per ml of milk |
| Antibiotic use | Antibiotic treatment (days/year/animal) and % of herd treated |
| Longevity | Annual herd replacement (%/year) |
| | Survival rate or deaths by age class (%) |
| | Rate of on farm deaths (%) |
| Lameness (relevance mainly to dairy cattle) | Locomotion score (1–5) |
| Fertility | Finally pregnant by insemination (%) |
| | Insemination period (days) |
| | Conception rate |
| Vitality | Body condition score (1–5) |

Source: the Sustainable Agriculture Initiative.[115]

of diseases. These numerical indicators can be used to track performance over the years, to set benchmarks and to steer improved management.

The Belgian Federal Agency for the Safety of the Food Chain has developed a tool to measure animal health throughout the food chain from suppliers to slaughterhouses.[125] Known as the Animal Health Barometer, this tool consists of a basket of 13 weighted animal health indicators covering foods produced in Belgium and for food imports. Both products and processes are included in the basket of indicators. The barometer includes indicators for prevention in terms of self-checking, compulsory notification and traceability, and recording of mortality for certain animal species. Specific examples of animal health indicators in this barometer include the duty to report notifiable animal diseases and bovine abortions, inspections of infrastructure, facilities and hygiene, inspections of traceability and animal welfare, antibiotic resistance in Escherichia coli indicator bacteria and parasitic liver damage in pigs.

This barometer measures the state of the general health of food production animals in Belgium on an annual basis, and compares this with findings from the previous year. The animal health barometer is an instrument to gain insight into the evolution of the general animal health through the years in an objective manner and to communicate about it in a simple way.

In Europe EFSA is working to develop a set of scientifically measurable animal welfare indicators for all farm species. These welfare indicators will support decision-making on the acceptable conditions for farmed animals and will be used to underpin monitoring and control programmes, implemented at farm level, to guarantee standards of animal health and welfare.[67] Certification schemes that aim to provide an assurance on animal welfare have been developed in many countries but there is no internationally agreed mechanism for recognising the equivalence of animal welfare schemes. These include the US Animal Welfare Approved programme and the UK's RSPCA Freedom Food programme. The lack of standardisation is a complication in international trade as the lack of clarity may impede demand for products from animals reared according to specified levels of welfare. An important first step is to define a credible best practice framework for animal welfare certification schemes that could apply in any country. Schemes may aim to provide assurance on minimum levels of welfare or may also aim to promote welfare improvement within their scheme membership.

## Economic indicators

### Financial share derived by food system actors

Food is a value-added item in the economic system. It delivers massive financial benefits to some but much less to others. The structure of the food system can be represented as an hourglass with high numbers of disparate actors at each end – farmers and consumers – and a highly concentrated and powerful centre made up of a relatively small number of multiple retailers, caterers and multinational processors.[126] According to the UK's Defra, currently almost half of the £196 bn that UK consumers spend on food and drink goes to retailers, manufacturers and caterers, with £9.2 bn (5%) going to primary growers.[127] Sixty years ago farmers in Europe and the USA received 45–60% of the money consumers spent on food, but retailers, processors and manufacturers are increasingly capturing the economic value of food. Farmers sell the basic commodities (squeezed by more powerful interests) and others add the value. The percentage share received by each group from farmers to manufacturers, caterers and retailers, or where the market is concentrated, can be used as an indicator to show where the money flows within the food system, shining a light on these huge disparities that make agricultural work unsustainable, particularly without the subsidies on which farmers may not be able to continue to rely indefinitely, and that leads to economic decline in rural areas.

### Food price

Food price to the consumer is another economic value within the food system. At a generic level food prices can be assessed on a number of different indicators. One indicator is a comparison of food prices across different regions and countries. This can be calculated according to the food price level.[128] The Domestic Food Price Level Index is calculated by dividing the Food Purchasing Power Parity (FPPP) by the General PPP, thus providing an index of the price of food in the country relative to the price of the generic consumption basket. Data are available for 2005 from the World Bank International Comparison Program.[129] It is then extended to other years by adjusting both numerator and denominator using the relative changes in Food Consumer Price Index (CPI) and General CPI as provided by the International Labour Organization (ILO).

Other indicators of food price are:

- food price as a percentage of household expenditure, over time and between countries;
- food price as a percentage of income;
- food price as a percentage of the cost of production, data on which are often difficult to find.

In the UK total household expenditure has increased by 97% over the period 1997 to 2013, while expenditure on food has grown by 78%, reducing its share in overall household spending from 10% in 1997 to 8.5% in 2007 before reaching 9.3% in 2013. Data are available from national or regional statistics offices, such as the Office for National Statistics (ONS) in the UK, Eurostat for the EU or USDA in the USA. Prices for individual food groups can also be illuminating, for example whether the price of foods perceived as healthy (for example, fruit and vegetables) are changing price at a different rate than foods perceived as unhealthy (for example, those high in fat and sugar). In the UK, since 2002, more healthy foods and beverages have been consistently more expensive than less healthy ones, with a growing gap between them.[130] Price volatility can make price a particularly sensitive social indicator anywhere.

### Externalised costs of the diet

A further possibility is to study the externalised costs of the diet. One study even decades ago assessed the external environmental and health costs of UK agriculture in 1996 to be equivalent to £208/hectare for arable and permanent pasture with significant costs arising from contamination of drinking water with pesticides (£120 m/year), nitrate (£16 m), Cryptosporidium (£23 m) and phosphate and soil (£55 m), from damage to wildlife, habitats, hedgerows and drystone walls (£125 m), from emissions of gases (£1,113 m), from soil erosion and organic carbon losses (£106 m), from food poisoning (£169 m) and from bovine spongiform encephalopathy (BSE) (£607 m).[131] A further study estimated the total cost of a per capita weekly food basket to be 11.8% more (£2.91) than the price in the shop (£24.79) if externalities and subsidies are included, with farm externalities (81p), domestic road transport (76p), government subsidies (93p) and shopping transport (41p) contributing the most. As knowledge grows, so do the figures.

In summary, the economic indicators that can be considered include:

- proportion of the consumer food spend retained by farmers;
- average net incomes of farmers, in particular small- and medium-sized farms;
- farmers receive market prices consistently above costs of production;
- farmers have fair access to markets and services such as credit and information;
- proportion of food spend captured by food retailers, manufacturers, processors and caterers;
- concentration of market held by top companies within a sector;

- proportion of food system workers receiving a fair and living wage;
- Food Consumer Price Index;
- food price level across countries and regions;
- food price as a percentage of household expenditure;
- food price as a percentage of income;
- price for individual food groups over time;
- food price as a percentage of the costs of production;
- cost of externalities (for example, health and environmental costs).

## Food security indicators

Food security matters immensely and is of interest to policy makers, practitioners and academics in large part because the consequences of food insecurity can affect almost every part of society. Food security matters from a public health perspective, a moral perspective and also for maximising economic capacity. It is also important for sustainable diets. No diet can be described as sustainable if there is food insecurity. The most commonly used definition of food security is based on the definition from the 1996 World Food Summit:

> Food security at the individual, household, national regional and global levels is achieved when all people, at all times, have physical and economic access to sufficient, safe and nutritious food to meet their dietary needs and food preferences for an active and healthy life.[132]

A range of different indicators, measures and tools, often with different approaches and purposes, are used to measure food security. This is partly because many different academic disciplines have engaged with it, including agriculture, anthropology, economics, nutrition, public policy and social science. Food security metrics may focus on food availability, access, utilisation, the stability of food security over time, or some combination of these domains. Measures have been developed for use at national, regional, household and/or individual levels.

Food security measures developed for use at the country level often emphasise food availability, which is measured by tools such as food balance sheets. Such data are used to create the FAO's core food security measure, the prevalence of undernourishment. Inaccuracies and differences in interpretation of data have led to varying estimates of the numbers of food insecure households and the FAO now publishes a set of additional food security indicators along with its estimate of the prevalence of undernourishment. These metrics examine variations in the dietary energy supply, protein of animal origin, food prices, food access and factors that determine food access. Other indices measuring one or more aspects of food security at national level include the Global Hunger Index developed by the International Food Policy Research Institute (IFPRI) and the Global Food Security Index designed by the Economic Intelligence Unit (one of several companies of the Economist Group, a publicly traded multinational).

National level measures of food security do not evaluate household food security. Household measures of food security are concerned with food security dynamics within and between households, and rely on data from household consumption and expenditure surveys, which can more accurately capture the 'access' component of food security than measures made at the national level. However, for household estimates of food security, these data may provide widely varying estimates of household food consumption, and they do not account for individual consumption, including vulnerable groups such as infants, children and pregnant women. Dietary food group diversity has gained considerable traction as an indicator of food security as it is associated with various measures of household socio-economic status that are commonly considered proxy indicators of household food security (for example, food and non-food expenditures, daily calorie availability per person, education and household income). Because the types of foods vary across cultural contexts, dietary diversity is difficult to define, and therefore to measure, across settings.

Other measures of household food security use a participatory approach in which respondents are asked a set of questions related to their experience of food insecurity. One example is the United Nations Food Insecurity Experience Scale (FIES) that was developed by the FAO. This is based on the US Household Food Security Survey module, which has also been adopted by Canada and variations of it have been used in Central and South American countries. For the FIES, eight questions are used relating to the qualitative and quantitative manifestations of food insecurity. Respondents are asked whether, during the past 12 months:

- You were worried you would run out of food because of a lack of money or other resources?
- You were unable to eat healthy and nutritious food because of a lack of money or other resources?
- You ate only a few kinds of food because of a lack of money or other resources?
- You had to skip a meal because there was not enough money or other resources to get food?
- You ate less than you thought you should because of a lack of money or other resources?
- Your household ran out of food because of a lack of money or other resources?
- You were hungry or did not eat because there was not enough money or other resources for food?
- You went without eating for a whole day because of a lack of money or other resources?

The answers are used to place respondents on a scale from mild ('experiencing anxiety about ability to procure adequate food') to severe ('experiencing hunger').

The FIES thus provides information about the degree of severity of food insecurity and, accordingly, how prevalent these levels of severity are in the population. When incorporated into larger-scale, representative surveys, food insecurity can be examined across gender, age and other individual parameters and sub-groups in the population that are particularly vulnerable can be identified. However, unlike the US and Canadian models, the UN FIES fails to differentiate between adults' and children's experiences.

## Social LCA

Life-cycle analysis (LCA) finds a particular use in the food system for measuring environmental impacts (see above) such as the GHG of specific products, foods and meals. However, LCA can also be used to measure socio-economic impacts within the food system. The usefulness of a social LCA lies in its ability to solve problems and improve the conditions of stakeholders within the product life-cycle. Social LCA methodology is relatively new and there are a number of different approaches used particularly in the range and weighting of indicators and choice of stakeholder categories and system boundaries.[133] Labour rights, human dignity and well-being are fundamental values within a social LCA.[134, 135] The United Nations Environment Programme/Society of Environmental Toxicology and Chemistry (UNEP/SETAC) has produced guidelines on social LCA. These guidelines provide a framework to assess social impacts across product life-cycles and are in line with ISO 14040 and 14044.[136] Danish researchers have developed a social LCA method based on each of four impact categories representing the labour rights according to the conventions of the International Labour Organization (ILO) covering: forced labour, discrimination, restrictions of freedom of association and collective bargaining and child labour.[137]

Every product may contain a huge number of production activities or unit processes and prioritisation is needed to ease data collection. The Social Hotspots Database (SHDB) is an overarching global database that eases the data collection burden in social LCA studies. Proposed 'hotspots' are production activities or unit processes in the supply chain that may be at risk for social issues to be present. The SHDB enables efficient application of social LCA by allowing users to prioritise production activities for which site-specific data collection is most desirable. Data for three criteria are used to inform prioritisation: (1) labour intensity in worker hours per unit process; (2) risk for, or opportunity to affect, relevant social themes or sub-categories related to human rights, labour rights and decent work, governance and access to community services; and (3) gravity of a social issue.[138]

The potential for social LCA in the food system is being evaluated but is still under construction. A study of cheese production in New Zealand identifies a range of social indicators relevant to the employee, the local community, future generations, the consumer and the company.[139] A study of salmon production systems made a distinction between quantitative indicators such as the costs of production, labour or industrial accidents, and qualitative or descriptive

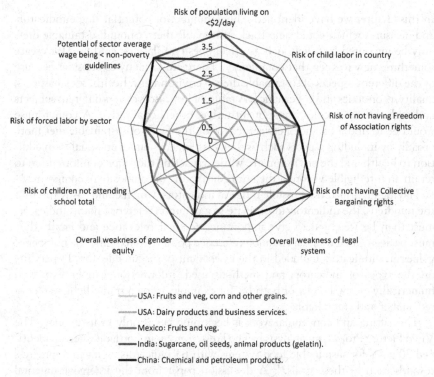

Figure 2.1 Potential social hotspots in the food supply chain

Source: Benoit-Norris et al., 2012.[138]

indicators, which could be the absence of forced labour, freedom of association, compliance with regulations, etc. Although quantitative indicators can be reflected in the functional unit chosen for the LCA, this is not the case for descriptive indicators.[140] A study of the strawberry yogurt supply chain found a multitude of social hotspots[138] and Figure 2.1 offers a visual representation of the most relevant ones. (The scale is defined as: 0 = no data or no evidence, 1 = low, 2 = medium, 3 = high and 4 = very high risk.)

The findings from this social LCA on strawberry yogurt indicate particular countries and sectors where the opportunity for social improvements exists, for example labour rights in the USA, child and forced labour and gender equity in some of the other countries involved in the supply chain.

Some studies have attempted to link social and economic aspects in LCAs. A Danish study linked social inventory indicators to impacts on human well-being and productivity and suggested that a common assessment unit such as quality adjusted life years (QALY) could be used to measure human well-being.[141] Nevertheless, much work still needs to be done to convert all impacts into QALY units.

## Multi-criteria indicators

In this chapter we have identified a huge number of potential single indicators and measures which could help track sustainable diets. Should sustainable diets only be measured by a few such as price, obesity, GHG or land use? Or create something new to keep that complexity? There are so many to consider because of the different aspects of sustainable diets – environment, health, social aspects, quality, economics and governance. A range of indicators covers different subjects and with different scales, some quantitative, others qualitative. A compromise would be to find a balance between covering the fields of sustainable diet more broadly by including aspects such as social issues, economics and quality in addition to health and the environment, while restricting the scope of information to retain an intelligible vision of the entire situation – a composite of composites?

Having identified the possible range of indicators, which could easily run into the hundreds, the indicators must relate to a common reference point. Indicators must then be weighted to give importance to their relevance and finally they must be aggregated round a common reference point so as to refine the number of values and indicators included in the assessment of sustainable diet. Depending on the types of indicators and methods used, information can be expressed numerically or graphically or both by, for example, using a traffic-light system of red, amber and green lights.

This sifting and conceptual work is beginning but is only in its infancy. The Vivid Picture Project, an analysis by EcoTrust, a group in Portland Oregon, identified 20 goals for sustainable food systems with 63 indicators to measure progress towards each of these goals.[142] A discussion paper from the intergovernmental CIHEAM group, which monitors the Mediterranean, collated a list of 60 indicators from four thematic areas with the aim of improving sustainability of diets and food systems in the Mediterranean region.[143] A process for developing metrics for sustainable diets has been developed by Thomas Allen (Bioversity International) and colleagues.[144] This involved making a long list of 1,500 indicators from the literature followed by shortlisting 36 of these indicators discussed during a focus group while gaining consensus through exchange of opinion using the Delphi technique.

It is possible to select and combine certain indicators to develop a composite or multi-criteria indicator (i.e., a score card or index), which can be used to try to take account of the multidimensional nature of sustainable diets. Nevertheless, this approach is less simple than it might appear because it requires consistency between the indicators for it to be meaningful. The challenge is to identify indicators from fields as diverse as health, the environment, socio-economics, quality and governance to be applicable within a coherent scientific framework. Any composite approach – merging or pooling indicators – is thus highly dependent on skilled judgement.

It is for this reason that we favour the multi-criteria approach – which Lang and colleagues on the UK Government's SDC termed the 'omni-standards' approach.[145] One example of a multi-criteria approach is the multidimensional poverty index (MPI), which is a measure that incorporates a range of indicators that capture the complexity of poverty.[146] Something similar could be developed for sustainable diets. A model based on the MPI illustrates four dimensions of sustainable diets including nutritional adequacy, environmental sustainability, cultural acceptability and low cost or accessibility to the urban poor and the rural poor.[147] In this, the rural poor have a more sustainable diet with higher scores in the four dimensions (see Figure 2.2). It is assumed that these four dimensions have several indicators that measure specific determinants and are weighted. Scores from 0 to 6 have been suggested with the higher number being the better score. The problem with composite indices is that they often mask more than they reveal. While these composite scores may be useful for communication, monitoring and advocacy, an absence of context and detail may render the score less than useful.

In 2013 WRAP's Product Sustainability Forum published another multi-criteria study, releasing a landmark set of industry-derived data.[149] It reviewed 150 different studies and collated tens of thousands of UK food products – donated by food companies wishing to improve their sustainability – against five criteria: embedded energy, waste, blue/green and grey water footprints, material use. Note that nutrition was not included. This was a weakness but nonetheless

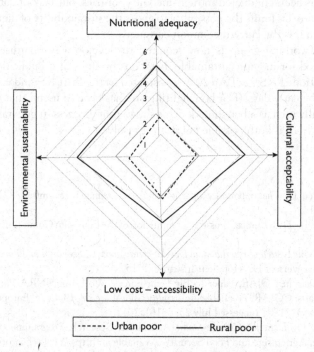

Figure 2.2  A multidimensional index for sustainable diet based on the MPI

Source: Alkire and Foster, 2011.[148]

this study edged towards the omni-standards or multi-criteria analysis required for measurement of sustainable diets.

Ethical Consumer, a UK NGO, produces reports on different types of food, including baked beans, breakfast cereals, margarines and spreads, nuts, pasta and so on, giving them a total ethical score that is made up of environmental ratings (for example, climate change, pollution, habitats and resources), animal testing, welfare and factory farming, human and workers' rights and irresponsible marketing, organic, fair trade, genetic engineering and anti-social finance.

## Conclusions

New measures are needed for both policy makers and the public on sustainable diets. Some are already available and well established from the past: measuring land use, carbon emissions, nutrients. Some have been developed for specific purposes such as embedded or virtual water but are of considerable value beyond their immediate rationale. Life-cycle analysis (LCA) has been much used in sustainability assessment of food products. It has become a, if not the, key procedure for product analysis, but it does not resolve all that is needed for sustainable diets. It measures product life-cycles rather than population impacts. In addition, the majority of LCA has been conducted in high-income countries, but lack of data in lower-income countries limits the possibility to assess the sustainability of diets globally.[68] That said, it is the current common currency.

A methodology working group is now required to develop a standardised multi-criteria method for judging sustainable diets, on the lines of a Publically Available Specification (PAS). A PAS 2050 was created by the British Standards Institute (BSI) in the early days of carbon auditing and has been so useful that it is now internationally used as a benchmark. This shows that progress in generating good robust methods is both possible but not yet resolved.

## References

1  Beyer MA, Laney D. *The Importance of 'Big Data': A Definition*. Stamford, CT: Garnter Inc., 2012

2  European Union. *Big Data Europe*. Brussels: Commission of the European Community, 2015

3  Spratt S, Baker J. *Big Data and International Development: Impacts, Scenarios and Policy Options*. London: Overseas Development Institute, 2015

4  Arnaud E. *Big Data in CGIAR*, paper to Big Data Europe Workshop, INRA Pars, 22 September. Paris: CGIAR. Available at: http://de.slideshare.net/BigData_Europe/big-data-in-cgiar-53151807 (accessed July 25, 2016), 2015

5  CGIAR, CIAT. *Big Data for Climate-Smart Agriculture*, Research Programme on Climate Change, Agriculture and Food Security. Available at: https://ccafs.cgiar.org/bigdata#.VrXQ4VJvDgk (accessed February 6, 2016). Montpellier: CGIAR, 2016

6  Prainsack B. Three Hs for health: the darker side of big data. *Bioethica Forum*, 2015; 8(2): 40–1

7 World Values Survey. *The World Values Survey*. Available at: www.worldvaluessurvey. org/ (accessed July 25, 2016), 2011

8 Weber M. *Economy and Society: An Outline of Interpretive Sociology* (Roth G, Wittich C, Eds). Berkeley, CA: University of California Press, 2013 [1922]

9 Rose G. *The Strategy of Preventive Medicine*. Oxford: Oxford University Press, 1992

10 Rose G. Sick individuals and sick populations. *International Journal of Epidemiology*, 2001; 30(3): 427–32

11 Australian Government. *Proposed Reforms to Country of Origin Food Labels: Overview*. Canberra: Australian Government Dept of Industry and Science, 2015

12 Finch J. Tesco labels will show products' carbon footprints. Available at: www.guardian. co.uk/environment/2008/apr/16/carbonfootprints.tesco?gusrc=rss&feed=networkfront (accessed July 6, 2008). *The Guardian*, Wednesday April 16, 2008

13 *Which? Making Sustainable Food Choices Easier: A Consumer Focused Approach to Food Labels*. London: Which?, 2010

14 Reddy S, Lang T, Dibb S. *Setting the Table: Advice to Government on Priority Elements of Sustainable Diets*. Available at: www.sd-commission.org.uk/publications.php?id=1033 (accessed October 18, 2013). London: Sustainable Development Commission, 2009

15 United Nations. *Sustainable Development Goals*, agreed at the UN Summit, September 27–29. Available at: https://sustainabledevelopment.un.org/post2015/summit (accessed July 26. 2016). New York: United Nations Department of Economic and Social Affairs, Division for Sustainable Development, 2015

16 UNFCCC. *UN Framework Convention on Climate Change (COP21)*, Paris, 30 November–11 December 2015. Available at: http://unfccc.int/secretariat/contact/items/2782.php (accessed January 18, 2016). Bonn, Germany: United Nations Framework Convention on Climate Change, 2015

17 European Environment Agency. *EEA Core Set of Indicators: Guide*. EEA Technical Report 1/2005. Available at: www.eea.europa.eu/publications/technical_report_2005_1 (accessed July 29, 2014). Luxembourg: Office for Official Publications of the European Communities, 2005

18 Defra. *Annex I: Sustainable Development Indicators, 2012*. Available at: http://sd.defra.gov.uk/documents/SDI-Consultation-Annex-I-proposed-SDIs.pdf (accessed August 3, 2014). London: Defra, 2012

19 WHO. *WHO Discussion Paper: A Comprehensive Global Monitoring Framework and Voluntary Global Targets for the Prevention and Control of NCDs*. Available at: www. who.int/nmh/events/2011/consultation_dec_2011/WHO_Discussion_Paper_FINAL. pdf?ua=1 (accessed October 28, 2014). Geneva: World Health Organization, 2011

20 WHO. WHO Global Infobase. Available at: https://apps.who.int/infobase (accessed August 4, 2014). Geneva: World Health Organization, 2011

21 World Obesity Federation. Obesity Data Portal. Available at: www.worldobesity.org/aboutobesity/resources/obesity-data-portal/ (accessed July 27, 2016). London: World Obesity Federation, 2016

22 Global Health Data Exchange. *Global Health Data Exchange*. Available at: http://ghdx.healthmetricsandevaluation.org/ (accessed October 27, 2014). Seattle: Institute for Health Metrics and Evaluation, 2013

23 CDC. *Centers for Disease Control and Prevention: Data and Statistics*. Available at: www. cdc.gov/DataStatistics/ (accessed October 27, 2014). *Secondary Centers for Disease Control and Prevention: Data and Statistics*. Available at: www.cdc.gov/DataStatistics/ (accessed October 27, 2014), 2014

24  Amine E, Baba N, Belhadj M, *et al. Diet, Nutrition and the Prevention of Chronic Diseases: Report of a Joint WHO/FAO Expert Consultation.* Geneva: World Health Organization, 2002

25  World Cancer Research Fund/American Institute for Cancer Research. *Food, Nutrition, Physical Activity, and the Prevention of Cancer: a Global Perspective.* Available at: www.dietandcancerreport.org/cancer_resource_center/er_full_report_english.php (accessed October 26, 2014). Washington, DC: American Institute for Cancer Research, 2007

26  The DHS Program. *Measure DHS: Demographic and Health Surveys.* Available at: http://dhsprogram.com/ (accessed October 27, 2014). *Secondary Measure DHS: Demographic and Health Surveys.* Available at: http://dhsprogram.com/ (accessed October 27, 2014), 2014

27  WHO. *WHO STEPwise Approach to Surveillance (STEPS).* Available at: www.who.int/chp/steps/en (accessed October 14, 2014). Geneva: World Health Organization, 2014

28  European Commission. *Eurobarometer Surveys,* European Commission Public Opinion. Available at: http://ec.europa.eu/public_opinion/index_en.htm (accessed October 27, 2014). Brussels: European Commission, 2015

29  UNICEF. *Multiple Indicator Cluster Survey (MICS),* UNICEF Statistics and Monitoring. Available at: www.unicef.org/statistics/index_24302.html (accessed October 27, 2014). New York: UNICEF, 2012

30  WHO. *WHO World Health Survey.* Available at: www.who.int/healthinfo/survey/en/ (accessed October 27, 2014). Geneva: World Health Organization, 2014

31  SHARE. *The Survey of Health: Ageing and Retirement in Europe (SHARE).* Available at: www.share-project.org/ (accessed October 27, 2014). Munich: SHARE-ERIC, 2011

32  Byrne D. *Nutrition & Diet for Healthy Lifestyles in Europe: Science & Policy Implications,* Eurodiet Core Report. Brussels: European Commission, 2000

33  GESIS. *International Social Survey Programme.* Available at: www.issp.org/ (accessed October 27, 2014). Mannheim, Germany: Secondary International Social Survey Programme, 2014

34  US FDA. Hazards Analysis Critical Control Point (HACCP). Available at: www.fda.gov/Food/GuidanceRegulation/HACCP/ (accessed August 2, 2016). Silver Spring, MD: United States Food and Drug Administration, 2015

35  Codex Alimentarius. *Recommended International Code of Practice: General Principles of Good Hygiene.* Rome: FAO and WHO Codex Alimentarius, 2003

36  Baert K, Van Huffel X, Wilmart O, *et al.* Measuring the safety of the food chain in Belgium: development of a barometer. *Food Research International,* 2011; 44(4): 940–50

37  Guenther PM, Casavale KO, Reedy J, *et al.* Update of the healthy eating index: HEI-2010. *Journal of the Academy of Nutrition and Dietetics,* 2013; 113(4): 569–80

38  Chiuve SE, Fung TT, Rimm EB, *et al.* Alternative dietary indices both strongly predict risk of chronic disease. *The Journal of Nutrition,* 2012; 142(6): 1009–18

39  McCullough ML, Feskanich D, Stampfer MJ, *et al.* Diet quality and major chronic disease risk in men and women: moving toward improved dietary guidance. *The American Journal of Clinical Nutrition,* 2002; 76(6): 1261–71

40  McCullough ML, Feskanich D, Rimm EB, *et al.* Adherence to the dietary guidelines for Americans and risk of major chronic disease in men. *The American Journal of Clinical Nutrition,* 2000; 72(5): 1223–31

41  McCullough ML, Feskanich D, Stampfer MJ, et al. Adherence to the dietary guidelines for Americans and risk of major chronic disease in women. *The American Journal of Clinical Nutrition*, 2000; 72(5): 1214–22

42  Patterson RE, Haines PS, Popkin BM. Diet quality index: capturing a multidimensional behavior. *Journal of the American Dietetic Association*, 1994; 94(1): 57–64

43  Huijbregts P, Feskens E, Rasanen L, et al. Dietary pattern and 20 year mortality in elderly men in Finland, Italy, and the Netherlands: longitudinal cohort study. *BMJ* (Clinical Research Ed.), 1997; 315(7099): 13–17

44  Trichopoulou A, Kouris-Blazos A, Wahlqvist ML, et al. Diet and overall survival in elderly people. *BMJ* (Clinical Research Ed.), 1995; 311(7018): 1457–60

45  Alkerwi A, Vernier C, Crichton GE, et al. Cross-comparison of diet quality indices for predicting chronic disease risk: findings from the Observation of Cardiovascular Risk Factors in Luxembourg (ORISCAV-LUX) study. *British Journal of Nutrition*, 2014: 1–11

46  Dernini S, Berry EM. Mediterranean diet: from a healthy diet to a sustainable dietary pattern. *Frontiers in Nutrition*, 2015; 2

47  USDA. *Food Availability (Per Capita) Data System*. www.ers.usda.gov/data-products/food-availability-(per-capita)-data-system.aspx (accessed October 29, 2014). Washington, DC: United States Department of Agriculture Economic Research Service, 2014

48  Defra. *Family Food 2012*. Available at: www.gov.uk/government/collections/family-food-statistics (accessed October 28, 2014). London: Department for Environment, Food and Rural Affairs, 2013

49  Defra. *Food Statistics Pocket Book*. Available at: www.gov.uk/government/uploads/system/uploads/attachment_data/file/526395/foodpocketbook-2015update-26may16.pdf (accessed June 15, 2016). London: Department for Environment, Food and Rural Affairs, 2016

50  Eisinger-Watzl M, Strassburg A, Ramunke J, et al. Comparison of two dietary assessment methods by food consumption: results of the German National Nutrition Survey II. *European Journal of Nutrition*, 2015; 54(3): 343–54

51  Castetbon K, Vernay M, Malon A, et al. Dietary intake, physical activity and nutritional status in adults: the French nutrition and health survey (ENNS, 2006–7). *The British Journal of Nutrition*, 2009; 102(5): 733–43

52  EFSA. Guidance of EFSA. Use of the EFSA Comprehensive European Food Consumption Database in Exposure Assessment. *EFSA Journal*, 2011; 9(3): 2097

53  de Boer EJ, Slimani N, van 't Veer P, et al. The European Food Consumption Validation Project: conclusions and recommendations. *European Journal of Clinical Nutrition*, 2011; 65 Suppl 1: S102–7

54  de Boer EJ, Slimani N, van 't Veer P, et al. Rationale and methods of the European Food Consumption Validation (EFCOVAL) Project. *European Journal of Clinical Nutrition*, 2011; 65 Suppl 1: S1–4

55  EFSA. Guidance of EFSA. General principles for the collection of national food consumption data in the view of a pan-European dietary survey. *EFSA Journal*, 7(12): 1435, 2009

56  Scottish Government Rural and Environment Research and Analysis Directorate. *Food Affordability, Access and Security: Their Implications for Scotland's Food Policy – a Report by Work Stream 5 of the Scottish Government's Food Forum*. Available at: www.scotland.gov.uk/resource/doc/277447/0083291.pdf (accessed October 31, 2014).

Edinburgh: Scottish Government Rural and Environment Research and Analysis Directorate, 2009

57  Swindale A, Bilinsky P. *Household Dietary Diversity Score (HDDS) for Measurement of Household Food Access: Indicator Guide (v.2)*. Washington, DC: FHI 360/FANTA, 2006. Available at: www.fantaproject.org/sites/default/files/resources/HDDS_v2_Sep06_0.pdf (accessed October 31, 2014). Washington, DC: Food and Nutrition Technical Assistance, 2006

58  Cummins S, Macintyre S. The location of food stores in urban areas: a case study in Glasgow. *British Food Journal*, 1999; 101(7): 545–53

59  Macdonald L, Ellaway A, Macintyre S. The food retail environment and area deprivation in Glasgow City, UK. *International Journal of Behavioral Nutrition and Physical Activity*, 2009; 6(1): 1

60  USDA. *Supplemental Nutrition Assistance Program (SNAP)*. Available at: www.fns.usda.gov/snap/supplemental-nutrition-assistance-program-snap (accessed August 2, 2016). Washington, DC: United States Department of Agriculture Food and Nutrition Service, 2016

61  Trussell Trust. *Trussell Trust foodbank use remains at record high with over one million three-day emergency food supplies given to people in crisis in 2015/16*. Available at: www.truselltrust.org/news-and-blog/latest-stats/ (accessed April 15, 2016). Salisbury: Trussell Trust, 2016

62  Cassidy ES, West PC, Gerber JS, *et al.* Redefining agricultural yields: from tonnes to people nourished per hectare. *Environmental Research Letters*, 2013; 8(3): 034015

63  Hastings G, Stead M, Macdermott L, *et al. Review of Research on the Effects of Food Promotion to Children*, Final Report to the Food Standards Agency by the Centre for Social Marketing, University of Strathclyde. London: Food Standards Agency, 2004

64  Hawkes C. *Marketing Food to Children: Changes in the Global Regulatory Environment 2004–6*. Geneva: World Health Organization, 2007

65  Rumbo JD. Consumer resistance in a world of advertising clutter: the case of Adbusters. *Psychology & Marketing*, 2002; 19(2): 127–48

66  Frazier WC, Harris JL. *Trends in Television Food Advertising to Young People: 2015 Update*. Hartford, CT: UConn Rudd Center for Food Policy and Obesity, 2016

67  Heller MC, Keoleian GA, Willett WC. Toward a life cycle-based, diet-level framework for food environmental impact and nutritional quality assessment: a critical review. *Environmental Science & Technology*, 2013; 47(22): 12632–47

68  Jones AD, Hoey L, Blesh J, *et al.* A systematic review of the measurement of sustainable diets. *Advances in Nutrition: An International Review Journal*, 2016; 7(4): 641–64

69  British Standards Institute. *PAS 2050: Assessing the Life Cycle Greenhouse Gas Emissions of Goods and Services*. British Standards Institute: London, 2008

70  Cuéllar AD, Webber ME. Wasted food, wasted energy: the embedded energy in food waste in the United States. *Environmental Science & Technology*, 2010; 44(16): 6464–9

71  Tukker A, Jansen B. Environmental impacts of products: a detailed review of studies. *Journal of Industrial Ecology*, 2006; 10(3): 159–82

72  Tukker A, Bausch-Goldbohm S, Verheijden M, *et al.* Environmental impacts of diet changes in the EU. Available at: http://ipts.jrc.ec.europa.eu/publications/pub.cfm?id=2359 (accessed December 19, 2015). Seville: Institute for Prospective and Technological Studies, Joint Research Centre, 2009

73  Tukker A, Goldbohm RA, De Koning A, *et al.* Environmental impacts of changes to healthier diets in Europe. *Ecological Economics*, 2011; 70(10): 1776–88

74 Collins A, Fairchild R. Sustainable food consumption at a sub-national level: an ecological footprint, nutritional and economic analysis. *Journal of Environmental Policy & Planning*, 2007; 9(1): 5–30

75 Van den Bergh JC, Verbruggen H. Spatial sustainability, trade and indicators: an evaluation of the 'ecological footprint'. *Ecological Economics*, 1999; 29(1): 61–72

76 Čuček L, Klemeš JJ, Kravanja Z. A review of footprint analysis tools for monitoring impacts on sustainability. *Journal of Cleaner Production*, 2012; 34: 9–20

77 Lang T. Locale/globale (Food Miles). *Slow Food* (Bra, Cuneo Italy), 19 May 2006, 94–7

78 Paxton A. *The Food Miles Report*. London: Sustainable Agriculture, Food and Environment (SAFE) Alliance, 1994

79 Pirog R, Benjamin A. *Calculating Food Miles for a Multiple Ingredient Food Product*. Ames, IA: Leopold Center for Sustainable Agriculture, Iowa State University Ames, 2005

80 Saunders C, Barber A, Taylor G. *Food Miles: Comparative Energy/Emissions Performance of New Zealand's Agriculture Industry*. Research Report 285. Christchurch, New Zealand: Agribusiness and Economics Research Unit, Lincoln University, 2006

81 Pretty JN, Ball AS, Lang T, *et al*. Farm costs and food miles: an assessment of the full cost of the UK weekly food basket. *Food Policy*, 2005; 30(1): 1–20

82 Smith A, Watkiss P, Tweddle G, *et al*. *The Validity of Food Miles as an Indicator of Sustainable Development: Final Report*, REPORT ED50254. London: Defra, 2005

83 Weber CL, Matthews HS. Food-miles and the relative climate impacts of food choices in the United States. *Environmental Science & Technology*, 2008; 42(10): 3508–13

84 Gaballa S, Abraham AB. *Food Miles in Australia: A Preliminary Study of Melbourne, Victoria*. East Brunswick, VIC: CERES, 2007

85 Boege S. *Road Transport of Goods and the Effects on the Spatial Environment*. Wuppertal, Germany: Wuppertal Institute, 1993

86 Owen B, Lee DS, Lim L. Flying into the future: aviation emissions scenarios to 2050. *Environmental Science & Technology*, 2010; 44(7): 2255–60

87 Coley D, Howard M, Winter M. Local food, food miles and carbon emissions: a comparison of farm shop and mass distribution approaches. *Food Policy*, 2009; 34(2): 150–5

88 IGD. *Sustainable Distribution in 2008*. Radlett Herts: Institute of Grocery Distribution, 2008

89 MacGregor J, Vorley B. *Fair Miles? The Concept of 'Food Miles' Through a Sustainable Development Lens*. London: International Institute for Environment and Development, 2006

90 Future Foundation. *Food Miles*, report to Somerfield, Chapter 4. London: Future Foundation, 2007

91 Animal Protection Institute, Compassion in World Farming. *Driving Pain: the State of Farmed-Animal Transport in the U.S. and Across Our Borders*. Sacramento, CA: API and CIWF, 2005

92 Allan A. *Virtual Water: Tackling the Threat to Our Planet's Most Precious Resource* (1st Ed.). London: IB Tauris, 2011

93 Hoekstra AY. The water footprint of animal products, in: J D'Silva, J Webster (Eds) *The Meat Crisis: Developing More Sustainable Production and Consumption*. London: Earthscan, 2010: 22–33

94 Vanham D, Hoekstra A, Bidoglio G. Potential water saving through changes in European diets. *Environment International*, 2013; 61: 45–56

95  Allan JA. Virtual water – the water, food and trade nexus: useful concept or misleading metaphor? *Water International*, 2003; 28: 4–11

96  World Resources Institute. *AQUEDUCT: The Water Risk Atlas*. Available at: www.wri.org/our-work/project/aqueduct/aqueduct-atlas (accessed 10 August 2016). Washington, DC: World Resources Institute, 2014

97  Millennium Ecosystem Assessment. *Ecosystems and Human Well-Being: Biodiversity Synthesis*. Washington, DC: World Resources Institute, 2005

98  Grid-Arendal U. *GLOBIO Modelling Human Impacts on Biodiversity*. Available at: www.globio.info/what-is-globio (accessed August 2, 2016). Arendal, Norway: UNEP Grid-Arendal, 2016

99  Convention on Biological Diversity. *Indicators*. Available at: www.cbd.int/2010-target/framework/indicators.shtml (accessed August 2, 2016). Montreal: Convention on Biological Diversity, 2016

100 Majer J, Beeston G. The biodiversity integrity index: an illustration using ants in Western Australia. *Conservation Biology*, 1996; 10(1): 65–73

101 Scholes RJ, Biggs R. A biodiversity intactness index. *Nature*, 2005; 434(7029): 45–9

102 Rouget M, Cowling RM, Vlok JAN, *et al.* Getting the biodiversity intactness index right: the importance of habitat degradation data. *Global Change Biology*, 2006; 12(11): 2032–6

103 Loh J, Green RE, Ricketts T, *et al.* The Living Planet Index: using species population time series to track trends in biodiversity. *Philosophical Transactions of the Royal Society B: Biological Sciences*, 2005; 360(1454): 289–95

104 Pauly D. The Sea Around Us Project: documenting and communicating global fisheries impacts on marine ecosystems. *Ambio*, 2007; 36(4): 290–5

105 van den Berg M, Bakkes J, Bouwman L, *et al.* *EU Resource Efficiency Perspectives in a Global Context*. Available at: http://ec.europa.eu/environment/enveco/studies_modelling/pdf/res_efficiency_perspectives.pdf (accessed December 9, 2014). The Hague: PBL Netherlands Environmental Assessment Agency, 2011

106 Alder J, Guénette S, Beblow J, *et al.* *Ecosystem-Based Global Fishing Policy Scenarios*. Fisheries Centre Research Reports 2007 Volume 15 Number 7. Available at: www.fisheries.ubc.ca/webfm_send/132 (accessed December 9, 2014). Vancouver, Canada: Fisheries Centre, University of British Columbia, 2007

107 Curran M, de Baan L, De Schryver AM, *et al.* Toward meaningful end points of biodiversity in life cycle assessment. *Environmental Science & Technology*, 2010; 45(1): 70–9

108 Souza DM, Teixeira RFM, Ostermann OP. Assessing biodiversity loss due to land use with Life Cycle Assessment: are we there yet? *Global Change Biology*, 2014; 21: 32–47

109 de Baan L, Alkemade R, Koellner T. Land use impacts on biodiversity in LCA: a global approach. *The International Journal of Life Cycle Assessment*, 2013; 18(6): 1216–30

110 Jeanneret P, Baumgartner D, Freiermuth Knuchel R, *et al.* Integration of Biodiversity as Impact Category for LCA in Agriculture, SALCA-Biodiversity, 6th International Conference on LCA in the Agri-Food Sector, 34–48. Available at: www.agroscope.admin.ch/agroscope/en/home/publications/publication-search.html (accessed May 19, 2015). Zurich: Agroscope Reckenholz-Tänikon Research Station ART, 2008: 12–14

111 Mueller C, de Baan L, Koellner T. Comparing direct land use impacts on biodiversity of conventional and organic milk: based on a Swedish case study. *The International Journal of Life Cycle Assessment*, 2014; 19(1): 52–68

112  Amundson R, Berhe AA, Hopmans JW, *et al.* Soil and human security in the 21st century. *Science*, 2015; 348(6235)

113  Roosevelt FD. *Statement on Signing the Soil Conservation and Domestic Allotment Act, March 1, 1936.* Santa Barbara, CA: University of California The American Presidency Project [online], 1936

114  Steinbeck J. *The Grapes of Wrath.* London: Penguin, 2000 [1939]

115  Kuneman G, Fellus E (Eds). *Sustainability Performance Assessment Version 2.0: Towards Consistent Measurement of Sustainability at Farm Level.* Available at: www.saiplatform. org/uploads/Modules/Library/spa-guidelines-2.0_saiplatform.pdf (accessed July 29, 2016). Etterbeek: Sustainable Agriculture Initiative Platform, 2014

116  Gustavsson J, Cederberg C, Sonnesson U, *et al. Global Food Losses and Food Waste: Extent, Causes and Prevention.* Rome: Food and Agriculture Organization, 2011

117  FAO. *Food Wastage Footprint: Full-Cost Accounting.* Available at: www.fao.org/3/a-i3991e.pdf (accessed October 27, 2014). Rome: Food and Agricultural Organization, 2014

118  WRAP. *Methods Used for Household Food and Drink Waste in the UK, 2012.* Available at: www.wrap.org.uk/sites/files/wrap/Methods Annex Report v2.pdf (accessed July 29, 2014). Banbury, England: Waste Resources Action Programme (UK), 2013.

119  Sharpe RS. PhD Thesis: 'A piecemeal way to save the world': investigating social sustainability in the UK's conventional food supply. Centre for Food Policy, City University London, forthcoming, 2017

120  ETI. *Ethical Trade Initiative: About Us.* Available at: www.ethicaltrade.org/ (accessed August 30, 2015). London: Ethical Trade Initiative, 2015

121  Harrison R, Carson R. *Animal Machines: The New Factory Farming Industry.* London: Vincent Stuart Ltd, 1964

122  FAWC. Farm Animal Welfare in Great Britain: Past, Present and Future. Available at: www.gov.uk/government/publications/fawc-report-on-farm-animal-welfare-in-great-britain-past-present-and-future (accessed October 23, 2014). London: Department for Environment, Food and Rural Affairs, 2014

123  Commission of the European Communities. *Animal Welfare: EU Action Plan, Evaluation and the Second Strategy on Animal Welfare 2011–15.* Available at: http://ec.europa.eu/food/animal/welfare/actionplan/actionplan_en.htm (accessed August 2, 2016). Brussels: Commission of the European Communities, DG Health and Consumers, 2011

124  Commission of the European Communities. *Animal Welfare: Summary of Lisbon Treaty's Amendment of 'Treaty on the Functioning of the European Union'.* Available at: http://ec.europa.eu/food/animals/welfare/index_en.htm (accessed August 2, 2016). Brussels: Commission of the European Communities, 2016

125  Federal Agency for the Safety of the Food Chain. *The Animal Health Barometer.* Available at: www.favv-afsca.fgov.be/scientificcommittee/barometer/animalhealth/measuring.asp (accessed October 27, 2014). Brussels: Federal Agency for the Safety of the Food Chain, 2011

126  Gereffi G, Lee J. Why the world suddenly cares about global supply chains. *Journal of Supply Chain Management*, 2012; 48: 24–32

127  Defra. *Agriculture in the United Kingdom 2013 (29 May 2014 Update), Table 14.1,* p. 94. Available at: www.gov.uk/government/uploads/system/uploads/attachment_data/file/315103/auk-2013-29may14.pdf (accessed October 26, 2014). London: Department for Environment, Food and Rural Affairs, 2014

128 FAO. *Food Security Indicators*. Available at: www.fao.org/economic/ess/ess-fs/ess-fadata/en/ -.UwOBffl_uCk (accessed 29 July 2016) and *Secondary Food Security Indicators*. Available at: www.fao.org/economic/ess/ess-fs/ess-fadata/en/ -.UwOBffl_uCk (accessed July 29, 2016), 2016

129 World Bank. *International Comparison Program*. Available at: http://web.worldbank.org/WBSITE/EXTERNAL/DATASTATISTICS/ICPEXT/0,,contentMDK:22377119~menuPK:62002075~pagePK:60002244~piPK:62002388~theSitePK:270065,00.html (accessed June 15, 2016). Washington, DC: World Bank, 2016

130 Jones NR, Conklin AI, Suhrcke M, *et al.* The growing price gap between more and less healthy foods: analysis of a novel longitudinal UK dataset. *PLoS ONE*, 2014; 9(10): e109343

131 Pretty JN, Brett C, Gee D, *et al.* An assessment of the total external costs of UK agriculture. *Agricultural Systems*, 2000; 65(2): 113–36

132 World Food Summit. *Rome Declaration on World Food Security and World Food Summit Plan of Action*. Rome, Italy: FAO, 1996

133 Jørgensen A, Le Bocq A, Nazarkina L, *et al.* Methodologies for social life cycle assessment. *The International Journal of Life Cycle Assessment*, 2008; 13(2): 96–103

134 Dreyer L, Hauschild M, Schierbeck J. Characterisation of social impacts in LCA. *The International Journal of Life Cycle Assessment*, 2010; 15(3): 247–59

135 Smith J, Barling D. Social impacts and life cycle assessment: proposals for methodological development for SMEs in the European food and drink sector. *The International Journal of Life Cycle Assessment*, 2014; 19(4): 944–9

136 Benoît C, Mazijn, B (Eds). *Guidelines for Social Life Cycle Assessment of Products*. Available at: www.cdo.ugent.be/publicaties/280.guidelines-sLCA.pdf (accessed November 1, 2014). Paris: United Nations Environment Programme, 2009

137 Dreyer L, Hauschild M, Schierbeck J. Characterisation of social impacts in LCA. Part 2: implementation in six company case studies. *The International Journal of Life Cycle Assessment*, 2010; 15(4): 385–402

138 Benoit-Norris C, Cavan DA, Norris G. Identifying social impacts in product supply chains: overview and application of the social hotspot database. *Sustainability*, 2012; 4(9): 1946–65

139 Paragahawewa U, Blackett P, Small B. *Social Life Cycle Analysis (S-LCA): Some Methodological Issues and Potential Application to Cheese Production in New Zealand*. Available at: www.saiplatform.org/uploads/Library/SocialLCA-FinalReport_July2009.pdf (accessed November 1, 2014). Hamilton, New Zealand: AgResearch, 2009

140 Kruse SA, Flysjö A, Kasperczyk N, *et al.* Socioeconomic indicators as a complement to life cycle assessment: an application to salmon production systems. *The International Journal of Life Cycle Assessment*, 2009; 14(1): 8–18

141 Weidema BP. The integration of economic and social aspects in life cycle impact assessment. *The International Journal of Life Cycle Assessment*, 2006; 11(1): 89–96

142 Feenstra G, Jaramillo C, McGrath S, *et al. Proposed Indicators for Sustainable Food Systems*. Ecotrust and Roots of Change Fund, 2008

143 Lacirignola C, Dernini S, Capone R, *et al. Towards the Development of Guidelines for Improving the Sustainability of Diets and Food Consumption Patterns: the Mediterranean Diet as a Pilot Study*. CIHEAM/FAO–Options Méditerranéennes, Series B: Studies and Research, N 70, 2012: 70

144 Allen T, Prosperi P, Peri I, *et al. Vulnerability and Resilience: Developing Metrics to Measure Sustainable Diets and Food Systems*. Resilience 2014, 7 May, Montpellier, France. Rome: Bioversity International, 2014

145 Lang T. From 'value-for-money' to 'values-for-money'? Ethical food and policy in Europe. *Environment and Planning A*, 2010; 42: 1814–32

146 Alkire S, Chatterjee M, Conconi A, *et al. Global Multidimensional Poverty Index 2014.* Oxford: Poverty and Human Development Initiative (OPHI), 2014

147 Fanzo J, Cogill B, Mattei F. *Metrics of Sustainable Diets and Food Systems.* Technical brief, Madrid Roundtable. Rome: Bioversity International, 2012

148 Alkire S, Foster J. Counting and multidimensional poverty measurement. *Journal of Public Economics*, 2011; 95(7–8): 476–87

149 WRAP Product Sustainability Forum. An initial assessment of the environmental impact of grocery products: latest review of evidence on resource use and environmental impacts across grocery sector products in the United Kingdom. Banbury: WRAP, March 2013

# Chapter 3

# Health

Nutrition science and the messy effects of diet on health

## Contents

## Core arguments

Food is essential for health. Health is an essential purpose of a sustainable diet. Some would say food's only purpose is to provide nutrients to maintain good health. In reality, poor diet is associated with over-, under- and mal-consumption; from obesity through to hunger and famine. Sustainable diets and the food system generally also have strong social and cultural impacts and inputs, and are a source of pleasure and human interaction. Diet's role in health can be both direct and indirect. This chapter reviews the links between diet and health, placing this as a key component of sustainability. An estimated 2 billion people in the world are overweight or obese while 795 million people are undernourished due to the inability to obtain sufficient food. The majority of non-communicable diseases, including type 2 diabetes, cardiovascular disease and some cancers, are related to diet. But diet-related health means more than nutrients. It is also affected by food safety, including microbial and chemical contamination, and the use of antibiotics in the food system, which is an increasing risk to human health due to the rise in antibiotic resistance. Also important for the sustainable diet debate are the health consequences for people working in the food system. Food is work and the work on food shapes people's health, not least through the level of wages received, if there are any. A sustainable diet should also be derived from a food system in which there is no or minimal harm to the health of the people working within it. The chapter concludes that a sustainable diet must adopt a broad sense of healthy. It must be accessible and affordable to everyone.

## Dietary links with health

Globally, there is considerable agreement on what constitutes a healthy dietary pattern. It is one based on plant foods, including grains, vegetables and fruits and nuts, with a small emphasis on animal-derived foods such as meat and dairy, if those are culturally appropriate. A healthy diet also means minimal amounts of sugary, fatty foods. This healthy dietary pattern should help to protect the environment because a low amount of meat and dairy seriously limits the diet's total greenhouse gas emissions. But eating a diet that is beneficial for the environment does not automatically mean it is healthy, in that high carbon-emitting animal foods, for example, can be replaced with foods high in fat, sugar and/or salt and of low micronutrient density. The health–environment links can be tricky.

Generally, diet is linked with health in a variety of ways. While a nutritious diet is essential for good health, poor diet contributes to a range of public health harms. Exposure to high-(saturated) fat, high-sugar, high-salt, energy-dense, micronutrient-poor foods, particularly in conjunction with low levels of physical activity, increases the risk of obesity and non-communicable diseases (NCDs) such as cardiovascular disease and type 2 diabetes mellitus.[1, 2] Worldwide, obesity has nearly doubled since 1980. In 2014 more than 2.1 billion people – nearly 30% of the global population – were overweight or obese.[3] The prevalence of overweight and obesity in different United Nations (UN) regions is shown in Figures 3.1 and 3.2 and the prevalence of type 2 diabetes is shown in Figure 3.3.

Alongside the problems related to over-nutrition, under-nutrition also remains significant. In 2014, 795 million people (11% of the world's population) remained undernourished[5] due to the inability to obtain sufficient food to meet their dietary energy requirements, and about 2 billion people, or 30% of the world's population, are affected by deficiencies of micronutrients, in particular that of vitamin A, iron

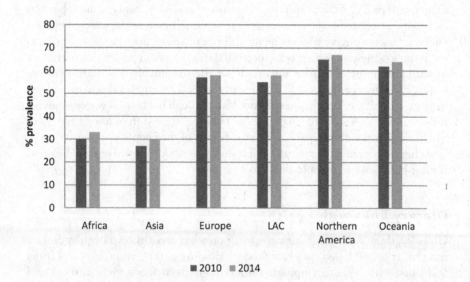

*Figure 3.1* Adult overweight and obesity by UN region 2010 and 2014

Source: *Global Nutrition Report*, 2016.[4]

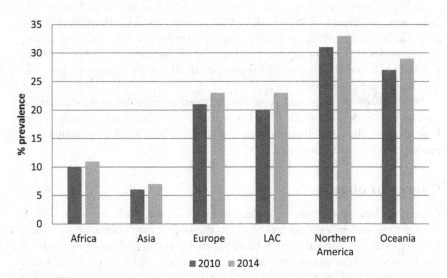

Figure 3.2 Adult obesity by UN region 2010 and 2014

Source: *Global Nutrition Report*, 2016.[4]

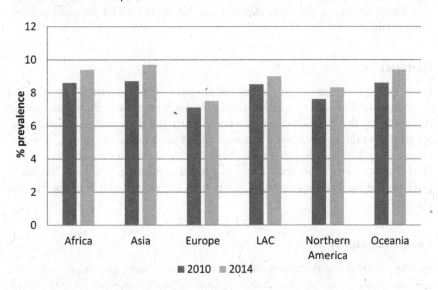

Figure 3.3 Adult diabetes (raised blood glucose) by UN region 2010 and 2014

Source: *Global Nutrition Report*, 2016.[4]

and iodine. The 2016 *Global Nutrition Report*[4] shows that 44% of countries with data available (57 out of 129 countries) experience serious levels of both under-nutrition and adult overweight and obesity, and that, despite good progress in some countries, the world is off track to reduce and reverse this trend.

A WHO report providing an overview of NCDs states that these conditions were responsible for 38 million (68%) of the world's 56 million deaths in 2012. More than 40% of them (16 million) were premature deaths among people under the age of 70 years. Almost three quarters of all NCD. deaths (28 million), and the majority of premature deaths (82%), occur in low- and middle-income countries.[2]

In rich, Western countries, poor dietary patterns make the greatest contribution to the burden of NCDs. The major dietary risks are low consumption of fruit, nuts, seeds, vegetables and whole grains and high intakes of sodium, fat, processed meats and trans fats.

## Causes of obesity

Obesity occurs when energy intake from food and drink consumption is greater than energy expenditure through the body's metabolism and physical activity over a prolonged period, resulting in the accumulation of excess body fat. However, there are many complex behavioural and societal factors that combine to contribute to the causes of obesity. Many reviews have pointed out this complexity factor. The UK Chief Scientist's *Foresight Report*, for example, referred to 'a complex web of more than 100 societal and biological factors that have, in recent decades, exposed our inherent human vulnerability to weight gain'.[6]

### Genetics

Some evidence suggests that genetics does play a role in obesity, with specific genes suggested to convey a higher risk of obesity if expressed.[7] However, during the period of the past 30–40 years when obesity has increased so significantly across the world, it is virtually inconceivable that a major population genetic change has taken place on that scale. Nevertheless, genes can sensitise individuals to environments that promote obesity. In this context, recent focus has been given to the food environment in an effort to understand the dramatic rise in obesity.

### Food availability

Increases in the rate of obesity in Western countries have coincided with substantial changes in the availability of food, food consumption and the food environment. These changes in turn have been influenced by changes in agricultural policies, technology, marketing and lifestyles. Available calories in Europe, Australia, New Zealand and North America increased considerably between 1980 and 2010 (Table 3.1).

A number of studies have explored how increased calorie levels in the food supply have translated into rising obesity rates. For example, individual studies

*Table 3.1* Available calories per day 1980 and 2010

|  | *1980* | *2010* |
| --- | --- | --- |
| Australia and New Zealand | 3,056 | 3,210 |
| Canada | 2,950 | 3,397 |
| UK | 3,116 | 3,405 |
| US | 3,178 | 3,659 |
| Western Europe | 3,306 | 3,515 |

Source: FAO, FAOSTAT. Food Balance Sheets.[8]

and systematic analyses have shown a strong association between consuming an excess amount of sugar, particularly from sugar-sweetened soft drinks, and weight gain.[9-12]

## Portion sizes

Portion sizes have increased considerably over the past 20 years, particularly for food eaten outside of the home. A 2002 US study found that portion sizes for hamburgers, French fries and sugar-containing fizzy drinks are two to five times higher than the originals, and that commonly available portions frequently exceed, sometimes greatly, the US Government recommended portion sizes.[13] A 2013 study by the British Heart Foundation looked at 245 food products within popular grocery stores in the UK. They found, for example, a chicken curry frozen meal was 53% larger than it was in 1993. Crumpets were 20–30% bigger. A 2013 US National Institutes of Health study estimates that most food portions have doubled and some have tripled over the past 20 years. Twenty years ago a bagel was three inches in diameter, today they are six inches while a medium bag of popcorn has increased from five to eleven cups. Other reports indicate that portion sizes in US restaurants have quadrupled since the 1950s. An analysis of Danish cookbook recipes found that energy intake from home-made meals had increased by 77% over the past 100 years.[14]

A number of studies have explored how increased portion size increases energy intake and food waste. In one study participants consumed 30% more energy at lunch when offered the largest portion of food compared with the smallest portion.[15] Larger bowl size has been shown to increase breakfast cereal consumption and food waste in children.[16] A study found that cinema goers who were given fresh popcorn ate 45% more popcorn when it was given to them in large containers. This container-size influence is so powerful that even when the popcorn was disliked, people still ate a third more popcorn when eating from a large container than from a medium-size container.[17] Another study found that people ate a greater quantity of a snack food when the same sized portion was presented in a large bowl compared with a medium and small bowl.[18]

### Energy density

The energy density of the diet has also been linked to higher body mass index, obesity and increased waist circumference.[19-23] The Dietary Guidelines for Americans encourage consumption of an eating pattern low in energy density to manage body weight, while the Revised Dietary Guidelines for Scotland 2013 recommend that the average energy density of the diet be lowered to 125 kcal/100g by reducing intake of high fat and/or sugary products and by replacing these with starchy carbohydrates (for example, bread, pasta, rice and potatoes), fruits and vegetables. A study in French adults found that more sustainable diets with lower GHG emissions had a below-average energy density and increased proportion of their energy intake from plants.[24]

Portion size and energy density also act cumulatively to promote higher energy intake in children[25] and adults.[26] Thus, reducing energy density through increasing the consumption of foods such as vegetables, soups and fruit at the expense of those high in sugar and fat reduces energy intake. [27, 28]

### Meat

A body of literature exists linking red and processed meat with obesity. A systematic review of 21 studies and meta-analysis of 18 studies showed that red and processed meat is a risk factor for obesity, higher body mass index (BMI) and higher waist circumference.[29]

### Food retailing

Food retailers, particularly supermarkets, have been evaluated in some studies for a link with obesity. Access to food stores can have a powerful influence on body weight, diet quality and other health outcomes, and inequitable access to healthy foods is thought to be one root cause of obesity. However, proximity to supermarkets or shopping at supermarkets *per se* does not appear to be associated with obesity.[30] Indeed, in the United States, living in close proximity to a 'full-service' supermarket is associated with healthier eating, lower BMI and lower incidence of obesity in adults. In this context, full-service supermarkets are distinguished from 'fast-food' outlets and convenience stores. Store size may also have an impact on obesity. Two studies, one from France involving 7,131 shoppers at 1,097 supermarkets[31] and another from Australia[32] involving 170 supermarkets in eight developed countries with Western-style diets, found that the larger the supermarket the greater the prevalence of obesity. Exposure to energy-dense snack foods and soft drinks in supermarkets was greater in socio-economically disadvantaged neighbourhoods.[33]

### Eating out

Eating out, which has been a growing trend during recent decades, has also been associated with weight gain.[34, 35] A study by the USDA Economic Research

Service found that eating one meal away from home each week translates to an additional weight gain of 1 kg each year or 134 kcals/day.[36] Exposure to take-aways and fast-food outlets has also been linked with greater BMI in children,[37] teenagers[38, 39] and adults,[34, 40] and poor dietary quality. Consumption of ready-made meals has also been implicated in higher energy intakes and an increased risk of obesity.[41]

### Food prices

Food prices and development of food preferences also play an important role in food purchasing and hence in food consumption and body weight. Lower price supermarkets[30, 42] and lower price food shopping baskets purchased in a super-market[43] are linked with a higher incidence of obesity, even after adjusting for socio-demographics. Less healthy foods are lower in price per 1,000 kcals than healthier foods and a UK study confirmed a growing gap between the price of healthier and less healthy foods.[44]

### Marketing

Evidence also suggests that marketing strategies contribute to an increased con-sumption of energy-dense food. In a study in Pittsburgh, USA, exposure to displays of sugar-sweetened beverages and foods high in saturated fats and added sugars, and price reduction of sugar-sweetened beverages, was associated with increased body mass index indicating that in-store marketing[45] is associated with body mass index among regular shoppers.[42] Some research indicates that food marketing has contributed to obesity by increasing the accessibility of bigger portions of inexpensive and energy-dense food.[46] Other research has shown that supermar-kets do not consistently promote foods that support healthy weight and healthy eating guidelines.[47] A UK study found that supermarkets do not offer promotions on less healthy foods more often than promotions on healthier foods but price promotions on less healthy foods generated a 35% increase in sales while price promotions on healthier foods generated only a 20% increase in sales.[48]

## Non-communicable diseases (NCDs)

A poor diet with exposure to high-fat, high-sugar, high-salt, energy-dense, micro-nutrient-poor foods increases the risk of non-communicable diseases (NCDs) such as cardiovascular disease (CVD), type 2 diabetes mellitus and some cancers.

### Cardiovascular disease

#### Dietary patterns

For CVD, there is strong evidence that dietary patterns rich in fruits, vegeta-bles, whole grains, low-fat dairy, fish and unsaturated oils, and low in red and processed meat, saturated fat, sodium, refined grains and sugar-sweetened foods and drinks, are associated with decreased risk of CVD. Regular consumption of nuts and legumes also contributes to a beneficial dietary pattern. In addition, research including specific nutrients within the context of dietary patterns indicates that dietary patterns lower in saturated fat, cholesterol and sodium and richer in fibre, unsaturated fat and potassium are beneficial for reducing cardiovascular risk.

Healthy dietary patterns also have a meaningful impact on cardiovascular risk factors such as blood pressure and blood lipids and CVD endpoints such as stroke and myocardial infarction.[45] There are a variety of specific dietary patterns. They include the Dietary Approaches to Stop Hypertension (DASH) sponsored by the US National Institutes of Health, which is low in saturated fat and sodium and high in fruit and vegetables. These, as well as the Mediterranean-style dietary pattern or the new Nordic diet and vegetarian dietary patterns, are associated with reduced blood pressure and improved lipid profile.[49-52] The DASH-style pattern shows consistent evidence of benefit. In addition, individuals whose diets mirror these healthy eating patterns have lower risk of CVD events such as stroke and heart attack and a lower CVD mortality.[50, 53-55] Results from the largest Mediterranean diet trial, PREDIMED, showed that a Mediterranean diet (plus extra virgin olive oil or nuts) had favourable effects in high-risk participants compared with the control groups who were advised to reduce dietary fat intake. An approximately 30% reduced risk of major CVD events was observed and the trial was stopped early because of the demonstrated benefits.[56] Greater adherence to the DASH-style diet has also been shown to reduce CVD, CHD and stroke.[54]

Consistent evidence also shows that vegetable and fruit intakes are inversely related to the incidence of myocardial infarction and stroke,[57, 58] with significantly larger positive effects when intakes are greater than five servings per day.[57, 59] Intake of whole grains[60] and low-fat dairy foods[61] have been inversely associated with CVD, and two servings per week of seafood containing omega-3 fatty acids is associated with lower cardiovascular mortality.[62]

## Fat

The relationship between fat, different types of dietary fat and risk of CVD has been extensively studied. It is well established that higher intakes of trans fat from partially hydrogenated vegetable oils is associated with increased risk of CVD and thus should be minimised in the diet.[63] Numerous controlled trials have demonstrated that, compared with polyunsaturated or monounsaturated fats or carbohydrates, saturated fat increases total and LDL cholesterol. Thus, limiting saturated fat has been a longstanding recommendation to reduce risk of CVD. UK and US dietary guidelines recommend consuming no more than 10% of daily energy from saturated fat.

However, recent meta-analyses of prospective observational studies did not find a significant association between higher saturated fat intake and risk of CVD in large populations.[64, 65] These data have re-ignited the debate regarding current recommendations to limit saturated fat intake. A central issue in the relationship between saturated fat and CVD is the specific macronutrients used to replace it because consuming unsaturated fats versus carbohydrates in place of saturated fat can have different effects on blood lipids and risk of CVD. Strong and consistent evidence from randomised controlled trials (RCTs) shows that replacing saturated fat with unsaturated fat, especially polyunsaturated fat, significantly reduces total and LDL cholesterol.[66] Replacing saturated fat with carbohydrates also reduces total and LDL cholesterol, but significantly reduces high-density lipoproteins (HDL) cholesterol and increases triglycerides.[67]

Strong and consistent evidence from RCTs and statistical modelling in prospective cohort studies shows that replacing saturated fat with polyunsaturated fat reduces the risk of CVD events and coronary mortality.[66, 65] Evidence is limited regarding whether replacing saturated fat with monounsaturated fat confers overall CVD benefits. This is partly because the main source of monounsaturates in typical Western diets is animal fat. The co-occurrence of saturated fat with monounsaturated fat in foods makes it difficult to tease out the independent relationship of monounsaturates with CVD. However, evidence from RCTs and prospective studies has demonstrated benefits of plant sources of monounsaturated fats, such as olives and nuts, on CVD risk.[68, 69]

Reducing total fat, and replacing total fat with carbohydrates, does not lower CVD risk because such diets are generally associated with hypertriglyceridaemia and low HDL cholesterol concentrations. Thus, dietary advice should put emphasis on optimising types of dietary fat, with an emphasis on replacing saturated fat with unsaturated fat, especially polyunsaturated fat, and not reducing total fat.

Moreover, when individuals reduce consumption of refined carbohydrates and added sugars, they should not replace them with saturated fat but with healthy sources of fats (for example, non-hydrogenated vegetable oils that are high in unsaturated fats and nuts and seeds) and healthy sources of carbohydrates (for example, whole grains, legumes, vegetables and fruits). The consumption of low-fat products with high amounts of added sugars or refined grains should be discouraged. A healthy dietary pattern that emphasises vegetables, fruit, whole grains, legumes and nuts, with the inclusion in moderate amounts, for people who wish to eat these foods, of low-fat dairy produce, lean meat and poultry and seafood, should be encouraged. Sugar-sweetened foods and beverages and, in rich countries, red and processed meat should be limited. Multiple dietary patterns can achieve these food and nutrient patterns and they should be tailored to people's nutritional needs and food preferences.

## Sugar

Moderate evidence from prospective cohort studies indicates that a higher intake of added sugars, especially in the form of sugar-sweetened beverages, is consistently associated with increased risk of hypertension, stroke and CHD in adults.[70]

Observational and intervention studies indicate a consistent relationship between higher intake of added sugars and higher blood pressure and serum triglycerides.

## Salt

Hypertension is a major risk factor for heart disease and stroke, the number one cause of death and disability globally. Higher sodium intakes are associated with increased blood pressure in both adults and children.[71] Conversely, higher potassium intakes are associated with decreased blood pressure.[72] The World Health Organization's (WHO) 2013 guidelines recommend that adults should consume less than 2,000 mg sodium (5 g salt) daily with recommendations for children reduced based on energy intake. Increased intakes of low-fat milk products and vegetable protein also are linked to lower blood pressure.

## Diabetes mellitus

Diet is a factor in type 2 diabetes, a major chronic disease that also is an independent risk factor for CVD. Higher consumption of added sugars, especially sugar-sweetened beverages, increases the risk of type 2 diabetes[73] among adults and this relationship is not fully explained by body weight. Saturated fatty acid intakes are associated with increased insulin resistance and risk of type 2 diabetes, and substitution of just 5% of saturated fats with monounsaturated fatty acids or polyunsaturated fatty acids can improve insulin response. Whole-grain intakes and low-fat dairy intakes are also associated with a reduced incidence of type 2 diabetes.

As for CVD, healthy dietary patterns higher in vegetables, fruits and whole grains, and lower in red and processed meats, high-fat dairy products, refined grains, sweets and sugar-sweetened drinks, reduce the risk of developing type 2 diabetes mellitus. In a meta-analysis of nine studies, the Mediterranean diet was associated with a significant reduction in the risk of developing diabetes.[74]

## Cancer

Strong evidence demonstrates that body fatness increases the risk of several cancers, including esophageal, pancreatic, colorectal, post-menopausal breast, endometrial and renal. For specific cancers, diets higher in red and processed meat and sources of sugar are linked with increased risk of colorectal cancer,[75, 76] while diets higher in vegetables, fruits, legumes, whole grains, lean meat, seafood and low-fat dairy are associated with reduced risk.[77] Data regarding this dietary pattern and cancers of the breast and lung point in the same direction.

## Dementia and depression

Evidence is also emerging, but is still limited, that a dietary pattern higher in vegetables, fruits, whole grains and nuts, and lower in meat and saturated fat, is associated with reduced risk of developing dementia and Alzheimer's disease, depression and, with the addition of dairy foods, favourable bone health outcomes including decreased risk of fracture and osteoporosis. However, definitive conclusions cannot be reached for these conditions due to the limited amount of research.

## Under-nutrition

Some 795 million people, or roughly 11% of the world's population, are under-nourished.[78] Under-nutrition, defined as being underweight for age, too short for age (stunted), dangerously thin for height (wasted) and deficient in vitamins and minerals, is estimated to contribute to more than a third of all child deaths worldwide, although it is rarely listed as the direct cause.

Under-nutrition is a narrower term than malnutrition. Malnutrition manifests itself in many different ways: as poor child growth and development; as individuals who are skin and bone or prone to infection; as those who carry too much weight or whose blood contains too much sugar, salt, fat or cholesterol; or those who are deficient in essential vitamins or minerals. The global prevalence of malnutrition is shown in Table 3.2. The 2016 *Global Nutrition Report* shows that one in three people in the world is malnourished.[4]

Lack of access to highly nutritious foods, especially in the recent context of rising food prices, is a common cause of under-nutrition. Poor feeding practices,

*Table 3.2* The global prevalence of malnutrition

| Indicator | Number of individuals | Current prevalence |
|---|---|---|
| Under-5 stunting | 159 million (in 2014) | 23.8 |
| | 255 million (in 1990) | 39.6 (in 1990) |
| Under-5 overweight | 41 million (in 2014) | 6.1 |
| | 31 million (in 1990) | 4.8 (in 1990) |
| Under-5 wasting | 50 million (in 2014) | 7.5 |
| Under-5 severe wasting | 16 million in 2014 | 2.4 |
| Anaemia in women (15–49 years, pregnant and non-pregnant) | 533 million in 2011 | 29 for non-pregnant women (in 2011); 33 in 1995 |
| | | 39 for pregnant women (in 2011); 43 in 1995 |
| Exclusive breast-feeding (under 6 months) | NA | 39 (in 2014) |
| Low birthweight | 20 million (in 2014) | 15 |
| Adult overweight (18+ years) | 1.9 billion (in 2014) | 39 |
| Adult obesity (18+ years) | 600 million (in 2014) | 13 |
| Adult diabetes (raised blood glucose) (aged 18+) | NA | 9 |

Source: *Global Nutrition Report*, 2016.[4]

such as inadequate breastfeeding, offering the wrong foods and not ensuring that a child gets enough nutritious food, contribute to under-nutrition. Infection – particularly frequent or persistent diarrhoea, pneumonia, measles and malaria – also undermines a child's nutritional status.

### Iron deficiency

Iron deficiency is the most common and widespread nutritional disorder in the world. As well as affecting a large number of children and women in developing countries, it is also prevalent in industrialised countries. The numbers are staggering: 2 billion people – over 30% of the world's population – are anaemic, many due to iron deficiency and, in resource-poor areas, this is frequently exacerbated by infectious diseases. Malaria, HIV/AIDS, hookworm infestation, schistosomiasis, and other infections such as tuberculosis, are particularly important factors contributing to the high prevalence of anaemia in some areas.

Iron deficiency affects more people than any other condition, constituting a public health condition of epidemic proportions. More subtle in its manifestations than, for example, protein-energy malnutrition, iron deficiency exacts its heaviest overall toll in terms of ill-health, premature death and lost earnings. Iron deficiency and anaemia reduce the work capacity of individuals and entire populations, bringing serious economic consequences and obstacles to national development. Overall, it is the most vulnerable, the poorest and the least educated who are disproportionately affected by iron deficiency, and it is they who stand to gain the most by its reduction.

### Vitamin A deficiency

Vitamin A deficiency is the leading cause of preventable blindness in children and increases the risk of disease and death from severe infections. In pregnant women vitamin A deficiency causes night blindness and may increase the risk of maternal mortality. Vitamin A deficiency is a public health problem in more than half of all countries, especially in Africa and South East Asia, hitting hardest in young children and pregnant women in low-income countries.

### Iodine deficiency

Iodine deficiency is the world's most prevalent, yet easily preventable, cause of brain damage. Iodine deficiency disorders, which can start before birth, jeopardise children's mental health and often their survival. Serious iodine deficiency during pregnancy can result in stillbirth, spontaneous abortion and congenital abnormalities such as cretinism, a grave, irreversible form of mental retardation that affects people living in iodine-deficient areas of Africa and Asia. However, of far greater significance is iodine deficiency's less visible, yet pervasive, mental impairment that reduces intellectual capacity at home, in school and at work.

## Micronutrient intakes in wealthy countries

In rich countries clinical micronutrient deficiencies are uncommon but risks of low intakes do occur. In the UK the latest data from the National Diet and Nutrition Survey (NDNS) indicated that intakes of several minerals and trace elements such as magnesium, zinc and iron fall below recommended intakes, particularly among young women.[79] Selenium intakes are low across most of the population due mainly to selenium deficient soils in parts of the UK. Vitamin D status as measured by blood levels is poor, particularly in northern Britain and in any population groups where exposure to sunlight is low.

A study that compared recent dietary survey data across several, mainly Western European, countries found, with the exception of vitamin D, there was a low risk of low intakes of vitamins across in all age and sex groups.[80] However, there was a risk of low intakes for several minerals, particularly in certain age groups. In Poland 55% of women and 48% of men had calcium intakes below the estimated average requirement (EAR). More than 50% of 11–17-year-old girls in Germany (59%), France (58%) and the UK (50%) had intakes below the EAR for iodine. Iron intakes were below the EAR in half of women aged 14–50 years in six of the studied countries. In all countries, the proportion of selenium intakes below the EAR was high: for women, between 55% in France and 87% in Denmark and, for men, between 59% in France and 86% in Denmark.

Similarly, in the USA most low micronutrient intakes are found in particular population groups. Non-Hispanic Black Americans and Mexican Americans are more likely to be low in vitamin D and folate compared with non-Hispanic white people. A report from the USDA's Agricultural Research Service examined the usual intake levels of 24 nutrients from food in 8,940 individuals using 2001–2002 NHANES data and compared these with the EARs.[81] The intakes of vitamins A, E, C and magnesium were marginally low across all population groups, whereas group-specific low intakes were seen for vitamin B6 among adult women, zinc for older adults and phosphorus for young women. The latest US data on phosphorus, magnesium, calcium and vitamin D also found low intakes of those nutrients.[82]

A study among adolescents in western Australia found that fewer than 50% of young women met the EAR for calcium, magnesium, folate or the adequate intake (AI) for vitamins D and E. Fewer than 50% of young men met the EAR for magnesium, potassium, pantothenic acid, folate or the AI for vitamins D and E.[83]

# Dietary guidelines

## Nutrient standards

A healthy diet is one that provides energy and nutrients (protein, vitamins, minerals, essential fatty acids) in amounts commensurate with good health and well-being. Healthy diets and nutrient intakes can be measured against various dietary standards and guidelines. Since the early 1960s, expert committees have established energy and nutrient intake standards. These standards are based on the best possible scientific evidence and reviewed regularly. They are intended for healthy individuals and have been expressed in the form of recommended dietary allowances (RDAs) or, more recently, in the form of dietary reference values (DRVs). DRVs are a complete set of nutrient recommendations and reference values, and include values such as population reference intakes, the average requirement, adequate intake level and upper and lower threshold intakes. The specific measures and outcomes used to establish the DRVs vary by nutrient, but all relate to nutritional status or functional indicators that report on the level of nutrient intake required to prevent diseases associated with a particular micronutrient deficiency (for example, scurvy and vitamin C deficiency), and/or to reduce chronic disease risk. Dietary reference values are therefore also set for components of food whose intakes should be limited (for example, saturated fat, sugar and salt) to reduce the risk of NCDs. Nutrient requirements can vary by population group and nutrient intake standards are generally set for a range of different ages, males and females and pregnancy and lactation. Dietary reference values can be used, for instance, as a basis for reference values in food labelling and for establishing food-based dietary guidelines (FBDG).

### Food-based dietary guidelines

Food-based dietary guidelines translate nutritional recommendations into messages about foods and diet, and can guide people on what to eat and help them make healthy dietary choices. Food-based dietary guidelines are defined by WHO/FAO as 'the expression of principles of nutrition education mostly as foods'.[84] The purpose of the guidelines is to educate the population and to guide national food and nutrition policies as well as the food industry. Food-based dietary guidelines are advocated as a practical method to reach nutrition goals set for the population, while considering the setting, including social, economic and cultural factors, as well as the physical and the biological environment. Food-based dietary guidelines avoid the use of numerical recommendations such as RDAs but provide a practical way of interpreting these into dietary advice for individuals within a population. So, if the population target for saturated fat is 10% of total energy, and the current intake is higher, messages will include those designed to reduce saturated fat intake, such as 'choose lean cuts of meat'. Food-based dietary guidelines also address public health concerns, such as chronic diseases, by targeting nutrients that may influence the disease outcome.

Following the call of the International Conference on Nutrition (ICN) in Rome in 1992, the WHO and FAO published guidelines for the development of FBDGs,[85] and a framework for FBDGs in the European Union was agreed in 2000 as part of the Eurodiet project and published in 2001.[86] The FAO and WHO organise regional training workshops for national government representatives from the health, nutrition and agricultural sectors, in order to support especially medium- and low-income countries in the development of FBDGs (and of national food and nutrition action plans). The WHO nutrition policy database monitors the development and implementation of national food and nutrition action plans and checks if countries have FBDGs. Presently, 27 out of 52 countries in the WHO European Region have FBDGs,[87] as do 22 out of 37 countries in the WHO Western Pacific Region.[88] When formulating FBDGs at national levels it is often difficult to separate the scientific from the political process, and therefore some countries opt to open the process for a stakeholder discussion or involve all stakeholders from the beginning in the formulation. The government may not be the leader in the dietary guidelines development, but it is important that it oversees the process and publicly endorses the dietary guidelines. An endorsement from the private sector may also be considered valuable for successful implementation. The development and revision processes of FBDGs have been subject to fierce debates and lobbying from the side of food producers and processors.[88]

Food-based dietary guidelines generally include advice about foods containing fat, foods containing sugar and the consumption of fruits and vegetables. They also often contain advice on eating protein-containing foods, foods rich in carbohydrates and dietary fibre, restricting salt, taking enough fluids, controlling alcohol intake and body weight, and other aspects of lifestyle such as getting enough physical activity and eating regular meals. Occasionally they have advice on food hygiene. Most countries have developed a graphic representation of FBDGs to illustrate the proportions of different foods with similar characteristics that should be included in a balanced diet, although they may have a list of dietary messages as well.

The most popular graphic representation of an FBDG is in the form of a pyramid. In Europe, Austria, Belgium, Finland, Greece, Ireland, Latvia, Spain, Germany and Switzerland are some of the countries that make use of such a food guide pyramid. The Irish food pyramid is typical in that it has five groups, each forming a layer. The base layer, across the widest part of the pyramid, is for the food group of which we should eat the greatest quantities, i.e. 'bread, cereal and potatoes', and the narrow top depicts the group of which we should eat the least, i.e. 'oils, fats and sugary foods'. Above the base layer are 'fruits and vegetables', the middle layer is 'milk, cheese and yogurt' and below the top layer is 'meat, fish and alternatives'. Advice to drink plenty of water is given close by. Some of the pyramids include physical activity. Germany uses a three-dimensional pyramid that provides qualitative (nutritional role of the food) as well as quantitative (how much of this food relative to others) advice on food consumption.

The other common graphical form used for FBDGs is a circle divided into segments like a cake. Each segment contains one food group similar to those used in the pyramids. Circles have been developed in the USA (MyPlate), Portugal, Sweden and the UK (depicted as a plate). Finland and Spain use a circle as well as the pyramid, and the German pyramid depicts a circle at the base of its 3D pyramid. The Netherlands have a wheel, the centre of which is used for food messages. Most circles are proportionally segmented in accordance with the recommended contributions from each food group. The Portuguese and German graphics have water at the centre of the circle, while the Spanish circle depicts both water and exercise at the centre.

## Microbiological foodborne illness

Illness caused by harmful microbiological organisms in food is a public health problem throughout the world. In the developing world, foodborne infection leads to the death of many children, and the resulting diarrhoeal disease can have long-term effects on children's growth as well as on their physical and cognitive development. In the industrialised world, foodborne infection causes considerable illness, with significant costs to individuals and healthcare systems.

Of course, this is not a new problem. A century and more ago, the main sources of microbiological foodborne illness were milk from infected cows and spoiled meat from sick animals. Public health measures we now take for granted, such as milk pasteurisation, have helped to eliminate typhoid fever, cholera and most lethal diarrhoeal diseases in industrialised countries.

Today, however, the modern food system continues to create favourable conditions for the dissemination of microbes – bacteria, protozoa and viruses. Such conditions include the concentration and consolidation of food production such as transporting large numbers of animals over long distances in close proximity, the preference for takeaways and the availability of partially cooked foods.

The US Center for Disease Control (CDC) estimates that 47.8 million illnesses, 127,839 hospitalisations and 3,037 deaths related to foodborne illness occur every year in the United States, which translate into 1 in 6 Americans becoming ill every year from consuming contaminated food. Known pathogens account for 9.4 million of these illnesses, 56,000 hospitalisations and 1,400 deaths,[89] illustrating that the burden from unknown agents is significant. Most (58%) illnesses were caused by norovirus, followed by non-typhoidal Salmonella spp. (11%), Clostridium perfringens (10%) and Campylobacter spp. (9%). Leading causes of hospitalisation were non-typhoidal Salmonella spp. (35%), norovirus (26%), Campylobacter spp. (15%) and Toxoplasma gondii (8%). Leading causes of death were non-typhoidal Salmonella spp. (28%), T. gondii (24%), Listeria monocytogenes (19%) and norovirus (11%).[89]

In the UK, the FSA monitors trends in foodborne disease caused by key pathogenic microbes, including Salmonella, Campylobacter, E. coli O157 and Listeria monocytogenes. About four out of five cases of Campylobacter in the UK come from contaminated poultry. A 12-month survey (2014–2015) tested 4,000 samples of whole chickens and their packaging bought from UK retailers and smaller independents and butchers. Almost three quarters (73%) tested positive for Campylobacter and 19% of chickens tested positive for the highest level of Campylobacter. Variation existed between retailers but none met the FSA target for reducing Camplylobacter.[90]

Foods of animal origin, in particular poultry and also beef, unpasteurised dairy produce and shellfish, contribute significantly to microbiological foodborne illness, while the impact arising from plant-based foods is lower. A 2011 study of 14 food-related pathogens in the Netherlands found that products of animal origin contributed over half (51%) to the costs of illness attributed to microbiological foodborne illness, with beef, pork, lamb and poultry having the greatest impact.[91] However, foodborne disease outbreaks associated with fruit and vegetables have been increasing worldwide. Some leafy green vegetables such as lettuces and spinaches and seed sprouts, and ready-to-eat salads made from these foods, have been shown to carry the potential risk of microbiological contamination due to the usage of untreated irrigation water.[92–94] Ready-to-eat foods, such as sandwiches and salads, are an increasing source of food poisoning, particularly where food handlers are infected.

## Chemical foodborne illness

The food system is also associated with a number of chemical substances, which may cause adverse effects in humans. These chemicals can be naturally present in the food (for example, allergens in wheat or milk) or contaminants (i.e., they are not expected to be present in food). Some contaminants have been known for many years while others have emerged as potentially problematic issues more recently. Examples of chemical contaminants include polychlorinated biphenyls (PCBs), polychlorinated dioxins/furans, heavy metals (for example, mercury, lead, arsenic, cadmium), aflatoxins, other mycotoxins, marine toxins, polybrominated diphenyl ethers, polyfluorinated carboxylates and sulphonates and perchlorate. Some of these are classified as persistent organic pollutants (POPs).

Foodborne outbreaks associated with chemical hazards are not widely reported. For example, 7% of foodborne outbreaks reported for 2012 in the United States had a confirmed or suspected chemical agent.[95] This represented about 1% of the foodborne illnesses reported. Over the longer time frame of 1998–2010, seafood-related agents were the most common chemical food safety issue, with scombroid toxin/histamine ciguatoxin, mycotoxins and paralytic shellfish poison identified as causing the majority of outbreaks.[96] Heavy metals, cleaning agents, neurotoxic shellfish poison, plant/herbal toxins, pesticides, puffer fish tetrodotoxin, monosodium glutamate, and other chemicals and natural toxins also were listed as causing at least one outbreak.

The effects of long exposures to low levels of chemicals through food or other environmental routes related to food production are not routinely surveyed for the general population in any country. The time lag makes the identification of associations difficult, so resources are typically prioritised to other surveillance activities that provide more accurate results. However, some studies have been conducted in specific populations that are exposed to higher levels of agrichemical residues through air or water, such as farmers, farm workers or those in farming communities.

Many chemicals used in food are associated with risk of endocrine system disruption. Endocrine disruptors are chemicals that may interfere with the body's endocrine system and produce adverse developmental, reproductive, neurological and immune effects in both humans and wildlife. A wide range of substances, both natural and synthetic, are thought to cause endocrine disruption, some of which may be found in food and food packaging, including plastics and metal cans. These include dioxin and dioxin-like compounds, polychlorinated biphenyls, pesticides, plasticisers such as bisphenol A and Di (2-ethylhexyl) phthalate (DEHP), which is used in a wide variety of food packaging.

Polychlorinated biphenyls and the chemically associated dioxins and furans are a class of synthetic compounds that were widely used commercially in the past, mainly in electrical equipment, but which were banned by many countries at the end of the 1970s due to environmental concerns. Because these compounds are very stable, they remain present in the environment and can be released from poorly maintained toxic waste sites. Food can be a source of PCB exposure, usually from fish and animal fat. Polychlorinated biphenyls can also accumulate in breast milk so nursing infants are at additional risk. Polychlorinated biphenyls have been associated in animals with cancers and effects on the reproductive and immune systems.[97] The effects of PCBs in humans are difficult to determine due to different levels of exposure and the presence of other toxins in the environment. Reduction in dietary exposure to PCBs and dioxins has been observed in both Europe and the USA since the end of the 1970s. Several national (for example, the USA and Australia) and regional (for example, the European Union[98]) governments set maximum PCB values for food and drinking water and monitor levels on an ongoing basis.

A 2012 WHO report, *The State of the Science of Endocrine Disrupting Chemicals*, pointed out that significant uncertainty exists regarding the potential risk of endocrine system disruption from many chemicals used in food. In humans, the contribution of these chemicals to the risk of endocrine-related diseases and human exposure levels from food and non-food sources are unclear.[99] Children and the developing foetus are more vulnerable to endocrine disruptors than are adults, again demonstrating that health outcomes related to the food supply can differ among human populations.

## Antibiotic use in the food system

Widespread antibiotic use for treatment of bacterial infection in humans began in the early twentieth century. Antibiotics have also been routinely used in farm animal production since the 1950s and some classes of antibiotics are used in both humans and food-producing animals.

Antibiotics are used mainly in intensively farmed animals for four main reasons: disease treatment, disease control, disease prevention and growth promotion. There have been real problems from illegal and inappropriate use.

- *Disease treatment.* Antibiotics are mostly used to treat respiratory and enteric infections in groups of intensively fed animals. Antibiotics are also used to treat infections in individual animals that are caused by a variety of bacterial pathogens. In particular, antibiotics are often used to treat mastitis in dairy cows,[100] which is a common infection in cows with a high milk output. The global increase in intensive fish farming has also been accompanied by bacterial infections that are usually treated with antibiotics added to fish foodstuffs and the application of antibiotics in aquaculture can be substantial.[101]
- *Disease control.* This refers to administration of antibiotics to intensively reared animals that may be at risk of infection because an infected animal has been discovered in a group. Thus, an entire herd of animals or flock of chickens receive an antibiotic as soon as an infection is seen in any single animal.
- *Disease prevention.* This refers to the administration of antibiotics to intensively reared animals thought to be at risk of infection before there is a clinical diagnosis of disease. Preventive antibiotics, often at low levels, are also given routinely to all animals at a certain stage of production at a farm – for instance in the early life stage of broiler chickens and weaning pigs. Preventive antibiotics are also frequently administered for long periods of time. This type of low-dose, long-duration administration of antibiotics to large groups of animals is, in practice, often indistinguishable from antibiotics for growth promotion.
- *Growth promotion.* The use of antibiotics as growth promoters was first advocated in the 1950s and became widespread as the cost of using them fell.[102] Low levels of antibiotics are administered to farm animals through their feed. This makes the animals grow faster with less feed, which is seen as favourable for greater production levels. This practice is banned in 51 countries but continues in the USA, although the USA is in the process of trying to phase out growth promotion uses.

Estimates vary regarding the relative quantity of antibiotics currently used in the food system versus those used in human medicine, and antibiotic use in food production varies substantially throughout the world.[102–106] In the USA, the total amount of antibiotics used in food-producing animals rose by 16% between 2009 and 2012 to 14.6 million kg per year, while data on human use in the USA from 2012 shows that Americans used 3.28 million kilograms of antibiotics that year. Data from Europe comparing antimicrobial consumption in animals and humans in 2012 also show that overall antimicrobial consumption was higher in animals than in humans, although contrasting situations were observed between countries.[107]

There is general agreement that antibiotic resistance is now widespread in both humans and the food system.[108] Resistance to antibiotics is a natural phenomenon and was anticipated to be a problem by Alexander Fleming in his Nobel Prize acceptance speech, and by other pioneers of their use.[109] As bacteria and other microbes are exposed to antibiotics, they will eventually develop resistance through random mutations and by transferring resistance genes among themselves.[103, 110] This has serious public health consequences. In Europe, an estimated 25,000 people die each year after becoming infected with antibiotic-resistant bacteria and related costs amount to over £1.5 billion euros in hospital admissions and productivity losses. Each year in the USA at least 2 million people become infected with bacteria that are resistant to antibiotics and at least 23,000 people die each year as a direct result of these infections. Many more people die from other conditions that were complicated by an antibiotic-resistant infection.[104]

Resistance can arise through the overuse, or improper use, of antibiotics in humans and animals.[111] In animals, concern centres on antibiotics being given to entire herds either to prevent disease or promote growth. In half the countries of the world, including the USA and Canada, antibiotics are still used as growth promoters. In North America there are very few regulations on antibiotic use in agriculture. However, the US Food and Drug Administration produced guidance in 2012 on the 'judicious use' of antimicrobials in the rearing of animals for food production.[112] If this guidance is followed, then a gradual phasing out of the use of antibiotics as growth promoters can be expected. In Europe, antibiotic use in animals is more tightly regulated and several European countries have set limits on antibiotic use in agriculture with annual targets to reduce the amounts used. In 1971, the UK withdrew authorisation for use of several substances as growth promoters, including tetracyclines and penicillin. Other countries followed suit and a comprehensive ban on the use of all antibiotics as growth promoters was eventually introduced in the European Union in 2006. Rational use of antibiotics in animals is part of the European Commission's action plan against antimicrobial resistance and the European Medicines Agency (EMA) announced in 2014 that sales of antibiotics for use in animals had fallen overall by 15% between 2010 and 2012.[113]

Resistance that arises in animals can affect humans in two ways. First, food-borne pathogens could develop their resistance in animals before going on to infect people via the food supply. Second, resistant genes could be transferred from animal bacteria to human pathogens through a process known as horizontal gene transfer, where genetic material is swapped between neighbouring bacteria. This transfer occurs via three mechanisms: transformation, transduction and conjugation. Transformation involves the uptake of naked DNA by competent bacterial cells, transduction involves the transfer of genetic material via bacteriophages and conjugation involves transfer of DNA via sexual pilus and requires cell-to-cell contact.

The relative contribution to resistance from the use of antibiotics in animals compared to that in humans is unclear. However, positive associations have been found between antimicrobial consumption in animals and resistance in bacteria from humans.[107] In particular, resistant strains of Campylobacter and Salmonella bacteria involved in human disease primarily come from farm animals. Evidence is also emerging that Staphylococcus aureus (including methicillin-resistant

Staphylococcus aureus) and Clostridium difficile also occur in food animals and can later be found in food products and environments shared with humans.[114]

The World Organization for Animal Health (OIE), an intergovernmental organisation responsible for improving animal health worldwide and preventing epizootics (animal diseases), publishes a list of antimicrobials that are critically important in animal health.[115] It complements a similar list for human health produced by WHO.[116] In its most recent list, published in 2011, WHO included veterinary drugs that fall into the same classes as those in the human medicines list so that veterinary medicines analogous to human medicines – which have a greater potential to impact resistance – can readily be identified. WHO recommends that carbapenems, lipopetides and oxazolidinones that have no veterinary equivalent, as well as any new classes of antibiotics developed for human therapy, should not be used in animals, plants or aquaculture. The OIE and the UK's Responsible Use of Medicines in Agriculture Alliance (RUMA) advocate the responsible use of antibiotics by trained professionals as well as vaccination and good hygiene practices to limit the spread of resistance from animals to humans. However, measures such as these can only slow the development of resistance, not stop it altogether. For this, new classes of drugs and treatments or alternative ways to treat and prevent disease are needed. However, few new classes of antibiotics have reached the market since the 1960s prompting many warnings of a post-antibiotic era.[111, 117, 118]

World leaders started to take notice.[116, 117] A former Goldman Sachs chief economist led an international commission to determine why no novel drugs have emerged in recent years, and argued that there need to be greater financial incentives as well as controls.[119] US President Obama created a task force, led by the secretaries of defence, agriculture, and health and human services, which developed a cross-government five-year action plan.[120, 121] The WHO declared antimicrobial resistance to be a global threat in its first surveillance report on the subject in April 2014.[122]

## Health effects for people associated with food production

Food production has recognised occupational health and safety risks. Modern agriculture involves the use of large machinery and potentially toxic inputs. Farming is a hazardous occupation. In the UK, one in a hundred workers (employees and the self-employed) work in agriculture, but it accounts for one in five fatal injuries to workers.[123] About 90 deaths per year are attributed to occupational carcinogens in the UK, the most significant of which is TCDD (2,3,7,8-Tetrachlorodibenzodioxin). Non-arsenical insecticides are also a significant carcinogen. About three quarters of the deaths are in general farming while most of the others are in horticulture. In 2004 there were about 135 new cancer registrations a year in the UK due to exposure to solar radiation. Nearly one in ten new cancers caused by sun exposure were in agriculture, although the agricultural workforce only accounted for about 1% of the UK workforce. [123]

In the USA the occupational fatality rate for workers in agriculture, forestry and fishing is significantly higher than all other industries.[124] Recognising the hazards in this industry, Congress in 1990 directed the National Institute for Occupational Safety and Health (NIOSH) to develop specific strategies to address the high risks of injuries and illness to agricultural workers and their families. Under the NIOSH portfolio, the agriculture, forestry and fishing sector has a number of strategic goals to guide research and partnership efforts targeting priority areas, including traumatic injury and hearing loss.

Chemical-related exposures are also important. In a study among US workers between 1998 and 2005,[125] the overall incidence of poisoning events was estimated to be 53.6/100,000 farm workers compared with 1.38/100,000 for non-farm workers. About a third of the affected workers were pesticide handlers and the rest were farm workers exposed to off-target drift of pesticide applications or exposed to treated plant or animal material. A wide array of signs and symptoms were reported (most of them low severity), with the most frequent being nervous or sensory symptoms, gastrointestinal irritation, eye problems, and skin and respiratory irritation. Acute poisoning is most frequent in processing and packing plant workers compared with other workers in agriculture. The scale of the problem is not easy to track as reporting of pesticide-related intoxication is not generally mandatory. In the USA, California, where large numbers of farm workers are employed, is the only state that requires mandatory reporting of pesticide-related intoxications.

Although farmers have a lower incidence of smoking, cancer and cardiovascular disease compared with non-farm workers, some evidence exists that they also experience high levels of anxiety, stress, depression and suicide.[126–129] Respiratory disorders, dermatitis and chronic pain associated with muscle and skeletal damage are also common. Dust from grain/cereal, animal feed or bedding (straw) is implicated as a significant cause of breathing or lung problems. Farmer's lung, which arises from the inhalation of dust or spores arising from mouldy hay, grain and straw, is the most common form of lung disease.[123] Agriculture is also unique among most industries in the significant levels of involvement of children and other family members who work and live on farms, which can lead to additional health and safety risks. Agricultural work may increase their risk of injury, illness and exposure to toxic chemicals.

Some chemical exposures occur through air or water. For example, residents living near Concentrated Animal Feeding Operations (CAFOs) are reported to have increased incidence of respiratory distress, digestive disorders and anxiety, depression and sleep disorders. Children living on farms raising swine were reported to have a higher incidence of asthma.[130] A report from Saxony also concluded that CAFOs contribute to respiratory illness.[131] Others are less convinced that health effects in communities can be attributed to emissions from CAFOs. A US review of existing studies funded by the National Soybean Board and the National Pork Board concluded that evidence of a small increase in self-reported disease in people with allergies or familial history of allergies was inconsistent.[132]

Likewise, ammonia pollution from agriculture has been cited as a major cause of health damage.[133] Ammonia, which can enter the atmosphere from fertiliser and from animal urine and manure, reacts with other components of air to create particles that can affect the lungs and cause asthma attacks, bronchitis and heart attacks.[134] When ammonia reacts with oxides of nitrogen and sulphur, it can form particulate matter that is less than 2.5 microns wide, a size considered most dangerous. Long-term reductions in particulate matter in the atmosphere have been related to increased life expectancy.[135]

## Is a healthy diet an environmentally friendly diet and vice versa?

Sustainable diets are not only those that contribute to public health – providing healthy, safe and nutritious food – but they are also those with low environmental impacts while also encompassing social and economic goals. Here we discuss the extent to which public health and environmental goals are compatible for food and diet.

Several studies have examined healthy dietary patterns, including Mediterranean-type diets, diets based on dietary guidelines, vegetarian and vegan diets, to find out whether there is synergy or conflict between health and environmental outcomes such as GHGs, acidification, eutrophication and land use. Meat intake is a focus of many of these studies due to its large impact on the environment.

A UK study used dietary intake data from the National Diet and Nutrition Survey (NDNS) to assess the potential benefits of reducing meat intakes on health and the environment.[136] Respondents were divided into fifths by energy-adjusted red and processed meat intake and vegetarians formed a sixth stratum. A feasible counterfactual UK population was specified, in which the proportion of vegetarians measured in the survey population doubled and the remainder adopted the dietary pattern of the lowest fifth of red and processed meat consumers. They found that sustained dietary intakes in the counterfactual population would reduce the risk of coronary heart disease (CHD), diabetes mellitus and colorectal cancer by 3–12% while reducing UK food and drink associated GHGs by approximately 3%, a significant figure given that cuts in emissions will have to come from diverse sources.

A further UK study, conducted in Scotland, aimed to find out whether a reduction in GHGs can be achieved while meeting dietary requirements for health.[137] The researchers created a database that linked nutrient composition and GHG data for 82 food groups. Linear programming was used iteratively to produce a diet that met the dietary requirements of an adult woman (19–50 year old) while minimising GHGs. Acceptability constraints were added to the model to include foods commonly consumed in the United Kingdom in sensible quantities. A sample menu was created to ensure that the quantities and types of food generated from the model could be combined into a realistic seven-day diet. Reductions in

GHGs of the diets were set against 1990 emission values. The first model, without any acceptability constraints, produced a 90% reduction in GHGs but included only seven food items, all in unrealistic quantities. The addition of acceptability constraints gave a more realistic diet with 52 foods, but reduced GHGs by a lesser amount of, in this case, 36%. This diet included meat products but in smaller amounts than in the current diet. The retail cost of the diet was comparable to the average UK expenditure on food.

Another UK study,[138] in this case from a group in Oxford, evaluated the impact of three counterfactual dietary scenarios designed by the Committee on Climate Change (CCC) to consider cardiovascular disease and cancer. The CCC had been established under the Climate Change Act to advise the UK Government on how it can meet its targets to reduce GHG emissions. The researchers found that a diet with a 50% reduction in total meat and dairy replaced by fruit, vegetables and cereals contributed the most to estimated reduced risk of total mortality and also had the largest potential positive environmental impact. This diet scenario increased fruit and vegetable consumption by 63% and decreased saturated fat and salt consumption; micronutrient intake was generally similar with the exception of a drop in vitamin B12.

A second study from Oxford demonstrated that incorporating the societal costs of GHGs into the price of food through tax can save lives, reduce GHGs and raise tax.[139] The researchers modelled two tax scenarios: (a) a tax of £2.72/tonne carbon dioxide equivalents/100 g product applied to all food and drink groups with above average GHG emissions, and (b), as for (a), but food groups with emissions below average are subsidised to create a tax neutral scenario. The first tax scenario results in 7,770 deaths averted and a reduction in GHG emissions of 18,683 $ktCO_2e$/year. Estimated annual revenue would be £2.02 billion. The second tax scenario results in 2,685 extra deaths and a reduction in GHG emissions of 15,228 $ktCO_2e$/year. This revenue neutral scenario indicates that health and environmental goals are not always aligned.

Research has also evaluated the environmental impact of the Dietary Approaches to Stop Hypertension (DASH) diet.[140] In this cross-sectional study of 24,293 adults aged 39–79 years from the Norfolk-UK cohort of the European Prospective Investigation into Cancer (EPIC), dietary intakes estimated from food-frequency questionnaires were analysed for their accordance with the eight DASH food- and nutrient-based targets. Associations between DASH accordance, GHGs and dietary costs were evaluated in regression analyses. Dietary GHGs were estimated with UK-specific data on carbon dioxide equivalents associated with commodities and foods. Dietary costs were estimated by using national food prices from a UK-based supermarket comparison website. Greater accordance with the DASH dietary targets was associated with lower GHGs. Diets in the highest quintile of accordance had a GHG impact of 5.60 compared with 6.71 kg carbon dioxide equivalents/d for least-accordant diets. Among the DASH food groups, GHGs were most strongly and positively associated with meat consumption and negatively with whole-grain consumption. In addition, higher accordance with the DASH diet was associated with higher dietary costs, with the mean cost of diets in the top quintile of DASH scores 18% higher than of diets in the lowest quintile.

A German study[141] evaluated the environmental impact of four dietary scenarios in Germany: (1) D-A-CH (official recommendations of the German Nutrition Society, valid for Germany, Austria and Switzerland); (2) UGB (alternative recommendations by the Federation for Independent Health Consultation with less meat, but more legumes and 42 vegetables); (3) ovo-lacto-vegetarian and (4) vegan, and compared these dietary scenarios with average diet/nutrition of 20 years previously. The vegan and vegetarian diets had the lowest environmental impacts followed by the UGB and D-A-CH recommendations. Within the separate environmental impacts measured, land use, $CO_2$ emissions, ammonia emissions, use of phosphorus and primary energy use followed the same trends across the four diets. Blue water use was, however, higher in the vegan and vegetarian scenarios presumably due to consumption of imported fruit, nuts and seeds from areas of water shortage. The study also found that women were nearer to an environmentally friendly diet than men and that environmental impacts compared with those associated with the diet 20 years previously (1986) were lower.

Researchers based in Germany, Pradhan and colleagues, examined 16 global dietary patterns that differed by food and energy content, grouped into four categories of low, moderate, high and very high energy intakes.[142] They assessed the relationship of these patterns to GHG emissions. Low energy diets provided less than 2,100 kcal/cap/day and were composed of more than 50% cereals or more than 70% starchy roots, cereals and pulses. Animal products were minor in this group (<10%). Moderate, high and very high energy diets had 2,100–2,400, 2,400–2,800 and more than 2,800 kcal/cap/day, respectively. Very high energy diets had high amounts of meat and alcoholic beverages. Overall, very high energy diets, common in the developed world and linked with obesity with consequences for health, exhibited high total per capita $CO_2$e emissions due to high carbon intensity and high intake of animal products; the low energy diets, on the other hand, had the lowest total per capita $CO_2$e emissions.

A Dutch study evaluated the health/nutritional and environmental impacts of six different diets: current average Dutch, official 'recommended' Dutch, semi-vegetarian, vegetarian, vegan and Mediterranean and produced a health score, a GHG index and land use index for each of these six diets.[143] The average Dutch diet had the lowest health score, while the vegan and Mediterranean diets had the highest health scores and the semi-vegetarian, vegetarian and recommended Dutch diets had almost the same health scores and fell in the middle. Compared with the current average Dutch diet, all five of the other diets scored better on both GHGEs and land use. The vegetarian and vegan diets performed the best on both environmental impact measures. However, a change from the average Dutch diet to the recommended diet gives an 11% reduction in GHG and a 38% reduction in land use. This reduction is substantial and due entirely to less meat and fewer extra products such as snacks, sweets and pastries. The lower impact of the Mediterranean and vegan diets are also partly explained by reduced dairy consumption. Drinks (alcohol, soft drinks, juices, tea and coffee) were also estimated to make a considerable environmental impact. Eating according to the Dutch recommended dietary guidelines scored better on both health and environmental indicators than the average Dutch diet. The vegan diet had the highest score on sustainability (GHG and land use) and the second highest score on health while the Mediterranean diet had the highest score on health and the third highest score on sustainability.

A Danish study evaluated the possibility for the new Nordic diet to reduce GHGEs.[144] The researchers compared the GHGEs of three diets: the average Danish diet (ADD); a diet based on the Nordic Nutritional Recommendations (NNR); and a new Nordic diet (NND), which contains locally produced Nordic foods where more than 75% is organically produced. NNR and NND include less meat and more fruit and vegetables than the ADD. All diets were adjusted to contain a similar energy and protein content. The GHG emissions from the provision of the NNR and NND were lower than for the ADD, by 8% and 7% respectively. If GHG emissions from transport (locally produced versus imported food) are also taken into account, the difference in GHG emissions between the NND and ADD increases to 12%. If the production method (organic versus conventional) is taken into account so that the ADD contains the actual proportion of organically produced food (6.6%) and the NND contains 80%, the GHG emissions for the NND are only 6% less than for the ADD. When the NND was optimised to be more climate friendly, the global warming potential of the NND was 27% lower than it was for the ADD. This was achieved by including less beef, and only including organic produce if the GHG emissions are lower than for the conventional version, or by substituting all meat with legumes, dairy products and eggs.

An Italian study examined three dietary patterns – vegan, vegetarian and omnivorous diets – both organically and conventionally grown, and compared the health and environmental outcomes of these diets with the normal Italian diet derived from conventionally grown food.[145] The organically grown vegan diet had the most potential health benefits, whereas the conventionally grown average Italian diet had the least. The organically grown vegan diet also had the lowest estimated impact on resources and ecosystem quality, and the average Italian diet had the greatest projected impact. Beef was the single food with the greatest projected impact on the environment; other foods estimated to have high impact included cheese, milk and seafood.

A Spanish study analysed the sustainability of the Mediterranean dietary pattern in the context of the Spanish population in terms of GHGEs, agricultural land use, energy consumption and water consumption.[146] The researchers also compared the current Spanish diet with the Mediterranean diet and with the Western dietary pattern, exemplified by the US food pattern, in terms of their corresponding environmental footprints. The environmental footprints of the dietary patterns studied were calculated from the dietary make-up of each dietary pattern and the specific environmental footprints of each food group. The dietary compositions were obtained from different sources, including food balance sheets and household consumption surveys. The specific environmental footprints of food groups were obtained from different available life-cycle assessments. The researchers found that the adherence of the Spanish population to the Mediterranean dietary pattern has a marked impact on all the environmental footprints studied, including a 72% reduction in GHGEs, a 58% reduction in land use, a 52% reduction in energy use and a 33% reduction in extent water use. On the other hand, the adherence to a Western dietary pattern implies an increase in all these descriptors of between 12 and 72%.

French workers examined dietary patterns with different indicators of nutritional quality and found that, despite containing large amounts of plant foods, not all diets of the highest nutritional quality were those with the lowest GHG emissions.[147] For this study the dietary pattern was assessed by use of nutrient-based indicators. High quality diets had an energy density below the median, a mean adequacy ratio above the median and a mean excess ratio (percentage of maximum recommended for nutrients that should be limited – saturated fat, sodium and free sugars) below the median. Four dietary patterns were identified based on compliance with these properties to generate one high quality diet, two intermediate quality diets and one low quality diet. In this study, the high quality diets had higher GHG emissions than did the low quality diets. Regarding the food groups, a higher consumption of starches, sweets and salted snacks, and fats was associated with lower diet-related GHG emissions, and an increased intake of fruit and vegetables was associated with increased diet-related GHG emissions. However, the strongest positive association with GHG emissions was still for the ruminant meat group. Overall, this study used a different approach from other studies to date, as nutritional quality determined the formation of dietary pattern categories.

This same French research group went on to evaluate specific foods, rather than diets, and to identify those that showed synergies in health, reduced environmental impact and cost to the purchaser.[148] Environmental impact indicators (i.e., GHGEs, acidification and eutrophication) were collected for 363 of the most commonly consumed foods in the national French food consumption survey. Prices were also collected. The nutritional quality of the foods was assessed by calculating the ratio of the score for the nutritional adequacy of individual foods (SAIN) to the score for disqualifying nutrients, such as saturated fatty acid and sugar (LIM). A sustainability score based on the median GHG emissions, price and SAIN:LIM ratio was calculated for each food; the foods with the best values for all three variables received the highest score. The environmental indicators were strongly and positively correlated. Meat, fish, eggs and dairy products had the strongest influence on the environment; starchy foods, legumes, fruits and vegetables had the least influence. GHG emissions were inversely correlated with SAIN:LIM and positively correlated with price per kilogram. The correlation with price per kilocalorie was null. This showed that foods with a heavy environmental impact tend to have lower nutritional quality and a higher price per kilogram but not a lower price per kilocalorie. Using price per kilogram, 94 foods had a maximum sustainability score, including most plant-based foods and excluding all foods with animal ingredients except milk, yogurt and soups. Using price per kilocalorie restricted the list to 42 foods, including 52% of all starchy foods and legumes but only 11% of fruits and vegetables (mainly 100% fruit juices). Overall, the sustainability dimensions seemed to be compatible when considering price per kilogram of food but were less compatible when considering price per kilocalorie.

A further study by the French group set out to evaluate the diet-related GHGEs for self-selected, rather than hypothetical, diets to see which are the most sustainable diets consumed in real life.[149] The study involved 1,918 adults participating in the cross-sectional French national dietary survey and described three types of diets. 'Lower-Carbon' diets were defined as having lower GHGEs than the overall median, 'Higher-Quality' diets were defined as having a probability of adequate nutrition intake according to the PANDiet score – an index of the probability of adequate intake of 24 nutrients[150] – and 'More Sustainable' diets were defined as having a combination of both criteria. Diet cost, as a proxy for affordability, and energy density were also assessed. 'More Sustainable' diets were consumed by 23% of men and 20% of women, and their GHGE values were 19% and 17% lower than the population average (mean) value respectively. In comparison with the average value, 'Lower-Carbon' diets achieved a 20% GHGE reduction and lower cost, but they were not sustainable because they had a lower PANDiet score. 'Higher-Quality' diets were not sustainable because of their above-average GHGEs and cost. 'More Sustainable' diets had an above-average PANDiet score and a below-average energy density, cost, GHGE and energy content. Plant foods provided a greater proportion of the energy intake in the 'More Sustainable' diet compared with that in the usual diet. Overall this study showed that reducing diet-related GHGE by 20% while maintaining high nutritional quality seems realistic. This goal could be achieved at no extra cost by reducing energy intake and energy density and increasing the share of plant-based products.

A study across the 27 countries of the European Union assessed the environmental impacts of changing to healthier diets by comparing the environmental impact of the European status quo with that of three simulated diet baskets.[151] Basket number 1 followed universal dietary recommendations, basket number 2 followed the same pattern as basket 1 but with reduced meat consumption, while basket 3 was a 'Mediterranean' pattern with reduced meat consumption. Production technologies, protein and energy intake were kept constant. Though this implies just moderate dietary shifts, impact reductions of up to 8% were possible in the reduced meat scenarios.

A further Europe-wide study examined the large-scale consequences in the European Union of replacing 25–50% of animal-derived foods with plant-based foods on a dietary energy basis, assuming corresponding changes in production.[152] The researchers found that halving the consumption of meat, dairy products and eggs in the European Union would achieve a 40% reduction in nitrogen emissions, 25–40% reduction in greenhouse gas emissions and 23% per capita less use of crop-land for food production. In addition, the dietary changes would also lower health risks. The European Union would become a net exporter of cereals, while the use of soymeal would be reduced by 75%. The nitrogen use efficiency (NUE) of the food system would increase from the current 18% to between 41% and 47%, depending on choices made regarding land use. As agriculture is the major source of nitrogen pollution, this is expected to result in a significant improvement in both air and water quality in the EU. The resulting 40% reduction in the intake of saturated fat would lead to a reduction in cardiovascular mortality.

In the USA, Pimentel and Pimentel compared the use of land and energy resources devoted to an average meat-based diet compared with a lacto-ovo-vegetarian (plant-based) diet.[153] In both diets, the daily quantity of calories consumed was kept constant at about 3,533 kcal per person. They concluded that both the meat-based average American diet and the lacto-ovo-vegetarian diet require significant quantities of non-renewable fossil energy to produce. Thus, both food systems are not sustainable in the long term based on heavy fossil energy requirements. However, the meat-based diet requires more energy, land and water resources than the lacto-ovo-vegetarian diet indicating from these environmental perspectives the lacto-ovo-vegetarian diet is more sustainable than the average American meat-based diet.

A study based in New York examined 42 different dietary patterns and land use in New York.[154] Dietary patterns ranged from low-fat, lacto-ovo-vegetarian diets to high-fat, meat-rich omnivorous diets. Across this range, the diets met US dietary guidelines when possible. Overall, increasing meat in the diet increased per capita land requirements. However, increasing the total dietary fat content of low-meat diets (i.e., vegetarian alternatives) increased the land requirements compared to high-meat diets. In other words, although meat increased land requirements, diets including meat could feed more people than some higher fat vegetarian-style diets.

A study in Brazil examined a high red and processed meat dietary pattern in relation to both diet quality (using the Brazilian Healthy Eating Index) and GHGs pattern.[155] The researchers used the World Cancer Research Fund recommendation of 71.4 g daily as the cut-off to estimate high red and processed meat daily and found that 81% of men and 58% of women consumed more meat than recommended. In this study, excessive meat intake was associated with poorer diet quality in men and also with increased projected GHG emissions from agriculture.

An Australian study[156] compared the GHG emissions from four dietary patterns: the average Australian diet in 1995; the average Australian diet with minimal inclusion of energy-dense, processed non-core foods; a diet consistent with the Australian dietary guidelines (the Total diet); and a recommended dietary pattern that meets the energy and nutrient requirements for the population containing only core foods (the Foundation diet). The average Australian diet as assessed in 1995 had the highest per capita GHGs and was the highest in energy. The Foundation diet had the lowest emissions – about 25% lower than the average Australian diet. The estimated emissions from the recommended Total diet and the average diet without non-core foods were similar, despite the recommended diet providing more energy. Overall, the recommended dietary patterns in the Australian Dietary Guidelines are nutrient-rich and have the lowest GHG emissions (~25% lower than the average diet). The average Australian diet did not meet the suggested dietary target for dietary fibre, vitamin A, folate, calcium and magnesium. However, when most non-core foods were removed from the average diet, nutrient intake was further compromised. Food groups that made the greatest contribution to diet-related GHGe were energy-dense, nutrient poor 'non-core' foods. Non-core foods accounted for 27% of the diet-related emissions. The findings from this research indicate that reducing energy-dense, processed non-core foods while sticking to the recommended portions of core foods could have benefits for both population health and the environment.

A New Zealand study modelled 16 diets with a focus on achieving nutrient requirements at the lowest costs while minimising GHGs.[157] Four of the diets focused on ensuring nutrient requirements but with variation such as the addition of porridge and more fruit and vegetables, while the second four diets had the same aims but minimised GHGs. Four of the diets aimed to model the Mediterranean and the Asian-style diet with and without GHG minimisation. The final four diets had the same aim as the first four diets (i.e., to meet nutrient requirements) but each of the four diets was based on a familiar meal (i.e., mince, sausages, tuna pasta bake and a Pacific-style meal). These 16 optimised diets met nutrient requirements and also had low GHG emission profiles compared with the estimate for the 'typical New Zealand diet'. All of the optimised low-cost and low-GHG dietary patterns had likely health advantages over the current New Zealand dietary pattern, i.e., lower cardiovascular disease and cancer risk. Health benefits were likely to be attributable to the higher ratio of polyunsaturated to saturated fat intake, less saturated fat from meat, lower sodium intake, higher potassium intake and higher fibre intake.

## Conclusions

A broad picture emerges. Diets with higher overall health scores, including vegan, lacto-ovo-vegetarian and pesco-vegetarian diets, as well as official dietary guidelines and Mediterranean-style dietary patterns, are associated with lower environmental impacts in terms of GHGs and land use and, for the most part, higher combined (health and environmental) sustainability scores. These synergies can be explained by a reduction in overall food consumption and by a reduction in the consumption of meat, dairy and extras.

Research conducted in the United Kingdom has shown that changing population food choices to meet dietary requirements could help towards mitigating climate change.[137] However, in Europe, modelling changes towards a healthier diet resulted in minimal reductions in environmental impacts. Within the French context, self-selected diets of the highest nutritional quality were not those with the lowest diet-related GHGEs.[147] In particular, the consumption of sweets and salted snack foods were negatively correlated with GHGEs, meaning they have low GHGEs. Therefore, proposals for sustainable diets must have a strong health perspective because not all diets that meet the dietary requirements for health will necessarily have lower GHGEs.

In terms of health, a barrier to recommending a vegan diet is the supply of some nutrients such as vitamin B12, vitamin D, iron and calcium as well as omega-3 fatty acids (EPA and DHA). This is, to some extent, also the case for vegetarians, whose diets score higher on nutrition if alternatives such as meat substitutes and fortified products such as soya milk are included. Oil seeds such as rapeseed and linseed provide an alternative source of omega-3 fatty acids although these sources are not so bioavailable as the long chain varieties found in fish. Other potential sources of omega-3 fatty acids are microalgae. If a portion of meat and/or fish is added to the vegetarian diet each week, the nutritional quality improves without significantly increasing the environmental impact. A tricky issue for those who think the answer to sustainable diets is veganism is that it may not fulfil the FAO definition of a sustainable diet: being both nutritionally adequate and culturally acceptable to the general public. The provision of vitamin B12, vitamin D, calcium and iron is lower than usual and the addition of fortified foods or supplements may not be acceptable to the general public. An entirely meatless diet is not necessary and not optimal when health and environmental considerations are combined.

If the inclusion of some meat is suggested in the diet, the question would be how much. Van Dooren in the Netherlands suggests one portion of meat and/ or fish each week.[143] In the 2012 modelling conducted for the UK Livewell diet, the suggested amounts of meat were 90 g each of cooked beef and cooked pork each week, 21 g of ham each week and 203 g of poultry. The diet also includes fish (119 g oily fish, 161 g white fish and 49 g shellfish each week).[158] Together with the rest of the foods in the diet, this quantity of meat and fish would meet the nutritional requirements for an adult (woman). Diets need modelling for all ages and population groups to ensure nutrient requirements are met as meat and animal produce is a bioavailable source of iron and zinc and, for milk, calcium.

Dietary guidelines produced by governments, health councils and nutrition associations have largely focused on nutrition and health issues in relation to food-related diseases in Western countries. Such guidelines, however, do not address the environmental concerns related to the food system (see Chapter 4) and there is a need for food-based dietary guidelines to address the issue of sustainability. In short, we see the case for new sustainable dietary guidelines. Some national bodies (for example, in Sweden, Germany, Kuwait, the Netherlands, Brazil) have developed guidance that includes environmental and, in the case of Brazil, social issues (see Chapter 8). The Italian Barilla Center has published a Double Pyramid, providing guidance on how to achieve diets that combine both

health and environmental benefits. And a working group of the UK's Green
Food Project, set up by the Department for the Environment, Food and Rural
Affairs, in 2011 drafted some guideline principles of a sustainable healthy diet.
Chapter 8 discusses these and other initiatives more. Meanwhile, this chapter
has set out the strong evidence for a health focus in sustainable diets. In the
next, we find the same for environment.

## References

1  WHO. *Global Status Report on Noncommunicable Diseases 2010*. Available at: www.
   who.int/nmh/publications/ncd_report2010/en/ (accessed April 15, 2016). Geneva:
   World Health Organization, 2011

2  WHO. *Global Status Report on Noncommunicable Diseases, 2014*. Available at: www.
   who.int/nmh/publications/ncd-status-report-2014/en/ (accessed January 19, 2015).
   Geneva: World Health Organization, 2014

3  Dobbs R, Sawers C, Thompson F, *et al*. *Overcoming Obesity: An Initial Economic
   Analysis*, Discussion paper. Available at: www.mckinsey.com/industries/healthcare-
   systems-and-services/our-insights/how-the-world-could-better-fight-obesity (accessed
   November 10, 2014). New York: McKinsey & Company, 2014

4  IFPRI. *Global Nutrition Report 2016: From Promise to Impact – Ending Malnutrition
   by 2030*. Available at: http://ebrary.ifpri.org/utils/getfile/collection/p15738coll2/
   id/130354/filename/130565.pdf (accessed June 19, 2016). Washington, DC:
   International Food Policy Research Institute, 2016

5  FAO, IFAD, WFP. *The State of Food Insecurity in the World 2014: Strengthening the
   Enabling Environment for Food Security and Nutrition*. Available at: www.fao.org/
   publications/sofi/2014/en/ (accessed November 5, 2014). Rome: Food and Agricultural
   Organization, 2014

6  Butland B, Jebb S, Kopelman P, *et al*. *Foresight. Tackling Obesities: Future Choices*.
   Project report. London: Government Office for Science and Department of Health,
   2007

7  Croquet H, Meyre D. Genetics of obesity: what have we learned? *Current Genomics*,
   2011; 12(3): 169–79

8  FAO. *FAOSTAT*. *Food Balance Sheets*. Available at http://faostat3.fao.org/download/
   FB/FBS/E (accessed February 2, 2015). Rome: Food and Agricultural Organization,
   2013

9  Malik VS, Pan A, Willett WC, *et al*. Sugar-sweetened beverages and weight gain in
   children and adults: a systematic review and meta-analysis. *The American Journal of
   Clinical Nutrition*, 2013; 98(4): 1084–102

10 Te Morenga L, Mallard S, Mann J. Dietary sugars and body weight: systematic review
   and meta-analyses of randomised controlled trials and cohort studies. *BMJ* (Clinical
   Research Ed.) 2013; 346: e7492

11 DeBoer MD, Scharf RJ, Demmer RT. Sugar-sweetened beverages and weight gain in
   2- to 5-year-old children. *Pediatrics*, 2013; 132(3): 413–20

12 Hu FB. Resolved: there is sufficient scientific evidence that decreasing sugar-
   sweetened beverage consumption will reduce the prevalence of obesity and obesity-
   related diseases. *Obesity Reviews*, 2013; 14(8): 606–19

13 Young LR, Nestle M. The contribution of expanding portion sizes to the US obesity epidemic. *The American Journal of Public Health*, 2002; 92(2): 246–9

14 Eidner MB, Lund AS, Harboe BS, *et al.* Calories and portion sizes in recipes throughout 100 years: an overlooked factor in the development of overweight and obesity? *Scandinavian Journal of Public Health*, 2013; 41(8): 839–45

15 Rolls BJ, Morris EL, Roe LS. Portion size of food affects energy intake in normal-weight and overweight men and women. *The American Journal of Clinical Nutrition*, 2002; 76(6): 1207–13

16 Wansink B, van Ittersum K, Payne CR. Larger bowl size increases the amount of cereal children request, consume, and waste. *The Journal of Pediatrics*, 2014; 164(2): 323–6

17 Wansink B, Kim J. Bad popcorn in big buckets: portion size can influence intake as much as taste. *Journal of Nutrition Education and Behavior*, 2005; 37(5): 242–5

18 Marchiori D, Corneille O, Klein O. Container size influences snack food intake independently of portion size. *Appetite*, 2012; 58(3): 814–17

19 Mendoza JA, Drewnowski A, Christakis DA. Dietary energy density is associated with obesity and the metabolic syndrome in US adults. *Diabetes Care*, 2007; 30(4): 974–9

20 Murakami K, Sasaki S, Takahashi Y, *et al.* Dietary energy density is associated with body mass index and waist circumference, but not with other metabolic risk factors, in free-living young Japanese women. *Nutrition*, 2007; 23(11–12): 798–806

21 Vernarelli JA, Mitchell DC, Hartman TJ, *et al.* Dietary energy density is associated with body weight status and vegetable intake in US children. *The Journal of Nutrition*, 2011; 141(12): 2204–10

22 Perez-Escamilla R, Obbagy JE, Altman JM, *et al.* Dietary energy density and body weight in adults and children: a systematic review. *Journal of the Academy of Nutrition and Dietetics*, 2012; 112(5): 671–84

23 Vernarelli JA, Mitchell DC, Rolls BJ, *et al.* Dietary energy density is associated with obesity and other biomarkers of chronic disease in US adults. *European Journal of Nutrition*, 2015; 54(1): 59–65

24 Masset G, Vieux F, Verger EO, *et al.* Reducing energy intake and energy density for a sustainable diet: a study based on self-selected diets in French adults. *The American Journal of Clinical Nutrition*, 2014; 99(6): 1460–9

25 Fisher JO, Liu Y, Birch LL, *et al.* Effects of portion size and energy density on young children's intake at a meal. *The American Journal of Clinical Nutrition*, 2007; 86(1): 174–9

26 Kral TV, Roe LS, Rolls BJ. Combined effects of energy density and portion size on energy intake in women. *The American Journal of Clinical Nutrition*, 2004; 79(6): 962–8

27 Ello-Martin JA, Ledikwe JH, Rolls BJ. The influence of food portion size and energy density on energy intake: implications for weight management. *The American Journal of Clinical Nutrition*, 2005; 82(1 Suppl): 236s–41s

28 Rolls BJ, Roe LS, Meengs JS. Reductions in portion size and energy density of foods are additive and lead to sustained decreases in energy intake. *The American Journal of Clinical Nutrition*, 2006; 83(1): 11–17

29 Rouhani MH, Salehi-Abargouei A, Surkan PJ, *et al.* Is there a relationship between red or processed meat intake and obesity? A systematic review and meta-analysis of observational studies. *Obesity Reviews*, 2014; 15(9): 740–8

30 Drewnowski A, Aggarwal A, Hurvitz PM, *et al.* Obesity and supermarket access: proximity or price? *American Journal of Public Health*, 2012; 102(8): e74–80

31 Chaix B, Bean K, Daniel M, *et al.* Associations of supermarket characteristics with weight status and body fat: a multilevel analysis of individuals within supermarkets (RECORD study). *PLoS ONE*, 2012; 7(4): e32908

32 Cameron AJ, Waterlander WE, Svastisalee CM. The correlation between supermarket size and national obesity prevalence. *BMC Obesity*, 1: 27. Available at: www.biomedcentral.com/2052-9538/1/1/27 (accessed June 19, 2015), 2014

33 Cameron AJ, Thornton LE, McNaughton SA, *et al.* Variation in supermarket exposure to energy-dense snack foods by socio-economic position. *Public Health Nutrition*, 2013; 16(7): 1178–85

34 Bezerra IN, Curioni C, Sichieri R. Association between eating out of home and body weight. *Nutrition Reviews*, 2012; 70(2): 65–79

35 Nago ES, Lachat CK, Dossa RA, *et al.* Association of out-of-home eating with anthropometric changes: a systematic review of prospective studies. *Critical Reviews in Food Science and Nutrition*, 2014; 54(9): 1103–16

36 McGuire S, Todd JE, Mancino L, Lin B-H. The impact of food away from home on adult diet quality. ERR-90, US Department of Agriculture, Econ. Res. Serv., February 2010. *Advances in Nutrition*, 2011; 2(5): 442–3

37 Patterson R, Risby A, Chan MY. Consumption of takeaway and fast food in a deprived inner London borough: are they associated with childhood obesity? *BMJ Open*, 2012; 2(3)

38 Fraser LK, Edwards KL, Cade JE, *et al.* Fast food, other food choices and body mass index in teenagers in the United Kingdom (ALSPAC): a structural equation modelling approach. *International Journal of Obesity*, (2005) 2011; 35(10): 1325–30

39 Larson N, Neumark-Sztainer D, Laska MN, *et al.* Young adults and eating away from home: associations with dietary intake patterns and weight status differ by choice of restaurant. *Journal of the American Dietetic Association*, 2011; 111(11): 1696–703

40 Burgoine T, Forouhi NG, Griffin SJ, *et al.* Associations between exposure to takeaway food outlets, takeaway food consumption, and body weight in Cambridgeshire, UK: population based, cross sectional study. *BMJ* (Clinical Research Ed.) 2014; 348: g1464

41 Alkerwi A, Crichton GE, Hebert JR. Consumption of ready-made meals and increased risk of obesity: findings from the Observation of Cardiovascular Risk Factors in Luxembourg (ORISCAV-LUX) study. *The British Journal of Nutrition*, 2014: 1–8

42 Ghosh-Dastidar B, Cohen D, Hunter G, *et al.* Distance to store, food prices, and obesity in urban food deserts. *American Journal of Preventive Medicine*, 2014; 47(5): 587–95

43 Lear SA, Gasevic D, Schuurman N. Association of supermarket characteristics with the body mass index of their shoppers. *Nutrition Journal*, 2013; 12: 117

44 Jones NRV, Conklin AI, Suhrcke M, *et al.* The growing price gap between more and less healthy foods: analysis of a novel longitudinal UK dataset. *PLoS ONE*, 2014; 9(10): e109343

45 Dietary Guidelines Advisory Committee. *Scientific Report of the 2015 Dietary Guidelines Committee.* Available at: www.health.gov/dietaryguidelines/2015-scientific-report/ (accessed May 11, 2015). Washington, DC: USDA and US Department of Health and Human Services, 2015

46  Chandon P, Wansink B. Does food marketing need to make us fat? A review and solutions. *Nutrition Reviews*, 2012; 70(10): 571–93

47  Martin-Biggers J, Yorkin M, Aljallad C, *et al.* What foods are US supermarkets promoting? A content analysis of supermarket sales circulars. *Appetite*, 2013; 62: 160–5

48  Nakamura R, Suhrcke M, Jebb SA, *et al.* Price promotions on healthier compared with less healthy foods: a hierarchical regression analysis of the impact on sales and social patterning of responses to promotions in Great Britain. *The American Journal of Clinical Nutrition*, 2015; 101(4): 808–16

49  Estruch R, Martinez-Gonzalez MA, Corella D, *et al.* Effects of a Mediterranean-style diet on cardiovascular risk factors: a randomized trial. *Annals of Internal Medicine*, 2006; 145(1): 1–11

50  Crowe FL, Appleby PN, Travis RC, *et al.* Risk of hospitalization or death from ischemic heart disease among British vegetarians and nonvegetarians: results from the EPIC-Oxford cohort study. *The American Journal of Clinical Nutrition*, 2013; 97(3): 597–603

51  Margetts BM, Beilin LJ, Armstrong BK, *et al.* A randomized control trial of a vegetarian diet in the treatment of mild hypertension. *Clinical and Experimental Pharmacology & Physiology*, 1985; 12(3): 263–6

52  Nunez-Cordoba JM, Valencia-Serrano F, Toledo E, *et al.* The Mediterranean diet and incidence of hypertension: the Seguimiento Universidad de Navarra (SUN) Study. *American Journal of Epidemiology*, 2009; 169(3): 339–46

53  Fung TT, Chiuve SE, McCullough ML, *et al.* Adherence to a DASH-style diet and risk of coronary heart disease and stroke in women. *Archives of Internal Medicine*, 2008; 168(7): 713–20

54  Salehi-Abargouei A, Maghsoudi Z, Shirani F, *et al.* Effects of Dietary Approaches to Stop Hypertension (DASH)-style diet on fatal or nonfatal cardiovascular diseases – incidence: a systematic review and meta-analysis on observational prospective studies. *Nutrition*, 2013; 29(4): 611–18

55  Schwingshackl L, Hoffmann G. Diet quality as assessed by the healthy eating index, the alternate healthy eating index, the dietary approaches to stop hypertension score, and health outcomes: a systematic review and meta-analysis of cohort studies. *Journal of the Academy of Nutrition and Dietetics*, 2015; 115(5): 780–800.e5

56  Estruch R, Ros E, Martinez-Gonzalez MA. Mediterranean diet for primary prevention of cardiovascular disease. *The New England Journal of Medicine*, 2013; 369(7): 676–7

57  He FJ, Nowson CA, MacGregor GA. Fruit and vegetable consumption and stroke: meta-analysis of cohort studies. *Lancet*, 2006; 367(9507): 320–6

58  Crowe FL, Roddam AW, Key TJ, *et al.* Fruit and vegetable intake and mortality from ischaemic heart disease: results from the European Prospective Investigation into Cancer and Nutrition (EPIC)-Heart study. *European Heart Journal*, 2011; 32(10): 1235–43

59  He FJ, Nowson CA, Lucas M, *et al.* Increased consumption of fruit and vegetables is related to a reduced risk of coronary heart disease: meta-analysis of cohort studies. *Journal of Human Hypertension*, 2007; 21(9): 717–28

60  Flight I, Clifton P. Cereal grains and legumes in the prevention of coronary heart disease and stroke: a review of the literature. *European Journal of Clinical Nutrition*, 2006; 60(10): 1145–59

61  Qin LQ, Xu JY, Han SF, *et al.* Dairy consumption and risk of cardiovascular disease: an updated meta-analysis of prospective cohort studies. *Asia Pacific Journal of Clinical Nutrition*, 2015; 24(1): 90–100

62  Mori TA. Dietary n-3 PUFA and CVD: a review of the evidence. *The Proceedings of the Nutrition Society*, 2014; 73(1): 57–64

63  Mozaffarian D, Aro A, Willett WC. Health effects of trans-fatty acids: experimental and observational evidence. *European Journal of Clinical Nutrition*, 2009; 63 Suppl 2: S5–21

64  Siri-Tarino PW, Sun Q, Hu FB, *et al.* Meta-analysis of prospective cohort studies evaluating the association of saturated fat with cardiovascular disease. *The American Journal of Clinical Nutrition*, 2010; 91(3): 535–46

65  Skeaff CM, Miller J. Dietary fat and coronary heart disease: summary of evidence from prospective cohort and randomised controlled trials. *Annals of Nutrition & Metabolism*, 2009; 55(1–3): 173–201

66  Mozaffarian D, Micha R, Wallace S. Effects on coronary heart disease of increasing polyunsaturated fat in place of saturated fat: a systematic review and meta-analysis of randomized controlled trials. *PLoS Medicine*, 2010; 7(3): e1000252

67  Mensink RP, Zock PL, Kester AD, *et al.* Effects of dietary fatty acids and carbohydrates on the ratio of serum total to HDL cholesterol and on serum lipids and apolipoproteins: a meta-analysis of 60 controlled trials. *The American Journal of Clinical Nutrition*, 2003; 77(5): 1146–55

68  Martinez-Gonzalez MA, Dominguez LJ, Delgado-Rodriguez M. Olive oil consumption and risk of CHD and/or stroke: a meta-analysis of case-control, cohort and intervention studies. *The British Journal of Nutrition*, 2014; 112(2): 248–59

69  Grosso G, Yang J, Marventano S, *et al.* Nut consumption on all-cause, cardiovascular, and cancer mortality risk: a systematic review and meta-analysis of epidemiologic studies. *The American Journal of Clinical Nutrition*, 2015; 101(4): 783–93

70  Xi B, Huang Y, Reilly KH, *et al.* Sugar-sweetened beverages and risk of hypertension and CVD: a dose-response meta-analysis. *The British Journal of Nutrition*, 2015; 113(5): 709–17

71  WHO. *Sodium Intake for Adults and Children.* Available at: www.who.int/nutrition/publications/guidelines/sodium_intake/en/ (accessed May 15, 2015). Geneva: World Health Organization, 2012

72  World Health Organization. *Potassium Intake for Adults and Children.* Available at: www.who.int/nutrition/publications/guidelines/potassium_intake/en/ (accessed May 15, 2015). Geneva: World Health Organization, 2012

73  Wang M, Yu M, Fang L, *et al.* Association between sugar-sweetened beverages and type 2 diabetes: a meta-analysis. *Journal of Diabetes Investigation*, 2015; 6(3): 360–6

74  Schwingshackl L, Missbach B, Konig J, *et al.* Adherence to a Mediterranean diet and risk of diabetes: a systematic review and meta-analysis. *Public Health Nutrition*, 2015; 18(7): 1292–9

75  Aune D, Chan DS, Vieira AR, *et al.* Red and processed meat intake and risk of colorectal adenomas: a systematic review and meta-analysis of epidemiological studies. *Cancer Causes & Control*, 2013; 24(4): 611–27

76  Chan DS, Lau R, Aune D, *et al.* Red and processed meat and colorectal cancer incidence: meta-analysis of prospective studies. *PLoS ONE*, 2011; 6(6): e20456

77  Bamia C, Lagiou P, Buckland G, *et al.* Mediterranean diet and colorectal cancer risk: results from a European cohort. *European Journal of Epidemiology*, 2013; 28(4): 317–28

78  FAO, IFAD, WFP. *State of Food Insecurity in the World, 2015 (SOFI):* Available at: www.fao.org/publications/card/en/c/c2cda20d-ebeb-4467-8a94-038087fe0f6e/ (accessed January 2, 2015). Rome: Food and Agricultural Organization, 2015

79  Bates B, Lennox A, Prentice A, *et al. National Diet and Nutrition Survey: Headline Results from Year 1, Year 2 and Year 3 (combined) of the Rolling Programme (2008/2009–2010/2011).* Available at: www.natcen.ac.uk/media/175123/national-diet-and-nutrition-survey-years-1-2-and-3.pdf (accessed May 20, 2015). London: Department of Health, 2012

80  Mensink GBM, Fletcher R, Gurinovic M, *et al.* Mapping low intake of micronutrients across Europe. *The British Journal of Nutrition,* 2013; 110(4): 755–73

81  Moshfegh A, Goldman J, Cleveland L. *What We Eat in America, NHANES 2001–2002: Usual Nutrient Intakes from Food Compared to Dietary Reference Intakes.* Available at: www.ars.usda.gov/SP2UserFiles/Place/80400530/pdf/0102/usualintaketables2001-02.pdf (accessed May 19, 2015). Beltsville, MD: US Department of Agriculture Agricultural Research Service, 2005

82  Moshfegh A, Goldman J, Ahuja J, *et al. What We Eat in America, NHANES 2005–2006: Usual Nutrient Intakes from Food and Water Compared to 1997 Dietary Reference Intakes for Vitamin D, Calcium, Phosphorus, and Magnesium.* Available at: www.ars.usda.gov/SP2UserFiles/Place/80400530/pdf/0506/usual_nutrient_intake_vitD_ca_phos_mg_2005-06.pdf (accessed May 19, 2015). Beltsville, MD: US Department of Agriculture Agricultural Research Service, 2009

83  Gallagher CM, Black LJ, Oddy WH. Micronutrient intakes from food and supplements in Australian adolescents. *Nutrients,* 2014; 6(1): 342–54

84  World Health Organization (WHO)/Food and Agriculture Organization of the United Nations. *Preparation and Use of Food-Based Dietary Guidelines.* WHO Technical Report Series No. 880. Available at: http://apps.who.int/iris/bitstream/10665/42051/1/WHO_TRS_880.pdf?ua=1&ua=1 (accessed July 31, 2016). Geneva: World Health Organization, 1998

85  FAO, WHO. *Preparation and Use of Food-Based Dietary Guidelines.* Report of a joint FAO/WHO consultation. Available at: www.fao.org/docrep/X0243E/x0243e00.htm (accessed May 26, 2015). Nicosia: World Health Organization, 1996

86  Gibney M, Sandström B. A framework for food-based dietary guidelines in the European Union. *Public Health Nutrition,* 2001; 4(2a): 293–305

87  WHO. *Food and Health in Europe: A New Basis for Action.* WHO Regional Publications, European Series No 96. Copenhagen: WHO Regional Office for Europe, 2004

88  Keller I, Lang T. Food-based dietary guidelines and implementation: lessons from four countries – Chile, Germany, New Zealand and South Africa. *Public Health Nutrition,* 2008; 11(8): 867–74

89  Scallan E, Hoekstra RM, Angulo FJ, *et al.* Foodborne illness acquired in the United States: major pathogens. *Emerging Infectious Diseases,* 2011; 17(1): 7–15

90  FSA. *A Microbiological Survey of Campylobacter Contamination in Fresh Whole UK Produced Chilled Chickens at Retail Sale – February 2014 to February 2015.* Available at: www.food.gov.uk/sites/default/files/full-campy-survey-report.pdf (accessed June 2, 2015). London: Food Standards Agency, 2015

91  Mangen MJ, Bouwknegt M, Friesema IH, *et al.* Cost-of-illness and disease burden of food-related pathogens in the Netherlands, 2011. *International Journal of Food Microbiology,* 2015; 196: 84–93

92  Mercanoglu Taban B, Halkman AK. Do leafy green vegetables and their ready-to-eat [RTE] salads carry a risk of foodborne pathogens? *Anaerobe*, 2011; 17(6): 286–7

93  Kozak GK, MacDonald D, Landry L, *et al*. Foodborne outbreaks in Canada linked to produce: 2001 through 2009. *Journal of Food Protection*, 2013; 76(1): 173–83

94  Sivapalasingam S, Friedman CR, Cohen L, *et al*. Fresh produce: a growing cause of outbreaks of foodborne illness in the United States, 1973 through 1997. *Journal of Food Protection*, 2004; 67(10): 2342–53

95  Centers for Disease Control. *Surveillance for Foodborne Disease Outbreaks, United States, 2012, Annual Report*. Available at: www.cdc.gov/foodsafety/pdfs/foodborne-disease-outbreaks-annual-report-2012-508c.pdf (accessed March 4, 2015). Atlanta, GA: Centers for Disease Control, 2014

96  Centers for Disease Control. Surveillance for foodborne disease outbreaks: United States, 2009–2010. *MMWR Morbidity and Mortality Weekly Report*, 2013, 62(3): 41–7. Atlanta, GA: Centers for Disease Control, 2013

97  Quinete N, Schettgen T, Bertram J, *et al*. Occurrence and distribution of PCB metabolites in blood and their potential health effects in humans: a review. *Environmental Science and Pollution Research International*, 2014; 21(20): 11951–72

98  EFSA. Update of the monitoring of dioxins and PCBs levels in food and feed. Available at: www.efsa.europa.eu/efsajournal (accessed January 6, 2015). *EFSA Journal*, 2012; 10(7): doi:10.2903/j.efsa.012.832

99  WHO. *State of the Science of Endocrine Disrupting Chemicals – 2012: An Assessment of the State of the Science of Endocrine Disruptors Prepared by a Group of Experts for the United Nations Environment Programme (UNEP) and WHO*, A Bergman, JJ Heindel, S Jobling, KA Kidd and R Thomas Zoeller (Eds). Geneva: World Health Organization, 2013

100  Oliver SP, Murinda SE. Antimicrobial resistance of mastitis pathogens. *The Veterinary Clinics of North America: Food Animal Practice*, 2012; 28(2): 165–85

101  Heuer OE, Kruse H, Grave K, *et al*. Human health consequences of use of antimicrobial agents in aquaculture. *Clinical Infectious Diseases* (an official publication of the Infectious Diseases Society of America), 2009; 49(8): 1248–53

102  Marshall BM, Levy SB. Food animals and antimicrobials: impacts on human health. *Clinical Microbiology Reviews*, 2011; 24(4): 718–33

103  Woolhouse ME, Ward MJ. Microbiology: sources of antimicrobial resistance. *Science*, 2013; 341(6153): 1460–1

104  Centers for Disease Control. *Antibiotic Resistance Threats in the United States*. Available at: www.cdc.gov/drugresistance/threat-report-2013/ (accessed January 7, 2015). Atlanta, GA: Centers for Disease Control, 2013

105  Teuber M. Veterinary use and antibiotic resistance. *Current Opinion in Microbiology*, 2001; 4(5): 493–9

106  Wellington EM, Boxall AB, Cross P, *et al*. The role of the natural environment in the emergence of antibiotic resistance in gram-negative bacteria. *The Lancet Infectious Diseases*, 2013; 13(2): 155–65

107  ECDC, EFSA, EMA. ECDC/EFSA/EMA first joint report on the integrated analysis of the consumption of antimicrobial agents and occurrence of antimicrobial resistance in bacteria from humans and food producing animals. *EFSA Journal*, 2015; 13(1): doi:10.2903/j.efsa.015.4006

108 Review on Antimicrobial Resistance (Chaired by Jim O'Neill). *Tackling Drug-Resistant Infections Globally: Final Report and Recommendations*. London: Review on Antimicrobial Resistance, 2016

109 Dubos RJ. The evolution of infectious diseases in the course of history. *Canadian Medical Association Journal*, 1958; 79(6): 445–51

110 Verraes C, Van Boxstael S, Van Meervenne E, *et al.* Antimicrobial resistance in the food chain: a review. *International Journal of Environmental Research and Public Health*, 2013; 10(7): 2643–69

111 Wallinga D, Rayner G, Lang T. Antimicrobial resistance and biological governance: explanations for policy failure. *Public Health*, 2015; 129(10): 1314–25

112 US Department of Health and Human Services Food and Drug Administration Center for Veterinary Medicine. *The Judicious Use of Medically Important Antimicrobial Drugs in Food-Producing Animals, 2012*. Available at: www.fda.gov/downloads/AnimalVeterinary/GuidanceComplianceEnforcement/GuidanceforIndustry/UCM216936.pdf (accessed February 26, 2015). Washington, DC: US Department of Health and Human Services Food and Drug Administration Center for Veterinary Medicine, 2012

113 European Medicines Agency. *Sales of Veterinary Antimicrobial Agents in 26 EU/EEA countries in 2012*. Available at: www.ema.europa.eu/docs/en_GB/document_library/Report/2014/10/WC500175671.pdf (accessed February 25, 2015). London: European Medicines Agency, 2014

114 WHO. *Tackling Foodborne Antimicrobial Resistance Globally Through Integrated Surveillance. Report of the 3rd Meeting of the WHO Advisory Group on Integrated Surveillance of Antimicrobial Resistance, June 2011*. Available at: http://apps.who.int/iris/bitstream/10665/75198/1/9789241504010_eng.pdf (accessed February 15, 2015). Geneva: World Health Organisation, 2012

115 World Organisation for Animal Health. *OIE List of Antimicrobials of Veterinary Importance*. Available at: www.oie.int/doc/ged/D9840.PDF (accessed February 25, 2015). Paris: World Organization of Animal Health, 2007

116 WHO. *Critically Important Antimicrobials for Human Medicine: 3rd revision, 2011*. Available at: http://apps.who.int/iris/bitstream/10665/77376/1/9789241504485_eng.pdf?ua=1 (accessed February 26, 2015). Geneva: World Health Organization, 2012

117 WHO. *Antimicrobial Resistance: Global Report on Surveillance*. Geneva: World Health Organization, 2014

118 World Economic Forum. *Global Risks Report 2013: Special Report – The Dangers of Hubris on Human Health*. Davos: World Economic Forum, 2013

119 DH/Defra. *UK Five Year Antimicrobial Resistance Strategy 2013 to 2018*. September 2013. Available at: www.gov.uk/government/uploads/system/uploads/attachment_data/file/244058/20130902_UK_5_year_AMR_strategy.pdf (accessed February 25, 2015). London: Department of Health and Department for Environment, Food and Rural Affairs, 2013

120 Obama B. *National Strategy for Combating Antibiotic-Resistant Bacteria*, September 18. Available at: www.whitehouse.gov/the-press-office/2014/09/18/executive-order-combating-antibiotic-resistant-bacteria (accessed February 26, 2015). Washington, DC, The White House: Office of the Press Secretary, 2014

121 President of the United States. *National Action Plan for Combating Antibiotic-Resistant Bacteria*. Washington, DC: The White House, Office of the US President, 2015: 62

122  WHO. *Antimicrobial Resistance: Global Report on Surveillance, 2014.* Available at: http://apps.who.int/iris/bitstream/10665/112642/1/9789241564748_eng.pdf?ua=1 (accessed February 25, 2015). Geneva: World Health Organization, 2014

123  HSE. *Health and Safety in Agriculture, Forestry and Fishing in Great Britain, 2014/2015.* Available at: www.hse.gov.uk/Statistics/industry/agriculture/agriculture.pdf (accessed June 2, 2015). London: Health and Safety Executive, 2015

124  United States Department of Labor. *Fatal Occupational Injuries, Total Hours Worked, and Rates of Fatal Occupational Injuries by Selected Worker Characteristics, Occupations, and Industries, Civilian Workers.* Available at: www.bls.gov/iif/oshwc/cfoi/cfoi_rates_2014hb.pdf (accessed March 3, 2016). Washington, DC: United States Department of Labor, 2014

125  Calvert GM, Karnik J, Mehler L, *et al.* Acute pesticide poisoning among agricultural workers in the United States, 1998-2005. *American Journal of Industrial Medicine,* 2008; 51(12): 883–98

126  Fraser CE, Smith KB, Judd F, *et al.* Farming and mental health problems and mental illness. *The International Journal of Social Psychiatry,* 2005; 51(4): 340–9

127  Freire C, Koifman S. Pesticides, depression and suicide: a systematic review of the epidemiological evidence. *International Journal of Hygiene and Environmental Health,* 2013; 216(4): 445–60

128  Roberts SE, Jaremin B, Lloyd K. High-risk occupations for suicide. *Psychological Medicine,* 2013; 43(6): 1231–40

129  Hounsome B, Edwards RT, Hounsome N, *et al.* Psychological morbidity of farmers and non-farming population: results from a UK survey. *Community Mental Health Journal,* 2012; 48(4): 503–10

130  Pavilonis BT, Sanderson WT, Merchant JA. Relative exposure to swine animal feeding operations and childhood asthma prevalence in an agricultural cohort. *Environmental Research,* 2013; 122: 74–80

131  Schulze A, Rommelt H, Ehrenstein V, *et al.* Effects on pulmonary health of neighboring residents of concentrated animal feeding operations: exposure assessed using optimized estimation technique. *Archives of Environmental & Occupational Health,* 2011; 66(3): 146–54

132  O'Connor AM, Auvermann B, Bickett-Weddle D, *et al.* The association between proximity to animal feeding operations and community health: a systematic review. *PLoS ONE,* 5(3): e9530 doi:101371/journalpone0009530 2010

133  Paulot F, Jacob DJ. Hidden cost of U.S. agricultural exports: particulate matter from ammonia emissions. *Environmental Science & Technology,* 2014; 48(2): 903–8

134  Stokstad E. Air pollution. Ammonia pollution from farming may exact hefty health costs. *Science,* 2014; 343(6168): 238

135  Pope CA 3rd, Ezzati M, Dockery DW. Fine-particulate air pollution and life expectancy in the United States. *The New England Journal of Medicine,* 2009; 360(4): 376–86

136  Aston LM, Smith JN, Powles JW. Impact of a reduced red and processed meat dietary pattern on disease risks and greenhouse gas emissions in the UK: a modelling study. *BMJ Open,* 2012; 2(5)

137  Macdiarmid JI, Kyle J, Horgan GW, *et al.* Sustainable diets for the future: can we contribute to reducing greenhouse gas emissions by eating a healthy diet? *The American Journal of Clinical Nutrition,* 2012; 96(3): 632–9

138 Scarborough P, Allender S, Clarke D, et al. Modelling the health impact of environmentally sustainable dietary scenarios in the UK. *European Journal of Clinical Nutrition*, 2012; 66(6): 710–15

139 Briggs AD, Kehlbacher A, Tiffin R, et al. Assessing the impact on chronic disease of incorporating the societal cost of greenhouse gases into the price of food: an econometric and comparative risk assessment modelling study. *BMJ Open*, 2013; 3(10): e003543

140 Monsivais P, Scarborough P, Lloyd T, et al. Greater accordance with the dietary approaches to stop hypertension dietary pattern is associated with lower diet-related greenhouse gas production but higher dietary costs in the United Kingdom. *The American Journal of Clinical Nutrition*, 2015, Jul; 102(1): 138–45

141 Meier T, Christen O. Environmental impacts of dietary recommendations and dietary styles: Germany as an example. *Environmental Science & Technology*, 2013; 47(2): 877–88

142 Pradhan P, Reusser DE, Kropp JP. Embodied greenhouse gas emissions in diets. *PLoS ONE*, 2013; 8(5): e62228

143 van Dooren C, Marinussen M, Blonk H, et al. Exploring dietary guidelines based on ecological and nutritional values: A comparison of six dietary patterns. *Food Policy*, 2014; 44(0): 36–46

144 Saxe H, Larsen TM, Mogensen L. The global warming potential of two healthy Nordic diets compared with the average Danish diet. *Climatic Change*, 2013; 116: 249–62

145 Baroni L, Cenci L, Tettamanti M, et al. Evaluating the environmental impact of various dietary patterns combined with different food production systems. *European Journal of Clinical Nutrition*, 2007; 61(2): 279–86

146 Saez-Almendros S, Obrador B, Bach-Faig A, et al. Environmental footprints of Mediterranean versus Western dietary patterns: beyond the health benefits of the Mediterranean diet. *Environmental Health: A Global Access Science Source*, 2013; 12: 118

147 Vieux F, Soler LG, Touazi D, et al. High nutritional quality is not associated with low greenhouse gas emissions in self-selected diets of French adults. *The American Journal of Clinical Nutrition*, 2013; 97(3): 569–83

148 Masset G, Soler LG, Vieux F, et al. Identifying sustainable foods: the relationship between environmental impact, nutritional quality, and prices of foods representative of the French diet. *Journal of the Academy of Nutrition and Dietetics*, 2014; 114(6): 862–9

149 Masset G, Vieux F, Verger EO, et al. Reducing energy intake and energy density for a sustainable diet: a study based on self-selected diets in French adults. *The American Journal of Clinical Nutrition*, 2014; 99(6): 1460–9

150 Verger EO, Mariotti F, Holmes BA, et al. Evaluation of a diet quality index based on the probability of adequate nutrient intake (PANDiet) using national French and US dietary surveys. *PLoS ONE*, 2012 7(8): e42155

151 Tukker A, Goldbohm RA, De Koning A, et al. Environmental impacts of changes to healthier diets in Europe. *Ecological Economics*, 2011; 70(10): 1776–88

152 Westhoek H, Lesschen JP, Rood T, et al. Food choices, health and environment: effects of cutting Europe's meat and dairy intake. *Global Environmental Change*, 2014; (26): 196–205

153  Pimentel D, Pimentel M. Sustainability of meat-based and plant-based diets and the environment. *The American Journal of Clinical Nutrition*, 2003; 78(3 Suppl): 660s–3s

154  Peters CJ, Wilkins JL, Fick GW. Testing a complete-diet model for estimating the land resource requirements of food consumption and agricultural carrying capacity: the New York State example. *Renewable Agriculture and Food Systems*, 2007; 22(02): 145–53

155  de Carvalho AM, Cesar CL, Fisberg RM, *et al.* Excessive meat consumption in Brazil: diet quality and environmental impacts. *Public Health Nutrition*, 2013; 16(10): 1893–9

156  Hendrie GA, Ridoutt BG, Wiedmann TO, *et al.* Greenhouse gas emissions and the Australian diet: comparing dietary recommendations with average intakes. *Nutrients*, 2014; 6(1): 289–303

157  Wilson N, Nghiem N, Ni Mhurchu C, *et al.* Foods and dietary patterns that are healthy, low-cost, and environmentally sustainable: a case study of optimization modeling for New Zealand. *PLoS ONE*, 2013; 8(3): e59648

158  Macdiarmid JI, Kyle J, Horgan GW, *et al. Livewell: A Balance of Sustainable and Healthy Food Choices.* Available at: http://assets.wwf.org.uk/downloads/livewell_report_corrected.pdf?_ga=1.98855454.1264079436.1469998857 (accessed May 20, 2015). Woking, UK: WWF-UK, 2011

# Chapter 4

# Environment
## Why food drives ecosystem stress

## Core concepts

Food and diets have a considerable environmental impact. Agriculture is estimated to be responsible for 30% of greenhouse gas emissions, use of 92% of global
water and about 38% of the earth's ice-free land, while being a major source
of biodiversity loss and land degradation. This chapter describes how and what
people eat influences the environment and how the environment shapes human
nutrition. The term 'environment' is taken to mean the biological environment
and its resources such as the atmosphere, land, water, soil and solar energy. These
enable the plants to photosynthesise and grow, on which diet and public health
depend. This understanding of the environment becomes central to the notion
of sustainable diets. Choice of diet affects the relationship between production
and consumption. What humans eat, and how the food system grows, processes,
moves and markets food, all have major impacts on climate change, energy use,
water, land use, soil, biodiversity and waste. This circularity is now of critical
importance to twenty-first-century prosperity and survival.

## The impact of food and diet on the environment

It is well established that food and diets have a considerable environmental impact.
Indeed, food consumption has been identified as one of the most important drivers
of environmental pressures.[1] According to the Food and Agricultural Organization,
agriculture occupies about 38% of the earth's ice-free land,[2] the largest use of land
on the planet. Globally, agriculture is estimated to be responsible for up to 30%
of greenhouse gas emissions, including methane ($CH_4$) emissions from livestock
and rice cultivation, nitrous oxide ($N_2O$) emissions from fertilised soils, energy use,
fertiliser production and agriculturally induced land-use change.[3, 4] Of particular
concern is that 92% of global water is devoted to agricultural production,[5] while
agriculture is a significant force behind loss of biodiversity and degradation of land.[6]
Footprint analyses suggest that North America and Europe consume biological
resources as though they inhabit multiple planets; the USA consuming as though
it inhabits five planets, Europe three.[7] Food and agriculture represent a major force
driving the environment beyond the planet's boundaries.[8]

Although there is broad agreement on the impact of food and diet on the
environment, there is less agreement on how to address these issues. This is partly
because the environmental perspective on food systems raises some serious questions about notions of progress generally and for food in particular. The pursuit
of economic progress has become tangled with consumerism (using ever more
'stuff') and has underplayed how economic development distorts the relationship
between human beings, their food consumption and the health of the planet.[9, 10]
However, given that human health depends on the health of ecosystems, on
which food is making such a considerable impact, this raises the question about
the sustainability of the current food system. It is why there is such political

pressure on policy makers to reduce the food system's environmental impact. At best, there is some awareness of food's impact on carbon emissions but far less attention to its impact on soil or biodiversity.

Future environmental health is likely to hinge to a considerable extent on whether food consumption and production can be made sustainable. Although much of the focus to date has been on improving the environmental efficiency of production through, for example, managing resource use and inputs more effectively, such approaches will not be sufficient to address environmental concerns. Diets will also have to change. What and how much we eat directly affects what is produced, how and where the environmental impacts are. A theme of this book is how a good food system must be multi-criteria, with lower environmental impacts (the subject of this chapter), improvements to public health (Chapter 3) and also social (Chapter 5), quality (Chapter 6) and economic (Chapter 7) dimensions.

We now explore some of food's major environmental features such as climate change, energy use, water, land use, soil, biodiversity and waste. Tackling all these is an awesome task. If society is to have truly sustainable diets, this requires more than just addressing diet and carbon.

## Climate change

Climate change is one of the major challenges for humanity over the next century. Since the late 1800s the planet's average temperature has risen by 0.65–1.06°C, with further rises predicted by 2100 of 0.3–4.8°C.[11] The majority of this change has occurred since the 1950s, although the impacts can be traced back to the beginnings of the Industrial Revolution and its reliance on burning fossil fuels. These changes are caused by the increasing release of GHGs, including carbon dioxide ($CO_2$), methane ($CH_4$) and nitrous oxide ($N_2O$), which trap heat. Methane is 24 times and $N_2O$ is 296 times more potent as a GHG than $CO_2$ and impact on climate is estimated by converting the total GHGs to carbon dioxide equivalents.

Global GHG emissions due to human activities have grown since pre-industrial times, with an increase of 70% between 1970 and 2004.[12] To meet international climate goals set to reduce the risk of adverse effects from climate change, global GHG emissions need to be cut by 50% globally and 80% in the developed world by 2050 compared with 1990.[13, 14] This will require substantial mitigation efforts on all fronts, including the food sector. In 2008, a report by the UK Food Climate Research Network (FCRN)[15] argued the need for a 70% reduction in GHG emissions from food. In 2014 Ripple et al.[16] argued that reduction in fossil fuels and large cuts in $CO_2$ emissions, although necessary, will not alone abate climate change and simultaneous cuts in non-$CO_2$ GHG emissions will be needed. In their view, cuts in the latter can be achieved in particular by reducing the number of ruminants.

The food system produces GHGs at all stages, from agriculture and its inputs, through to food manufacture, distribution, refrigeration, retailing, food preparation in the home and waste disposal. However, the greatest impacts occur at the agricultural stage. At the farm stage, the dominant GHGs are $N_2O$ released from soil and livestock processes, including manure, urine and applications of nitrogen fertilisers, and $CH_4$ from ruminant digestion, rice cultivation and anaerobic soils. $CO_2$ emissions, arising from fossil fuel combustion to power machinery, for the manufacture of synthetic fertilisers and from the burning of biomass, also contribute, albeit to a lesser extent. $CO_2$ and $CH_4$ resulting from agriculturally induced land-use change including forest clearance can add considerably to farm-stage impacts. Beyond the farm gate, $CO_2$ from fossil fuel use, resulting from processing and distribution, dominates, with refrigerant gases making a contribution.

While there appear to be no studies that quantify GHG emissions arising from the entire global food system, estimates suggest that the direct impact of agriculture is about 10–12% of global emissions.[14, 17] However, this figure rises up to 30% when additional emissions from fuel use, fertiliser production and agriculturally induced land-use change are included.[18, 19] Land-use change alone accounts for 6–17% of global GHG emissions.[20]

In high-income countries studies show that food consumption contributes between 15 and 31% to national GHG emissions.[1, 19, 21] One regional analysis for Europe found that food accounts for 31% of the EU-25's total GHG impacts, with a further 9% arising from the hotel and restaurants sector,[1] while a UK study indicated that direct emissions from the UK food system are about 20% of the currently estimated consumption emissions, rising to 30% when land-use change emissions is included.[19] One fifth of UK food system emissions arise outside of the UK (50% when land-use change is included),[19] a figure that is expected to rise as imported emissions increase, offsetting a reduction in domestic emissions.[22] Indeed a 2016 analysis found that, while the UK is currently importing over 50% of its food and feed, 70% and 64% of the associated cropland and GHG impacts, respectively, are located abroad.[23] These results imply that the UK is increasingly reliant on external resources and that the environmental impact of its food supply is increasingly displaced overseas. In food, as with other consumables, there's a danger of countries apparently lowering their GHGs (or other impacts) when they have simply transferred production to other countries. A 2013 report from the UK's Committee on Climate Change (CCC) shows the need to cut imported as well as domestic emissions and recommends the monitoring of consumption-based emissions.[24]

EU nations have made some progress in the reduction of GHGs from agriculture over recent years.[25] However, global emissions continue to rise, with China, Brazil, India and the USA being the biggest net emitters of non-$CO_2$ GHGs where the impact of agriculture is particularly high (particularly $N_2O$ from soils and $CH_4$ from animals).[26]

## Meat and animal produce

Meat and meat products (including meat, poultry, sausages or similar) are identified as the food group responsible for most GHG emissions attributable to the food sector.[3, 27–29] Livestock is an important emitter of GHG. It is currently estimated to emit 7.1 gigatonnes of carbon dioxide equivalent ($CO_2e$) per annum, representing 14.5% of all human-induced emissions,[30] a figure that has been revised downwards since 2006.[31] There is a large variation between producers and regions of the world with, for example, South Asia's total livestock emissions at the same level as that of North America and Western Europe, but its protein production is only half the size. Beef and cows' milk production account for the majority of emissions, respectively contributing 41% and 19% of the sector's emissions, while pig meat and poultry meat and eggs contribute, respectively, 9% and 8% to the sector's emissions. A UK study found that emissions from livestock rearing account for over 57% of agricultural emissions.[19] The main sources of emissions are: feed production and processing (45% of the total – with 9% attributable to the expansion of pasture and feed crops into forests), enteric fermentation from ruminants (39%), and manure decomposition (10%). The remainder is attributable to the processing and transportation of animal products.

Differences exist in the ecological impact of different meat types.[1, 19, 32–36] A variety of studies have concluded that, per kilogram of meat, beef and lamb have the largest ecological impact at European and global level, on the basis of GHG emissions and also of land use (see Table 4.1), followed by pork and chicken. The lower GHG emissions per kg associated with pork and chicken are partly due to the fact that, unlike cattle and sheep, they are not ruminants so produce less $CH_4$. They also have a faster reproductive cycle and a more efficient conversion of feed to edible meat and protein.[37] However, these ecological improvements are not necessarily accompanied by improvements in animal welfare (see Chapter 5) and, depending on the production system, a switch from beef to pork and chicken can also increase arable land use overseas.[19]

Table 4.1 shows the results of an analysis from 52 life-cycle analysis studies of animal sources of protein in terms of carbon footprint ($CO_2e$) per kg weight and, to give one indication of nutritional value, per kg of protein.[36] For comparison, two plant-based protein-containing alternatives (pulses and soya) are included.

The production of extensively farmed beef appears to be linked to higher GHG emissions than does the production of intensively farmed beef per kg of product. In intensive systems the nutrients in the feed are relatively efficiently converted into meat and dairy because the animals do not have to (or cannot) walk about much to find their food.

The production of milk appears to be linked to lower GHG emissions than the production of chicken per kg but, if considered as an alternative source of protein and expressed per kg of protein rather than per kg of product, the GHG impact of milk is higher than that of chicken and broadly similar to that of pork. Eggs have a lower GHG impact than cheese. Entirely plant-based meat substitutes are associated with similar or slightly lower GHG emissions than the production of chicken, but their cultivation and preparation for consumption can have significant environmental impact.[19]

*Table 4.1* GHG emissions ($CO_2$ equivalents) of protein-rich food products per kg or product and per gram of protein from 52 life-cycle analyses

| Food product | GHG $CO_2$ equivalents/kg | GHG $CO_2$ equivalents/kg protein |
|---|---|---|
| Beef (20% protein) | 9–129 | 45–640 |
| Feedlot systems | 14–40 | 45–210 |
| Mixed systems/dairy calves | 9–42 | 114–250 |
| Meadow systems/suckler herds | 23–52 | 58–643 |
| Extensive pastoral systems | 12–129 | 60–640 |
| Culled dairy cows | 9–12 | 45–62 |
| Pork (20% protein) | 4–11 | 20–55 |
| Poultry (20% protein) | 2–6 | 10–30 |
| Cheese (25% protein) | 6–22 | 28–68 |
| Eggs (13% protein) | 2–6 | 15–42 |
| Mutton and lamb (20% protein) | 10–150 | 51–750 |
| Milk (3.5% protein) | 1–2 | 28–43 |
| Seafood from fisheries (16–20% protein) | 1–86 | 4–540 |
| Seafood from aquaculture (17–20% aquaculture) | 3–15 | 4–75 |
| Meat substitutes (egg or milk protein) (15–20% protein) | 3–6 | 17–34 |
| Meat substitutes (vegetable protein: e.g., soya) (8–20% protein) | 1–2 | 6–17 |
| Pulses (20–36% protein) | 1–2 | 4–10 |

Source: Nijdam et al. [36]

## Plant foods

Other foods such as bread, potatoes, cereals, rice, pasta, vegetables, fruit and snacks make a smaller contribution to GHG emissions than animal foods, although rice grown in paddies generates high levels of $CH_4$,[38] and field-grown fruit and vegetables such as brassicas, root vegetables, tubers and hard fruits such as apples and pears generate relatively low emissions compared with those grown in hot houses because of the high energy input (and therefore GHG emissions) needed for artificial heating and lighting.

Table 4.2 compares the contribution made by animal products and non-animal foods to GHG emissions, derived from estimates across three European countries: the UK, the Netherlands and Sweden. The figures for all food groups show some variation across the three countries, although the estimates for the non-animal-based foods show a greater spread than the animal-based foods and fish, which is partly because different studies have different underlying assumptions and different numbers and products are included in the product groups. Estimates for the GHG emissions associated with food are associated with some uncertainty although the greater GHG impact of animal compared with plant foods is clear in all studies.

*Table 4.2* The contribution to total GHG emissions made by different food product groups (expressed as a proportion of all food groups combined)

| Food product group | UK | The Netherlands | Sweden |
|---|---|---|---|
| Meat, meat products and fish | 38 | 28 | 35 |
| Dairy | 15 | 23 | 15 |
| Bread, biscuits, cakes and flour | 5 | 13 | 10 |
| Potatoes, fruit and vegetables | 6 | 15 | 19 |
| Fats and oils | 10 | 3 | 4 |
| Drinks and sweetened products | 20 | A | 15 |
| Other foods | 3 | 3 | 17 |

Source: Health Council of the Netherlands[39] (data from[32, 34, 40, 41]).

Note: A = falls into the category of other foods.

*Table 4.3* Estimated GHG emissions from the supply of food from primary production and after the regional distribution centre (RDC) for the UK (kilotonnes)

| Primary production | Direct emissions | Attributed land-use change emissions | Total |
|---|---|---|---|
| Red meat (beef, sheep, goat and pig meat) | 19,400 | 76,607 | 96,007 |
| Milk | 17,200 | 9,416 | 26,616 |
| White meat (poultry) | 10,900 | 4,629 | 15,529 |
| Cereals including brewing and distilling | 9,750 | 3,711 | 13,461 |
| Vegetables and legumes | 5,380 | 1,682 | 7,062 |
| Oil-based crops | 4,060 | 2,365 | 6,425 |
| Salad crops | 3,580 | 126 | 3,706 |
| Fish | 2,780 | - | 2,780 |
| Grapes and wine | 2,610 | 584 | 3,174 |
| Temperate and Mediterranean fruit | 2,220 | 450 | 2,670 |
| Rice | 1,860 | 185 | 2,045 |
| Exotic fruit | 1,780 | 102 | 1,882 |
| Eggs | 1,650 | 113 | 1,763 |
| Sugar | 1,200 | 325 | 1,525 |
| Beverages | 1,180 | 714 | 1,894 |
| Nuts | 254 | 326 | 580 |
| Miscellaneous, including spices | 79 | 93 | 172 |
| Sub-total for primary food production | 85,883 | 101,408 | 187,291 |
| Post regional distribution centre (processing, distribution, retail preparation) | 66,300 | 0 | 66,300 |
| Totals | 152,183 | 101,408 | 253,591 |

Source: data from Audsley et al.[19]

Few studies have evaluated the GHG impact across the whole of a product's life from production through to distribution, processing, consumer behaviour and waste processing. A UK study estimated total GHG emissions from the supply of foods for the UK,[19] including direct emissions from primary production, emissions attributed to land-use change and emissions arising after processing, distribution and retail preparation (see Tables 4.3 and 4.4). This study again shows the high GHG impact of animal products. Estimated total GHG emissions arising from processing, distribution, retail and preparation of food for UK consumption are considerably less than the emissions associated with primary production but, accounting for 26% of the total in this study, they are not insignificant.

Climate change is predicted to have an overall adverse impact on agriculture and hence food supply. Increased evaporation and ocean storm surges, greater numbers of gales, floods, rains and cyclones, as well as drought and reduced rainfall in other areas, are predicted to lead to poor crop yields, increased and new animal diseases, damage to the habitat of some species, increase in pests and destruction of crops through loss of land, fires, floods, drought and storm damage. Some parts of the world are expected to be more affected than others. World Bank projections suggest that India and Mexico will be the most significantly affected countries with predicted decreases of agricultural output of 38% and 35%. The USA and Germany, by contrast, are projected to decrease by 6% and 3% respectively.[42]

Climate impacts on agriculture may affect both the quantity and quality of food produced. A reduced availability of some main staple foodstuffs will lead to

Table 4.4 Estimated GHG emissions from processing, distribution, retail and preparation of food consumption in the UK (kilotonnes $CO_2$/year)

|  | Home consumption | Eating out | Total |
| --- | --- | --- | --- |
| Cooking | 11,100 | 4,410 | 15,510 |
| Manufacturing | 12,200 | 2,720 | 14,920 |
| Food storage energy | 11,200 | 2,170 | 13,370 |
| Refrigerants | 4,630 | 1,270 | 5,900 |
| Electricity | 4,530 | 1,090 | 5,620 |
| Landfill of food waste | 2,550 | 928 | 3,478 |
| Washing up | 1,970 | 257 | 2,227 |
| Road fuel and oil | 1,380 | 271 | 1,651 |
| Travel to outlet | 1,330 | 113 | 1,443 |
| Packaging | 719 | 136 | 855 |
| Landfill | 488 | 155 | 643 |
| Carrier bags and takeaway containers | 391 | 51 | 441 |
| Food storage refrigerants | 61 | 180 | 241 |
| Total | 52,549 | 13,751 | 66,300 |

Source: data from Audsley et al.[19]

increased prices with major implications for food security in many areas of the world. Those most at risk through food shortages and high prices would be the most economically disadvantaged, but high prices can also impact on the quality of food. For example, poorer weight gain in livestock may lead to lower quality meat, lower nitrogen in wheat crops may make it less suitable for bread and pasta making, and poorer quality fruit and vegetables may have reduced storage capacity and be more vulnerable to pest damage. Findings from a US meta-analysis from seven experimental locations in the USA, Australia and Japan and involving 143 comparisons between edible portions of crops grown in normal and elevated $CO_2$ suggest that the $CO_2$ levels expected in the second half of this century will likely reduce the levels of zinc, iron and protein in wheat, rice, peas and soybeans.[43] Some two billion people live in countries where citizens receive more than 60% of their zinc or iron from these types of crops.

Several researchers have evaluated the potential to reduce GHG emissions by improving the environmental efficiency of food production or changing food consumption or both. The environmental efficiency approach, i.e., producing more food with less impact, often known as sustainable intensification, has been the focus of industry and policy in recent years, but there is a growing acknowledgement of the need for both consumption and production approaches.[35, 44–47] The United Nations Conference on Trade and Development (UNCTAD) argues for a change in dietary pattern towards more climate-friendly food and a profound transformation of agriculture with a 'rapid and significant shift from conventional monoculture based on high external input dependent industrial production towards mosaics of sustainable regenerative production that also considerably improve the productivity of small scale farmers'.[47]

Increasingly, several studies[4, 19, 48–50] and reviews[3, 15, 46, 51, 52] conclude that improvements in food production efficiency alone will be insufficient to avert absolute increases in GHG emissions. An FAO report also suggests that, while much can be done to improve the environmental efficiency of livestock production, it is 'unlikely that emission intensity gains, based on the deployment or current technology will entirely offset the inflation of emissions related to this sector's growth'.[30] A Swedish study by Hedenhus et al. concluded that reduced ruminant meat and dairy consumption will be indispensable for reducing global GHG emissions to keep the global average surface temperatures from increasing by more than 20°C above the pre-industrial level.[50]

From the perspective of GHG emissions alone, this all suggests that, without a technological breakthrough, people who eat a lot of meat will need to eat less. How much less requires a consideration of the nutritional role of meat in the diet and the implications for human nutrition and public health (see Chapter 3). Another issue is the mode of production. The common scientific view from recent evidence is that beef is far 'worse' than other meats, with beef production requiring 28, 11, 5 and 6 times more land, irrigation water, GHGs and RN than other animals.[53] Differences emerge between pasture-fed, intensively fed and mixed-mode-fed animals. Intensive rearing means shorter lives for the animals and therefore less input, while ranged meat takes longer to get to 'killing' weight or status. Those who favour pasture-reared animals argue that this means meat is more expensive, which is a good thing, as the price signals then encourage low meat consumption.[54]

## Energy use

Energy is an essential resource across the entire food production cycle.[53] It is estimated that an average of 7–10 kcal of energy input is required in the production of 1 kcal of food. This varies dramatically depending on the food, from an average energy input of 3 kcal for plant crops to 35 kcal in the production of beef. A British study found that energy use in animal food production varied between 2.7 gigajoules (GJ) per ton of milk to 17 GJ per ton of poultry and 30 GJ per ton of beef. Equivalent figures for potatoes were 1.4 GJ and for bread wheat 2.5 GJ.[55]

Overall, the food sector accounts for 30% of the world's energy consumption, of which primary farm and fisheries production accounts for around one fifth, which is equivalent to 6% of the total global energy consumption.[56] Higher-income countries use a significant portion of this energy for processing and transport while, in low-income countries, cooking consumes the greatest share.

Much of this energy comes from fossil fuels, which are used throughout the food system from the manufacture and application of agricultural inputs such as fertilisers and irrigation, through to crop and livestock production, processing and packaging, distribution, such as shipping and cold storage, the running of refrigeration, preparation and disposal equipment in food retailing and food service establishments and in domestic kitchens. Oil accounts for between 30% and 75% of energy inputs of UK agriculture, depending on the cropping system.[55] The average American diet is estimated to be underpinned by 2,000 litres of oil equivalents per year, which accounts for 19% of total US energy use.[57] In this study, agricultural production as well as food processing and packaging accounted for 14%, while transportation and preparation contributed 5%. In two other pieces of US research, the processing industry energy use for cooking, cooling and freezing was found to contribute an average share of 15–20% of total US food system energy use, with inputs to packaging and transport relatively small.[58, 59]

On farms, the availability of cheap and plentiful petroleum has been a key factor in the twentieth-century increase in productivity. Mechanisation replaced animals as motive power, releasing not just horses and oxen but also humans from hard labour; this happened earlier in the USA than Europe and is still underway around the world. For example, instead of the 1,200 hours of labour needed in the USA to produce 1 hectare of maize in the past, nowadays only 11 hours is needed.[57] However, this process has occurred rather unevenly across the world. A 2003 analysis highlighted by Mrema et al.[60] showed that in Europe there was one tractor for 45 hectares, compared with one tractor for 67 hectares in Latin America and one tractor for 2,113 hectares in Africa. Despite the benefits of mechanisation, the extensive use of machines in farming places substantial claims on energy. Although energy efficiency increased during the twentieth century, the total amount of energy required for agriculture is still growing.

In addition to agricultural machinery, the production of fertilisers and pesticides also uses much energy. Generally, fertilisers contain nitrogen compounds together with varying proportions of compounds containing potassium and phosphorus. Although potash and phosphate compounds are typically obtained by mining minerals, nitrogen compounds are manufactured from ammonia using the Haber process. In this process atmospheric nitrogen is combined with hydrogen obtained largely from natural gas, though other hydrocarbon sources such as coal (particularly in China) and oil are also used. Since 950m$^3$ of natural gas is required to produce each tonne of ammonia (global production of fertiliser is currently some 178 million tonnes per year), the fertiliser manufacturing industry consumes about 3–5% of the world's annual natural gas supply or 1–2% of the world's energy supply.[61] Nitrogen fertilisers can account for 50% or more of total energy use in commercial agriculture.[55, 62] With the expected increase in the amount of land under modern farming methods by 2030, the total annual demand for fertiliser has been estimated to increase 25% by 2030 to 223 million tonnes, of which some 62% would be nitrogenous.[63]

Food processing also uses large amounts of energy and can be remarkably inefficient in terms of the energy consumed relative to the energy delivered to the consumer. Energy usage in food processing depends on the specific food and can be highly variable even for one food product. Few studies have evaluated the energy used in producing one food product, but a Swedish analysis of a typical fast-food burger found that it typically uses 3–8 times more energy in its production and distribution than it delivers to the consumer in food.[64]

Dependence on energy in the food system raises the question of the impact of high or volatile energy prices on the price of food as well as of domestic food security and the nation's reliance on imported energy. Intensive energy use also makes the food system an important contributor to GHG emissions. With food production anticipated to increase by 25% between now and 2030, sustainable energy sourcing will become an increasingly major issue. Given also that the production of animal foods requires more energy than the production of plant foods, the question then arises as to what the fossil fuel requirements would be for human diets made up of various combinations of animal and plant foods. An analysis based on data for various foods produced in the United States evaluated the fossil fuel requirements of a vegan diet, a vegetarian diet containing milk and eggs and a mixed diet containing meat.[65] The diet containing meat involves an energy input almost twice as high as that for the vegetarian and the vegetarian diet is more energy-intensive than the vegan diet. Eating less meat and more plant foods is therefore likely to be more economical in terms of fossil fuel energy than a diet with a higher meat intake. It also restores farm animals to their ecological niche.

# Water

Over the past century, fresh water abstraction for human use has increased at more than double the rate of population growth. Currently about 3.8 trillion m$^3$ of water is used by humans each year. Food production is not possible without water and a pure safe water supply is also essential for public health. An estimated 780 million people worldwide currently lack access to safe drinking water. About 70% of the planet is composed of water, but most of this is salty and food systems require salt-free water.

Agriculture is the greatest user of water worldwide, accounting for 70–80% of human water withdrawals,[66] with agriculture and food production in total accounting for an estimated 92% of the global water footprint.[67] Water use will continue to rise over the coming decades and, depending on how food is produced and the validity of forecasts for demographic trends, the demand for water in food production could reach 10–13 trillion m$^3$ annually by mid-century. This is 2.5 to 3.5 times greater than the total human use of fresh water today.[68] A distinction is now made between 'blue' water (fresh surface and groundwater); 'green' water (precipitation on land that does not run off or recharge the groundwater but is stored in the soil or temporarily stays on top of the soil or plants); and 'grey' water (an indicator of freshwater pollution that can be associated with the production of a product over its full supply chain).[69]

Many countries rely heavily on water resources elsewhere. For example, European countries such as Italy, Germany, the UK and the Netherlands have external water footprints contributing 60% to 95% of their total water footprint. On the other hand, some other countries such as Chad, Ethiopia, India, Niger, DR Congo, Mali, Argentina and Sudan have very small external water footprints, smaller than 4% of the total footprint.[67]

A 2016 analysis traced, quantified and mapped the UK's direct and indirect water needs and assess the 'imported water risk' by evaluating the sustainability of the water consumption in the source regions.[70] In this analysis, half of the UK's global blue water footprint – the direct and indirect consumption of ground and surface water resources behind all commodities consumed in the UK – is located in places where the blue water footprint exceeds the maximum sustainable blue water footprint. About 55% of the unsustainable part of the UK's blue water footprint is located in six countries: Spain (14%), USA (11%), Pakistan (10%), India (7%), Iran (6%) and South Africa (6%). This analysis also shows that about half of the global consumptive water footprint of the UK's direct and indirect crop consumption is inefficient, which means that consumptive water footprints exceed specified water footprint benchmark levels. About 37% of the inefficient part of the UK's consumptive water footprint is located in six countries: Indonesia (7%), Ghana (7%), India (7%), Brazil (6%), Spain (5%) and Argentina (5%). In some source countries, like Pakistan, Iran, Spain, USA and Egypt, unsustainable and inefficient blue water consumption coincide. The authors concluded that, by lowering overall consumptive water footprints to benchmark levels, the global blue water footprint of UK crop consumption could be reduced by 19%.

Water scarcity is a growing problem. The United Nations Environment Programme estimated in 2007 that, by 2025, 1.8 billion people will be living in regions with absolute water scarcity and, by 2050, 54 countries would be in absolute water stress, affecting 40% of the future population.[71] Those prognoses still hold. Water availability is susceptible to impacts from climate change. The Intergovernmental Panel on Climate Change has warned that as soon as 2020 some African countries may witness decreases in yields of up to 50% from rain-fed agriculture owing to climate change.[12]

Livestock makes a significant claim on the planet's water resources. Research by Mekonnen and Hoekstra shows that nearly 30% of the water footprint of humanity is related to the production of animal products.[72] The global water footprint of animal production amounts to 2,422 billion m$^3$ per year. A third of this total is related to beef cattle, another 19% to dairy cattle. Among the commonly consumed meats, in general, beef has a higher water footprint than sheep, which in turn has a higher water footprint than pork, with poultry having the lowest water footprint.[73] By far the greatest proportion of the total water footprint of all animal products comes from growing the feed.

Per ton of product, animal products generally have a larger water footprint than crop products (Table 4.5). The same is true for the water footprint per calorie. The average water footprint per calorie for beef is 20 times larger than that for cereals and starchy roots. With regards to the water requirements for protein, it has been found that the water footprint per gram of protein for milk, eggs and chicken meat is about 1.5 times larger than for pulses. For beef, the water footprint per gram of protein is six times larger than for pulses. In the case of fat, butter has

Table 4.5 The water footprint of some selected food products from vegetable and animal origin

| | litre/kg | litre/kcal | litre/gram protein | litre/gram fat |
|---|---|---|---|---|
| Sugar crops | 197 | 0.69 | 0.0 | 0.0 |
| Vegetables | 322 | 1.34 | 26 | 154 |
| Starchy roots | 387 | 0.47 | 31 | 226 |
| Fruits | 962 | 2.09 | 180 | 348 |
| Cereals | 1,644 | 0.51 | 21 | 112 |
| Oil crops | 2,364 | 0.81 | 16 | 11 |
| Pulses* | 4,055 | 1.19 | 19 | 180 |
| Nuts | 9,063 | 3.63 | 139 | 47 |
| Milk | 1,020 | 1.82 | 31 | 33 |
| Eggs | 3,265 | 2.29 | 29 | 33 |
| Chicken meat | 4,325 | 3.00 | 34 | 43 |
| Butter | 5,553 | 0.72 | 0.0 | 6.4 |
| Pig meat | 5,988 | 2.15 | 57 | 23 |
| Sheep/goat meat | 8,763 | 4.25 | 63 | 54 |
| Bovine meat | 15,415 | 10.19 | 112 | 153 |

Source: Mekonnen and Hoekstra (2012).[72]

*Table 4.6* Embedded water in some common foods and drinks

| Food or drink | Quantity | Embedded water/litre |
| --- | --- | --- |
| One pint of beer | 568 ml | 170 |
| Glass of milk | 200 ml | 200 |
| Cup of tea | 250 ml | 35 |
| Cup of coffee | 125 ml | 140 |
| Cup of instant coffee | 125 ml | 80 |
| Glass of wine | 125 ml | 120 |
| Glass of orange juice | 200 ml | 170 |
| Glass of apple juice | 200 ml | 190 |
| Orange | 100 g | 50 |
| Apple | 100 g | 70 |
| Tomato | 70 g | 13 |
| Slice of bread | 30 g | 40 |
| One egg | 40 g | 135 |
| Potato | 100 g | 25 |
| One bag of potato crisps | 200 g | 185 |
| One hamburger | 150 g | 2,400 |

Source: Chapagain and Hoekstra, 2004;[74] Williams *et al.*, 2002.[75]

a relatively small water footprint per gram of fat, even lower than for oil crops. All other animal products, however, have larger water footprints per gram of fat when compared to oil crops. From a freshwater resource perspective, it is more efficient to obtain calories, protein and fat through crop products than animal products.

Much of the water consumed in food is hidden and known as 'embedded' or virtual water. Table 4.6 shows the embedded water in various food and drink products. A cup of black coffee represents 140 litres of pure water to create it: on the farm, processing, packing and finally delivery to the consumer. If milk is added, embedded water increases to 200 litres. A 150 g Dutch hamburger has 2,400 litres of embedded water: water to grow grain and grass, water drunk by the animal and used by services for the animal (cleaning, etc.). Life-cycle analyses show considerable disparities in products.

People's dietary habits greatly influence their overall water footprint. In industrialised countries it has been estimated that 3,600 litres of water a day are required to produce food for a mixed diet in which it is assumed that around a third of the energy comes from animal products, while for a vegetarian diet, in which it is assumed that around 9% of energy still comes from dairy products, 2,300 litres of water a day will be needed.[76] An EU 28 (EU 27 plus Croatia) water footprint analysis of the current diet and three alternative diets containing less meat found that all three alternative diets resulted in a substantial reduction in water footprint. Compared with the current diet, a healthy diet (as recommended by the German Nutrition Society) had a 23% lower water footprint, a vegetarian diet (including milk and milk products) had a 30% lower water footprint and a combined diet (combination of a healthy diet and a vegetarian diet) had a 38%

lower water footprint; the reduction in meat intake contributed most to water footprint reduction.[77]

Due to the international trade in feed, live animals and animal products, international virtual water flows are huge, adding up to 272 billion m$^3$ per year relating to animals and animal products and 1,766 m$^3$ per year for crops and crop products, a substantial amount of which must relate to feed.[67] Within Europe, millions of farm animals are taken on long journeys while the USA imports millions of cattle and pigs each year, mainly from Mexico and Canada. Given the projected doubling of meat production in the period 2000 to 2050,[31] the relationship between animal products and water use is worthy of the attention of policy makers.

## Land use

Land is essentially a finite resource. One can vary its use or take marginal lands into food use, treat it well or badly, but overall land is a fixed asset. Population growth in combination with increasing wealth and more resource-demanding lifestyles are driving an increase in competition for global land resources. Land use is essential for food production, yet some forms of land use are causing declines in biodiversity, degradation of soil and water and increasing GHG emissions with implications for food production and food security.

Agriculture occupies about 38% of the earth's terrestrial surface and is the largest use of land on the planet.[2] Croplands cover 1.53 billion hectares (about 12% of the earth's ice-free land) while pastures cover another 3.38 billion hectares (about 26% of the earth's ice-free land). The livestock sector uses 70% of agricultural land overall (including grazing and land to grow feed) and a third of the total land surface across the planet. As such, livestock, and therefore meat consumption, plays a leading role in $CO_2$ release and biodiversity loss from deforestation. For example, cattle ranching and soya production (grown for animal feed) are the key drivers of deforestation in the fragile Amazon region. There are calls to stop using animals reared on soy grown on Amazonian cleared land.[78]

As populations become wealthier, dietary patterns change, which usually involves higher meat and dairy consumption. Meat and milk consumption in China has more than doubled since the 1990s[79] and is projected to double again by the 2030s. Some Brazilian soya goes to China for feeding both humans and pigs. Dietary consumption patterns, more than population growth, will increasingly have a significant impact on land requirements globally.[80]

A diet based on wheat has been estimated to require six times less land than that for an existing affluent diet with meat.[81, 82] One hectare of land can produce rice or potatoes for 19–22 people per annum, while the same area will produce enough lamb or beef for only one or two people.[68] Dutch studies have shown that beef production per kg requires almost three to four times as much land as chicken and 15 times as much land as cereals.[82, 83]

Table 4.7 shows the results of an analysis from 52 life-cycle analysis studies of animal sources of protein in terms of land area used per kg weight and, to give one indication of nutritional value, per kg of protein.[36] For comparison, two plant-based protein-containing alternatives (pulses and soya) are included. The range in land use is very large, particularly per gram of protein produced, varying from 10m²/year/kg of protein for plant products and meat substitute containing egg protein to over 2,000 m²/year/kg of protein for beef from extensively farmed cattle.

Some studies have evaluated the potential impact of diets and dietary change on land requirements for food production. A UK study[21] evaluated the impact on land use of changing food consumption according to three scenarios. First, a 50% reduction in livestock product consumption (with meat maintained at 36% of animal produce consumption) balanced by increases in plant foods; second, a shift from red meat (beef and lamb) to white meat (pork and poultry) with red meat consumption reduced by 75% and, third, a 50% reduction in white meat consumption balanced by increases in plant commodities. Energy intakes were the same across all three dietary scenarios. All three dietary scenarios reduce

Table 4.7 Land requirements of protein-rich food products per kg or product and per gram of protein from 52 life-cycle analyses

| Food product | Land use (m²/year/kg) | Land use (m²/year/kg equivalents/kg protein) |
|---|---|---|
| Beef (20% protein) | 7–420 | 37–2,100 |
| Industrial systems | 15–29 | 75–143 |
| Meadow systems/suckler herds | 33–158 | 164–788 |
| Extensive pastoral systems | 286–420 | 1,430–2,100 |
| Culled dairy cows | 7 | 37 |
| Pork (20% protein) | 8–15 | 40–75 |
| Poultry (20% protein) | 5–8 | 23–40 |
| Cheese (25% protein) | 6–17 | 26–54 |
| Eggs (13% protein) | 4–7 | 29–52 |
| Mutton and lamb (20% protein) | 20–33 | 100–165 |
| Milk (3.5% protein) | 1–2 | 26–54 |
| Seafood from fisheries (16–20% protein) | Bottom trawling could have effect on large areas of seabed | 10–540 |
| Seafood from aquaculture (17–20% aquaculture) | 2–6 (land used for feed) | 13–30 (land used for feed) |
| Meat substitutes (egg or milk protein) (15–20% protein) | 1–3 | 8–17 |
| Meat substitutes (vegetable protein, e.g., soya) (8–20% protein) | 2–3 | 4–25 |
| Pulses (20–36% protein) | 3–8 | 10–43 |

Source: Nijdam et al.[36]

the estimated total amount of land required to support the UK food system. A switch from red to white meat increases the need for overseas arable land for pig and poultry feed, although a larger area of UK land that can be tilled is released. Under a reduction scenario, the amount of extra land required for the direct consumption of plant products is less than the amount of arable land released from livestock feed production. A 50% reduction in livestock product consumption opens up the opportunity to release about half of UK land currently used for UK food supplies if remaining production is concentrated on the more capable land.

A further modelling study conducted by researchers in Sweden[84] pointed to the importance of changing diets as well as improving livestock production efficiency. According to this study, improving livestock productivity could decrease the FAO's projected global agricultural land use of 5.4 billion ha in 2030 to 4.8 billion ha. Combining the higher productivity growth with a substitution of pork and/or poultry for 20% of ruminant meat reduces land use further to 4.4 billion ha. In another scenario, applied mainly to high-income regions, that assumes a minor transition towards vegetarian food (25% decrease in meat consumption) and a somewhat lower food wastage rate, land use in these regions would further decrease by about 15%.

A US study showed that a low carbohydrate and high protein diet, such as the Atkins diet, required nearly twice as much land (80% more) than a diet based on the US My Pyramid model.[85] A study among 389 young Dutch women evaluated the effect on land requirements and two nutritional indicators (iron and saturated fatty acids) of replacing meat and dairy products with plant-based products.[86] When all meat and dairy foods were replaced, land use reduced by more than half from a mean of 3.7 to 1.8 (m² year/day). In this 100% replacement scenario the major foods contributing to land use were brewed coffee and eggs. Iron intake increased from 9.5 to 12.0 mg/d with almost all iron being derived from non-haem iron sources compared with the meat-containing diet in which 10% of iron was haem (more highly bioavailable) iron. When 30% of the animal produce was replaced, the changes were in the same direction but less pronounced.

A study measuring the impact of fat and meat consumption on the land requirements of food production in New York State found a nearly five-fold difference (0.18–0.86 ha) in per capita land requirements across typical diets (containing 0–381 g/day of meat and eggs and providing 20–45% of total dietary energy as fat).[87] As would be expected, increasing meat in the diet increased per capita land requirements. However, the analysis also demonstrated an interaction between availability of land, meat and dietary fat: a diet containing no meat or one where low-fat meat and low-fat milk is favoured requires that additional oil seed is made available to ensure an adequate energy supply, so increasing the land requirement of a low meat or otherwise low fat diet. Some high-fat vegetarian diets can therefore require more land than a diet containing some meat. Moreover, avoided fat from animal produce will not likely be discarded but will be transferred to other foods and other populations so creating a nutritional problem alongside an environmental one. According to this model, a diet containing more meat and where the fat content of the diet is sufficient to provide adequate energy does not require the availability of more oil seed for dietary fat and therefore avoids the need for additional land. A meat-containing diet makes use of forage and pastureland that would not be used for crops while, at the same time, increasing the energy supply for the human population. Mathematical modelling of the carrying capacity of the New York State agricultural land for the entire range of meat and fat consumption suggested that a diet providing 63 g of meat and 27% of dietary energy as fat would support the same population as a vegetarian diet providing 31% fat. Similarly, a diet providing 126 g of meat and 34% fat could support the same population as a vegetarian diet providing 41% of dietary energy as fat. No overlap with the vegetarian diet occurred at meat intakes higher than 126 g a day.

In the context of competition for land, international trade, including that for food, involves trade in virtual land, particularly from low-income to rich countries, which can have an impact on environmental degradation and societal disturbance in low-income countries. Research by Meier et al.[88] evaluated different dietary scenarios in Germany from a virtual land flow perspective, based on representative consumption data for Germany in the years 2006 and 1985-9. In 2006 the usual German diet led to a virtual land import of $707m^2$ per person per year, representing 30% of the total nutrition-induced land demand, while virtual land from food exports amounted to $262m^2$ per person per year. The researchers show that the resulting net import of virtual land could be balanced by shifting to the officially recommended diet for Germany and reducing consumption of beverages (cocoa, coffee, green/black tea, wine). Such a shift could lead to maintained or improved competitiveness and environmental and public health benefits. Shifting to a vegetarian or vegan diet would lead to a positive virtual land balance (even with maintained consumption of beverages).

## Soil

The connection between soil, food and nutrition seems indisputable but is easily forgotten in the rush to food modernity: soil-less growing systems, artificial media and urbanised food cultures that barely know how food grows. The importance of maintaining a fertile soil for the continuance of civilisation with healthy crops, healthy animals and healthy human beings has been recognised for centuries.[89, 90] Healthy soil lies at the heart of a nourishing diet. Soil forms over time from the rocks below it and the plants above it. The rocks weather away, breaking down into small particles – the sand, silts and clays that make up soil. Plants provide the organic matter that binds these particles together, producing soil that provides homes and sustenance for a huge variety of microscopic and larger animal life. Just a small spoonful of soil contains millions of organisms such as bacteria and fungi. There are an estimated 12 quadrillion (12,000 trillion) 'meso' fauna – i.e., small soil animals, mainly springtails, mites and nematodes – which keep the plants healthy by grazing their roots and breaking down the dead matter so that it is not washed away (as occurred when higher plants first evolved in the late

Devonian period). The soil is a complex and little-understood web of organic and inorganic matter, water and water vapour that undergoes many chemical reactions, which support plant roots and plant growth.[91] Getting society's relationship with soil wrong can be devastating. Ancient Rome's granaries in North Africa being destroyed by deforestation and climate change and the USA's dustbowl in the 1930s are two examples.

Agricultural productivity has increased substantially in recent decades due to a combination of increased scientific knowledge and investment, notably through application of manufactured fertilisers and pesticides, and minerals including phosphorus and potassium, to compensate for soil deficiencies.

Although modern agriculture has been successful in increasing food production, it has also caused extensive soil degradation.[6] Soil degradation refers primarily to reduced soil quality due to loss of soil nutrients (soil mining), erosion, waterlogging or salinisation and compaction (an increasing problem as the machines get larger and larger). Overgrazing, deforestation, soil mining and inappropriate water management are the main contributors to soil degradation, which are leading to loss of arable land worldwide and, hence, lost production. Soil degradation is of major concern over much of the world's agricultural land, from Australia to Africa, from the mid-west of the United States to East Anglia in the UK.[91]

According to the UN's Global Environment Facility (GEF) and International Fund for Agriculture (IFAD), in the second half of the twentieth century an estimated 1,035 million hectares of land with food growing potential was affected by human-induced soil degradation,[92] which varies by region (see Table 4.8). This has been mainly due to wind erosion (45%) and water erosion (42%) but also chemical damage (10%). In China alone, between 1957 and 1990, the area of arable land was reduced by an area equal to all the cropland in Denmark, France, Germany and the Netherlands combined, mainly because of land degradation.

Some land degradation is irreversible and leads to desertification. Each year 12 million hectares are lost to deserts, enough land to grow 20 million tonnes of grain.

Table 4.8 Regions affected by land degradation

| Region affected | Area affected (millions of hectares) | | | | |
| --- | --- | --- | --- | --- | --- |
| | Water erosion | Wind erosion | Chemical deterioration | Physical deterioration | Total |
| North America | 38.4 | 37.8 | 2.2 | 1.0 | 79.4 |
| South America | 34.7 | 26.9 | 17.0 | 0.4 | 79.0 |
| Europe | 48.1 | 38.6 | 4.1 | 8.6 | 99.4 |
| Africa | 119.1 | 159.9 | 26.5 | 13.9 | 319.4 |
| Asia | 157.5 | 153.2 | 50.2 | 9.6 | 370.5 |
| Australasia | 69.6 | 16.0 | 0.6 | 1.2 | 87.4 |
| Total | 467.4 | 432.4 | 100.7 | 34.7 | 1,035.2 |

Source: GEF-IFAD Partnership.[92]

Given that more than 99.7% of human food (calories) comes from the land, with less than 0.3% derived from the sea and other aquatic sources,[93] maintaining and augmenting global food supply depends on the quality and productivity of the soils. Techniques are available to reduce soil erosion, including zero tillage methods, leaving the last crop as a cover for the next one, use of biomass mulches and crop rotations, although zero tillage methods may increase weed and pest problems in some cases.

Efforts to maintain soil fertility could be considered a public good, to be paid for or subsidised by governments, particularly if there are societal costs or benefits over and beyond the costs or benefits captured by the farmer.

## Phosphorus

Phosphorus is mined from mineral deposits in rock and is increasingly seen as a limit on modern food production because its use as a fertiliser has increased dramatically yet non-renewable sources of phosphorus are becoming scarce. The supply of phosphorus is finite; there are no substitutes and we cannot produce more than exists on the earth. The increased use of phosphorus is related to changes in the global food system including increased food production, changes in the diet to more phosphorus-intensive products, and changes in agricultural methods, including intensification of fertiliser input to increase yields. Moreover, excessive phosphorus is lost from the soil to aquatic ecosystems through run off and soil erosion, causing the eutrophication of many lakes and coastal waters. Phosphorus footprints vary considerably between countries. North America, Australia, New Zealand and countries in South America have the highest phosphorus footprint although, between 1961 and 2007, the phosphorus footprint of China increased by 417%.[94] Consumption of animal food is the most important factor affecting phosphorus footprint and accounts for 72% of the global phosphorus footprint.[94] Beef has the greatest impact.

# Biodiversity

## Agricultural biodiversity

Agricultural biodiversity encompasses the variety and variability of living organisms (plants, animals and microorganisms) that are involved in food and agriculture and is the result of deliberate interaction between humans and natural ecosystems and the species they contain.[95] The connection between agricultural and marine biodiversity and human nutrition and health is complex and costly.[96] Biodiversity has a positive influence on food production through contributing to environmental services such as adaptation to climate change, soil protection, crop pollination and pest control and minimises stresses experienced in monocultures, allowing for longer sustainability in food production.[97] Food production systems require (and exploit) ecosystems, which is why an estimated 52% of land in agricultural use worldwide is 'moderately or severely affected by land degradation and desertification'.[96] Soil and sea health are thus a concern for human health, a matter easily lost in consumer culture.

Biodiversity is important for dietary diversity, but is not sufficient in and of itself to ensure that diets are diverse.[97] One could have a restricted diet amidst plentiful biodiversity, or a diverse diet raiding and wrecking biodiversity. Thus biodiversity becomes a cultural factor for food security.[98, 99] In 2015 the FAO specifically recommended the need to 'maintain or improve the natural resource base' of food production to improve nutrition. This is the policy route known as 'nutrition-sensitive' agriculture.[100]

That biodiversity is an important feature of food sustainability and that nutritional diversity is essential for human health are both positions strongly supported by the literature.[101–106] The connection between them, however, can be loose. Studies show that consumers may or may not have nutritional diversity despite living or even growing biodiversity themselves.[101, 102] As Tim Johns and Bhuwon Sthapit suggested in 2004, socio-cultural and income factors are important intervening variables. Culinary knowledge as well as purchasing power shape the connection between nutritional health and biodiversity conservation,[98] hence the use of the term 'ecological nutrition' in the sub-title of this book.

Eating a diversity of foods is an internationally accepted recommendation for a healthy diet because it is associated with positive health outcomes such as reduced incidence of cancer[107–109] and of mortality.[110] As long as energy intakes are appropriate to maintain a healthy body weight, biologically diverse diets have been shown to be more likely to be nutritionally complete than diets low in variety in both high- and low-income countries.[110, 111] Lack of dietary diversity is a severe problem among poor populations in the developing world where diets are based predominantly on starchy staples.[112]

Given the positive influence of biodiversity on food production and its potential for improving the quality and hence sustainability of the diet, it is of significant concern that agricultural biodiversity has declined.[100] Industrial agriculture, including use of pesticides and synthetic fertilisers to achieve higher productivity, has brought monocultures, producing a single crop over a wide area, and a declining biodiversity. Palm oil is one example of a crop associated with reduced biodiversity, largely because of forest clearance.[113, 114] A Dutch study has linked pesticide use with reduced biodiversity in Europe and has recommended minimal use of these products.[115]

The FAO estimates that since the early 1900s some 75% of plant genetic diversity has been lost as multiple local varieties have been replaced by genetically uniform high-yielding varieties.[116] In human history about 7,000 plants have been cultivated for consumption. Indigenous people have survived and prospered due to their knowledge of how to use this range for consumption.[117–119] With economic development, that knowledge is often lost or systematically erased by forced social change. This is why some policy makers, lawyers and scientists began to champion indigenous people's food knowledge within the Right to

Food legal framework.[120] Whether through 'push' or 'pull' socio-economic forces, humans have reduced use to only about 150 edible plant species. Thirty crops provide 95% of human food energy needs, and four of these (rice, wheat, maize and potato) are responsible for more than 60% of our energy intake. A similar story of genetic erosion can also be extended to domesticated animals as a few highly productive breeds, which have been selected for their ability to convert feed to meat and milk, are disseminated worldwide, displacing local varieties. A major global review of biodiversity in farm crops from 1961–2009 and its impact concluded that, although food supplies had increased the output of protein, calories, fat and weight, there was an increasing homogeneity of what was grown.[103] The same 'big' crops had tended to spread everywhere they could be grown; food supplies 'became more similar in composition' for all the variables the researchers studied. This contributed, the researchers noted, to 'reductions in human oral and gut microbiota'. Others have noted that 'just three crops – rice, maize and wheat – provide nearly two-thirds of global dietary intake'.[104]

This erosion of agricultural biodiversity is associated with how the current food system has tended to industrialise and increase in scale, and to see biodiversity as the enemy of food production rather than as its friend.[121] The success of this productionist agriculture has been to provide increased accessibility to a narrow range of inexpensive agricultural commodities, but this leads to simplification of human diets, with a risk of nutrient deficiency, particularly among poor communities, and excess energy consumption. Until recently, loss of biodiversity has been viewed, if at all, mainly as an environmental loss but, increasingly, it is also seen as an issue for food and food security.[122] Pioneering nutrition scientists began to champion this issue – resurrecting the old but too-long submerged tradition of environmental and ecological nutrition.[123] Maintaining biodiversity is vital as this forms the building blocks from which plant scientists may need to draw in the future to develop new varieties capable of withstanding, for example, warmer temperatures, different pests and salinised water. It is becoming increasingly important to find a policy framework through which this genetic material can be preserved by, for example, saving seeds as well as sustaining the cultural knowledge of traditional plants and foods. Somehow, sustainable diets must factor in both the protection and enhancement of biodiversity in the field not just at the edge of the field.

## Marine biodiversity

The sea constitutes 90% of the habitable space on the planet and an estimated 50–80% of all life on the planet is found in the sea. UNESCO estimates that by the year 2100, without significant changes, more than half of the world's marine species may be on the brink of extinction.[124] Today, 60% of the world's major marine ecosystems that underpin livelihoods have been degraded or are being used unsustainably.

The threat to marine biodiversity comes from several sources in parallel. First, commercial overexploitation of the world's fish stocks is so severe that it has been estimated that up to 13% of global fisheries have 'collapsed'. Although recent work suggests that depletion of fisheries may have turned the corner, these findings are based on better managed, developed world fisheries. A 2013 review confirms the previous dismal picture, that serious depletions are the norm world-wide, management quality is poor and catch per effort is still declining.[125] A 2014 FAO report suggests that 30% of the world's wild fish stocks are being fished unsustainably, which is an improvement over recent years. Although the report says that 70% of wild fish stocks are being fished within biologically sustainable levels, fully fished stocks – meaning those at or very close to their maximum sustainable production – account for over 60% and under-fished stocks about 10%. This means that there is no room for complacency.[126]

Second, agricultural practices, coastal tourism, port and harbour developments, damming of rivers, urban development and construction, mining, fisheries, aquaculture and manufacturing, among others, are all sources of marine pollution threatening coastal and marine habitats. Third, excessive nutrients from sewage outfalls and agricultural runoff have contributed to the number of low oxygen (hypoxic) areas, known as dead zones, where most marine life cannot survive, resulting in the collapse of some ecosystems. There are now close to 500 dead zones covering more than 245,000 km² globally, equivalent to the surface of the United Kingdom. Fourth, increase in atmospheric $CO_2$ is resulting in acidification of the sea. Ocean acidification is corrosive to coral reefs and the shells of many marine organisms and may also threaten plankton, which is key to the survival of larger fish. Fifth, ocean warming is having pronounced impacts on the physiology, composition and distribution of marine species.[127] Many tropical regions are expected to have a large reduction in their maximum catch by 2050 whereas higher latitude regions may gain.[128, 129] Sixth, removal of mangroves and other coastal systems such as salt marshes and sea grass meadows has led to loss of critical marine habitats (contributing to the devastating effects of the 2004 Indian Ocean tsunami on Sri Lanka, for example). These coastal systems have the ability to sequester carbon at rates up to 50 times those of the same area of tropical forest. Total carbon deposits in these coastal systems may be up to five times the carbon stored in tropical forests. The ocean has been shielding the earth from the worst effects of rapid climate change by absorbing excess $CO_2$ but this is driving the damaging trio of acidification, warming and deoxygenation, which are increased by the effects of other human impacts, such as pollution, eutrophication and overfishing.[130]

Aquaculture provides 40% of the world's fish.[131] Fish farming involves the use of technologies and breeding programmes to generate species that are more practical and economic to produce. Potential environmental and genetic hazards exist if modified species are released into the wild where they may spread parasites and disease.[132] For example, the sea louse is a parasite affecting farmed and subsequently wild salmon.[133] There is also an increased risk of predation and altered marine population in that the modified fish may become established where that particular species was not previously present. Other environmental impacts of aquaculture include organic pollution and eutrophication, a build-up of nutrients (primarily organic nitrogen and phosphorus) and wastes. These factors can cause depletion of oxygen, reduction in water quality, death of coral and destruction of habitat but, through good management, they can often be contained locally. The use of prophylactic antibiotics in aquaculture, especially in developing countries, to forestall bacterial infections resulting from sanitary shortcomings in fish rearing has resulted in the emergence of antibiotic-resistant bacteria in aquaculture environments, in the increase of antibiotic resistance in fish pathogens, in the transfer of these resistant bacteria to bacteria of land animals and to human pathogens and in alterations of the bacterial flora both in sediments and in the water column. The use of large amounts of antibiotics that have to be mixed with fish food also creates problems for industrial health and increases the opportunities for the presence of residual antibiotics in fish and fish products.[134] Farmed fish often use other fish harvested from the sea, a reason there is growing interest in aquaculture using plant feeding fish such as tilapia.

Fish is, however, recognised to be a valuable human food. Compared with meat, poultry and eggs, fish is low in saturated fatty acids and a good source of protein and selenium; oily fish in particular is an excellent source of long-chain omega-3 fatty acids.[135] Fish accounts for 17% of the world's protein; in some coastal and island countries it can be more than 70%.[126] In rich countries much attention is being given to the related health benefits of fish, and official recommendations for Europeans and North Americans are to eat more fish. For much of the world's population, in contrast, fish contributes to nutrition because it is part of the established food economy. However, the demand for fish in some regions, including Europe, is increasingly being met by diverting fish towards affluent markets rather than local ones, with consequences for the food security of poorer nations, islands and coastal communities.[136] This calls into question the morality of advice in developed countries to increase fish consumption.

## Local food

Locally produced and consumed food has been claimed to be ecologically friendlier than food that is transported from further afield. However, evidence to date for this claim is weak. First, there is no clear definition of local food.[137] Only a few studies have evaluated the environmental impacts of home produced versus imported food. A UK Defra-commissioned study compared the environmental footprint of some meat, vegetables and fruits produced in the UK or elsewhere for the UK market.[138] Lamb produced in the UK had a higher environmental footprint than lamb produced in New Zealand and transported for consumption in the UK. There is considerable room for debate about these findings and the study provided no estimate of physical variability in each country and no explicit measure of the uncertainty. This research also considered the case of Brazilian (export) poultry and UK poultry meat production. Pre-farm gate, the GHG burden of chicken breast production was broadly similar in Brazil and the UK, although energy use was 25% in Brazil due to the shorter distance of transporting soya, which is the main feed. Energy used for processing was higher in Brazil than in the UK; transport accounted for 65% of post-farm gate energy in UK chicken breast and 80% in the Brazilian product. Overall, the energy use to produce the Brazilian chicken was about 12% higher than that for the UK product, but the global warming potential of the Brazilian product was slightly lower as the majority of the energy in the Brazilian system was derived from renewable sources. This same study also attempted to compare beef for export from Brazil compared with beef produced in the UK but, at the time of the study, the two systems were considerably different, which makes comparison difficult. Nevertheless, one basic finding was that emissions of GHGs are greater from the Brazilian beef systems, mainly because of enteric $CH_4$, reflecting the relatively slow growth and reproductive rates of Brazilian cattle compared with cattle in the UK.

Other UK research has found that GHGEs of some fruit and vegetables produced out of season in the UK, for example lettuce, strawberries and tomatoes in heated glass houses, are higher than the same food grown naturally in a warmer climate such as Spain and transported to the UK.[138–140] A comparison of raspberries grown in the UK or Spain found relatively small differences in GHG impacts but the water stress placed on the country was significantly higher in Spain.[141] Some foods grown abroad, such as apples in New Zealand, can have a lower GHG impact if transported to the UK and consumed after minimum storage than apples produced in the UK and stored for consumption out of season.[142] Energy needed for freezing can also make home-grown frozen products ecologically less friendly than fresh produce grown elsewhere, as demonstrated in a British study that compared broccoli grown and frozen in the UK with fresh broccoli grown in Spain and transported to the UK.[143]

Although some of these findings might appear counter-intuitive because of an expectation that transporting food across the world will have a higher GHG cost than home-grown produce, UK statistics show that 58% of transport emissions come from heavy goods vehicles and vans distributing food around the UK and consumers driving their cars to and from food shops.[144] In the UK it has been estimated that consumer car transport to and from shops is responsible for half of the kilometres travelled by food.[145] While it is true that buying certain foods from a nearby farm can reduce the transport-related emissions of GHGs, a UK study comparing the carbon emissions resulting from operating a large-scale vegetable box system delivered to the customer's home with those from a supply system where the customer travels to a local farm shop suggests that if a customer drives a round trip distance of more than 6.7 km in order to purchase their organic vegetables, their carbon emissions are likely to be greater than the emissions from the system of cold storage, packing, transport to a regional hub and final transport to customer's doorstep used by large-scale vegetable box suppliers.[146] Figure 4.1 gives the proportion of $CO_2$ emissions for different modes of food transport: air, car, heavy goods vehicles (HGV), sea, van.[144]

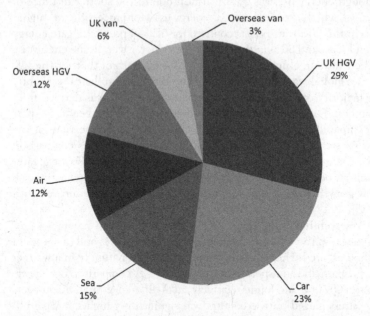

*Figure 4.1* Proportions of $CO_2$ emissions from different forms of transport used within the UK food system

Source: Defra, 2012.[144]

The differences in GHG emissions between home grown and imported food become very apparent, however, when considering fresh produce that is flown in to the UK. Although airfreight of food accounts for only 1% of food imports to the UK, it accounts for 12% of the food transport $CO_2$ equivalent emissions.[144] By contrast, 99% of food imports to the UK travel by sea, which accounts for 15% of food transport emissions. Analyses of green beans grown in Kenya[147] and pineapples grown in Mauritius[148] suggest that the emissions from flying these products from their points of production to the UK form the greatest proportion of the overall carbon footprint of the products (89% and 98%, respectively) and, in the case of beans, the overall footprint of Kenyan produce is 10 times greater than UK-grown produce.

Although the issue of local and seasonal food continues to be debated, overall, for fruit and vegetables, produce that is fragile (for example, salads and berries), grown in protected conditions (for example, tomatoes and cucumbers in hot houses), requires refrigeration (for example, salads) and/or rapid and energy-intensive modes of transport such as air (for example, green beans, mangetout, mangoes, berries from the southern hemisphere) is likely to be more GHG intensive than seasonal fruits and vegetables grown with no heat, consumed without prolonged storage and not transported by air.[149, 150]

Combining several environmental criteria, Jungbluth *et al.* compared different dietary scenarios (for example, becoming vegetarian, reducing food waste, reducing obesity, eating local food, organic food, a more balanced diet, eating seasonal food) and, of all these, eating seasonal food was found to have the smallest benefit.[151]

## Organic food

Organically grown food is often stated to be more environmentally friendly than conventional food. Organic agriculture does not allow synthetic fertilisers and restricts the use of pesticides, so is potentially less dependent on oil-based inputs. In general, organic farming aims to conserve biodiversity and foster recycling of resources by growing and rotating a mixture of crops, adding organic matter such as compost or manure and using clover or beans as cover crops to fix nitrogen from the atmosphere. Compared with non-organic systems, well-managed organic systems generally have higher soil organic matter, (carbon) and nitrogen,[152] which helps to conserve soil and water resources and confer resilience in the face of extremes of weather such as drought, while crop rotation and cover cropping can reduce soil erosion, pests and pesticide use.[153] Animal welfare is also given a high priority and the routine use of antibiotics and other medicines is minimised.[154]

The environmental impacts of organic agriculture are contested by some sections of conventional agricultural science. Moreover, the majority of studies on organic agriculture have been conducted in developed countries, yet almost a third of the world's organically managed land is located in developing countries and almost half of the world's organic producers are in Africa.[155]

Organic farming often scores better than conventional farming on GHG emissions when emissions are quantified for a whole farm or per area of land. However,

*Table 4.9* Comparison of land-use needs of selected organic and conventionally produced animal and plant foods

| Food | Production quantity | Organic production land use | Non-organic production land use | Land use needs of organic vs. non-organic production (%) |
|---|---|---|---|---|
| Milk | 10,000 litres | 1.98 ha | 1.19 ha | 65 |
| Pork | 1 ton | 1.28 ha | 0.74 ha | 73 |
| Beef | 1 ton | 4.2 ha | 2.3 ha | 83 |
| Poultry | 1 ton | 1.64 ha | 0.40 ha | 119 |
| Eggs | 20,000 eggs | 1.48 ha | 0.66 ha | 124 |
| Lamb and mutton | 1 ton | 3.12 ha | 1.28 ha | 126 |
| Tomatoes | 1 ton | 55 m$^2$ | 29 m$^2$ | 90 |
| Potatoes | 1 ton | 0.022 ha | 0.058 ha | 160 |

Source: Williams *et al.*, 2006.[158]

Table 4.10 Most beneficial method of food production (organic or non-organic) in terms of environmental impacts for selected animals and plants

| Environmental impact | Beef | Pork | Lamb and mutton | Poultry | Milk | Eggs | Bread wheat | Potatoes | Tomatoes |
|---|---|---|---|---|---|---|---|---|---|
| Global warming potential ($CO_2$ equivalents) | NON-ORG | ORG | ORG | NON-ORG | NON-ORG | NON-ORG | ORG | ORG | NON-ORG |
| Energy used | ORG | ORG | ORG | NON-ORG | ORG | NON-ORG | ORG | NS | NON-ORG |
| Land used | NON-ORG | NON-ORG | NON-ORG | NON-ORG | NON-ORG | NON-ORG | NON-ORG | NON-ORG | NON-ORG |
| Erosion and land degradation | NON-ORG | NS | NON-ORG | NS | | NS | | NS | NS |
| Water used | ORG | NS | NS | NS | NS | NS | | ORG | NON-ORG |
| Eutrophication | NON-ORG | ORG | NON-ORG | NON-ORG | NON-ORG | NON-ORG | NON-ORG | NS | NON-ORG |
| Acidification | NON-ORG | ORG | NON-ORG | NON-ORG | NON-ORG | NON-ORG | NS | ORG | NON-ORG |
| Pesticides used | ORG | ORG | ORG | ORG | ORG | ORG | ORG | ORG | ORG |
| Nitrogen loss | NON-ORG | NON-ORG | NON-ORG | NON-ORG | NON-ORG | NON-ORG | NON-ORG | ORG | ORG |

Source: Williams et al., 2006.[158]

Notes: ORG = organic; NON-ORG = non-organic; NS = No significant difference.

organic crops and livestock may require more land than their conventionally produced counterparts because of lower yields, with the result that this positive effect of organic farming on GHG emissions is less pronounced, not present at all or is negative.[152, 156, 157] A UK government report found a greater land use for organic foods ranging from 65% more for milk to 160% more for potatoes[158] (see Table 4.9). It has been argued that differences in yields between organic and conventional farms are context-related, with estimates ranging from 5–34% depending on the farming system and the site characteristics.[159]

In general, higher land use associated with organic food production may result in other environmental impacts such as increased nitrogen losses (nitrogen leaching, ammonia and nitrous oxide emissions), eutrophication (water pollution) and increased acidification on a per product weight basis.[157, 158] However, energy use tends to be lower in organic food production.

Organic agriculture does have a positive impact on biodiversity.[152, 160-2] A meta-analysis of 184 observations garnered from 94 studies found that the size of the effect on biodiversity varies with the crop, species and the landscape studied.[162]

In general, it appears to be more ecologically friendly to raise pigs organically while the environmental impacts for poultry and eggs are mostly lower when they are produced non-organically (see Table 4.10). The energy requirement for producing organic animal produce appears to be lower, with the exception of poultry and eggs where the energy cost of the feed is high. Although less water is needed to produce organic than non-organic beef, this should be seen in the light of the vast amounts of water required to produce animal protein. On a weight for weight basis it takes one hundred times more water to produce animal protein than grain protein so the 10% saving found in this study for organic cattle is not significant.

In summary, available evidence suggests that the environmental impacts of organic foods are mixed. In trying to come to an overall view on the relative environmental performance of organic and non-organic food it is also necessary to attribute relative importance to difference types of environmental impacts. This would imply the adoption of some sort of multi-criteria analysis that introduces an implicit or explicit weighting of environmental importance to each type of impact.[157] Currently, there remains insufficient evidence available to fully quantify the environmental impact of organic food compared with non-organic food.

## Waste

Food waste has a significant impact on the environment. It is estimated that 30–50% (or 1–2 billion tonnes) of food produced worldwide is not consumed due to poor practices in harvesting, storage and transportation, as well as market and consumer wastage.[68, 163] In less-developed countries wastage tends to occur at the farming end of the food system, with harvesting, inadequate local transportation and poor infrastructure resulting in inappropriate handling and storage. As the development level of a country increases, so the food loss problem generally moves further along the supply chain, with deficiencies in regional and national infrastructure having the largest impact. In South East Asian countries for example, losses of rice can range from 37–80% of total production depending on development stage, which amounts to total wastage in the region of about 180 million tonnes annually. In China, a country experiencing rapid development, the rice loss figure is about 45%, whereas in less-developed Vietnam, rice losses between the field and the table can amount to 80% of production.

In developed countries such as the UK, more efficient farming practices and better transport, storage and processing facilities ensure that a larger proportion of the food produced reaches markets and consumers. However, characteristics associated with modern consumer culture mean produce is often wasted through retail and customer behaviour. Major supermarkets, in meeting consumer expectations, will often reject entire crops of perfectly edible fruit and vegetables at the farm because they do not meet exacting marketing standards for their physical characteristics, such as size and appearance. For example, up to 30% of the UK's vegetable crop is never harvested as a result of such practices. Globally, retailers generate 1.6 million tonnes of food waste annually in this way. Of the produce that does appear in the supermarket, commonly used sales promotions frequently encourage customers to purchase excessive quantities, which, in the case of perishable foodstuffs, inevitably generate wastage in the home.

Overall between 30% and 50% of food bought in developed countries is thrown away by the purchaser. The per capita food waste by consumers in Europe and North America is estimated to be 95–115 kg/year, but this figure in sub-Saharan Africa and South/South East Asia is only 6–11 kg per year.[163] In 2012 waste in the UK was estimated to be 260 kg per household per year, a reduction of 19% from 320 kg per year in 2007; avoidable food waste had reduced by 24% from 210 to 160 kg per year.[164] A larger proportion of vegetables, fruits and bread is wasted in comparison to other food groups.[165]

Large amounts of land, energy, fertilisers and water are lost in the production of foodstuffs that end up as waste. Produced but uneaten food occupies almost 1.4 billion hectares of land, representing close to 30% of the world's agricultural land area.[166] An EU study showed that overall savings in land use of reducing food waste by households and in retail in the EU are considerable: 28,940 km$^2$ – close to the land area of Belgium (approximately 1.6% of EU agricultural lands in 2020).[167] The largest contributions to land-use savings from waste reduction are from meat and dairy due to the high land requirement for livestock and vegetables and fruits for which EU wastage is relatively large. A US study found that the energy embedded in wasted food is approximately 2% of annual energy consumption in the United States.[59] Production of lost and wasted food accounts for 23% of global fertiliser use.[168] Globally, the blue water footprint of food wastage – the consumption of surface and groundwater resources – is about 250 km$^3$, which is equivalent to the annual water discharge of the Volga river, or three times the volume of Lake Geneva.[166]

Waste's climate impact is also significant. An FAO estimate suggests that, without accounting for GHG emissions from land-use change, the carbon footprint of food produced and not eaten is estimated at 3.3 gigatonnes of $CO_2$ equivalent.[166] As such, food wastage ranks as the third top GHG emitter after the USA and China. In the UK, GHG emissions associated with wasted food by grocery retail and manufacturers are estimated to be 250,000 tonnes $CO_2$e.[165] While it is difficult to estimate its impact on biodiversity at global level, food wastage unduly compounds the negative impact that monocropping and agriculture expansion into wild areas have on loss of biodiversity, including mammals, birds, fish and amphibians.

Resources are also required to deal with food waste. Of the 15 million tonnes of food wasted in the UK each year, 40% ends up as landfill where it contributes to GHG production and hence to climate change. A report setting out to reduce food waste to zero in the UK aims to prevent 27 gigatonnes of GHGs entering the atmosphere, save the UK economy £27 million a year and return over 1.3 million tonnes of nutrients to the soil.[169]

## Packaging

A visible manifestation of the normalisation of elements of the Western diet is packaging. Packaging is itself a microcosm of highly contested issues: litter, hygiene, marketing, contaminants, pollution of the soil and particularly of the seas. Figure 4.2 gives an overview of how packaging is associated with levels of economic development.[170] It contrasts the use of packaged and non-packaged food by country income level: high, upper middle, low middle and low.

In high-income countries, a far higher proportion of packaged compared with fresh foods is consumed than in low-income countries. Low-income countries do

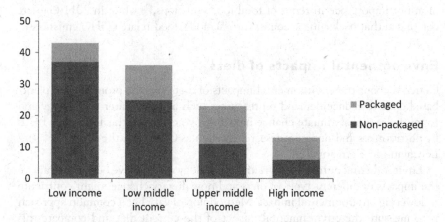

*Figure 4.2* Overall expenditure on food, contrasting use of packaged/non-packaged foods, by country income level

Source: Regmi and Gelhar, 2005.[170]

more cooking from raw food ingredients; their consumers also waste less food.[171] High-income countries have more food pre-cooked in factories. Retail sales of categories such as ready-meals have grown consistently in the USA and UK.

Food packaging – whether plastic, paper, glass or metal – has a significant impact on the environment. While food packaging helps to keep food safe and fresh, can extend shelf life and reduce food waste, can protect food during transport, delivery and storage and can provide information on nutrition, storage and cooking, it also consumes natural resources, fills rubbish containers and landfills and pollutes beaches, rivers, lakes and seas. According to a 2015 Worldwatch Institute report approximately 10–20 million tons of plastic, some of which is food packaging, end up in the sea each year. This plastic debris results in an estimated $13 bn-a-year loss from damage to marine ecosystems, including financial losses to fisheries and tourism, as well as time spent cleaning beaches.[172] Food packaging can also transfer chemicals into food with potential health effects that are gaining greater attention from researchers and regulators.[173, 174] In 2014, 311 metric tonnes (mt) of plastic was produced globally (not all for food). This is expected to rise to 1,124 mt by 2050.[175] This is not all for food of course, but, since only about 10% is recycled, too much of this vast flood of oil-based plastic ends up in the sea where it does already affect foodways. There it accumulates in vast slowly circulating plastic islands gyrating in the seas globally. Some of this breaks down into tiny fragments and gets eaten by fish. If anything illustrates how human activity damages ecological feedback loops in nature, this is it.

Food packaging production can be energy-intensive and is thus responsible for GHGEs. Information on GHGEs from food packaging is scarce and difficult to interpret. It may include manufacture of packaging materials, the process of packaging and a portion of refrigeration costs associated with the cold chain. In 2000 Jungbluth and colleagues stated that, for both vegetables and meat, packaging is of minor importance in terms of total food emissions,[176] while in 2011 Garnett concluded that packaging accounts for 7% of UK food-related GHG emissions.[3]

## Environmental impacts of diets

Concern about the environmental impacts of diets and the promotion of plant-based diets to reduce demand on resources such as land, water and energy and to minimise global climate change have been voiced since the 1960s and 1970s by nutritionists and nutrition researchers such as Gussow in the USA,[177, 178] and Leitzmann in Germany.[179]

Environmental nutrition and nutrition ecology studies have begun to evaluate the impacts of different types of diets and how dietary change might contribute to lowering environmental impact. Methodologies vary but a common approach is to measure the environmental impact of the current diet and compare this with the environmental impact of another type of diet such as, for example, a healthy diet that meets official guidelines like the Eatwell plate in the UK or the MyPlate guidance for North Americans, a diet with no or low animal food content, or identifiable diets such as the Mediterranean or new Nordic diets. Impacts measured usually include GHG emissions but may also include land and water. Life-cycle analysis is generally used to measure environmental impact and the most commonly measured impacts are GHG emissions but, increasingly, land use and sometimes energy and water use have been measured. Most studies to date have modelled and evaluated 'idealised' diets but a few researchers are now beginning to look at the environmental impacts of 'real' diets.

As would be expected, diets containing a greater proportion of animal foods translate into a greater impact on the environment. An Italian study that evaluated a range of environmental impacts from omnivorous diets concluded that the most dramatic impact of these diets was on water use, which accounted for 41–46% of the overall impact, while consumption of fossil fuels accounted for 20–26%, damage from inorganic chemical compounds for 15–18%, land use for 5–13%, with 3–4% of the overall impact due to eutrophication.[180]

Reducing intakes of animal foods reduces various environmental impacts, including GHG emissions,[48, 50, 180–195] land use,[86, 180, 182, 186, 188, 189, 191, 195, 196] water use[180, 191, 197] and water pollution,[180, 189] energy use[180, 189] and phosphorus demand.[94, 186] A study by Peters and colleagues reviewed the carrying capacity of US agricultural land.[198] They showed that dietary choice had a considerable impact on how many people the USA could feed. Comparing vegan, ovo-vegetarian, lacto-vegetarian and a different version of the 'healthy' diet promulgated by the US Government, they showed that the less meat consumed, the greater the land's carrying capacity.[198] Or, to put it the other way round, if US consumers ate differently and healthier, the USA could have a higher population and/or produce more food for areas with more pressured land–population ratios. This reinforced findings in other parts of the world.[82, 199, 200] Peters and others have cautioned, however, against demonising livestock production; in some terrains, it produces food that otherwise could not be produced. But the drift of the implications are nonetheless becoming ever more clear from the accumulation of studies. More plant-based diets should enable environmental protection of biodiversity.

A study by Popp and colleagues found that global agriculture non-$CO_2$ GHG emissions will rise until 2055 if food energy and diet preferences remain the same as in 1995, and will rise even more if increasing energy consumption and changing dietary preferences with higher income, like more meat and milk, are taken into account. They also found, however, that with reduced meat and dairy demand, non-$CO_2$ emissions would decrease even compared with the levels of 1995.[48] Stehfest and colleagues found that the cost of reaching stringent climate targets would be significantly lower if consumption of livestock products stopped, and this would also mean that significant areas of pasture and cropland could be abandoned, resulting in a large carbon uptake from re-growing vegetation.[182] Hedenhus and colleagues also concluded from a modelling exercise that reduced ruminant and dairy consumption will be indispensable for reaching the 2°C temperature target.[50]

Estimates of emissions reduction vary according to the studies and the types of diet involved. An analysis of diets in the 27 countries of the European Union compared the current diet with three healthier diets. The adoption of officially recommended guidelines for a healthy diet produced no change in environmental impact because it focuses mainly on increasing fruit and vegetable intake without reducing meat. However, both a healthy diet with less meat and a Mediterranean diet based on plant foods had the capacity to reduce the impacts related to food consumption by 8%.[190]

Four British studies have calculated the GHG impacts of different types of diets. Aston *et al.*[192] used red and processed meat intake data from the UK National Diet and Nutrition Survey (NDNS) and, using life-cycle analysis, modelled the GHG emissions of each quintile of meat intake, with an added scenario of doubling the proportion of vegetarians in the survey with the remainder adopting the dietary pattern of the lowest quintile of meat intakes. The expected reduction in GHG emissions from the additional scenario was calculated to be 3% of current emissions. In the second study Berners-Lee *et al.* estimated that potential GHG savings of 22% and 26% can be made by changing from the current UK-average diet to a vegetarian or vegan diet, respectively.[183] Scarborough and colleagues compared three dietary scenarios with the current UK diet: first, a 50% reduction in meat and dairy replaced by fruit, vegetables and cereals, which produced a 19% reduction in GHG emissions; second, a 75% reduction in beef, lamb and mutton replaced by pigs and poultry (9% reduction in GHG emissions); third, a 50% reduction in pigs and poultry replaced with fruits, vegetables and cereals (3% reduction in GHG emissions).[185] The Livewell study commissioned by WWF takes an alternative and very detailed approach: it starts with nutritional recommendations and adopts a linear optimisation approach to specify how these recommendations might be met for a 25% less GHG cost and in ways that are deemed culturally acceptable.[184] In an extension to this approach, lower impact diets from four countries (France, Spain, Sweden, UK), each with different food cultures, were modelled. This time, the diets needed to be culturally acceptable and no more expensive than the current average.[29] In all cases, emission reductions could only be achieved by lowering the meat component and increasing the plant components of the diet.

A 2016 Carbon Trust analysis commissioned by Public Health England evaluated the environmental impact of the refreshed UK Eatwell Guide compared with the current UK diet. The findings from this analysis were that dietary consumption according to the Eatwell Guide resulted in an appreciably lower environmental impact than the current UK diet.[201] A number of dietary choices contribute to the reduction such as increasing potatoes, fish, wholemeal and white bread, vegetables and fruit while reducing amounts of dairy, meat, rice, pasta, pizza and sweet foods. The analysis looked at the impact on GHGs, and land and water use, but it ignored biodiversity, is weak on culture and is not openly costed for socio-economic groups. Another report from the Carbon Trust concluded that achieving greater levels of protein diversity by replacing some meat with other protein sources would have a positive impact on both the environment and health.[202]

A few studies have been distinctive in measuring the environmental impacts of self-selected diets. First, a US study evaluated the environmental impacts (land use, water use and GHG emissions) from three alternatives to the US diet in 2008.[191] A 75% decrease in meat intake reduced land requirements by 25%, water requirements by 32% and GHG emissions by 44%. Respective figures for a 75% reduction in meat with no beef were 32% for land, 36% for water and 48% for GHG emissions. Maintaining the same meat consumption as in the 2008 US diet but without any beef reduced land requirements by 14%, water requirements by 18% and GHG emissions by 48%. Cassidy has also obtained data from 240,000 participants in a Healthy Food Programme. Participants increased the purchase weight of their fruit (by 5.4%) and vegetable (by 8.8%) and reduced their pork (by 10%) and beef (by 16%). These food purchase changes would be expected to reduce land requirements by 8–13%, water footprint by 7–12% and GHG emissions by 8–10%. Second, a French study estimated the GHG emissions associated with self-selected diets and then reduced the dietary energy intake to meet individual energy needs, which reduced the diet-associated GHGEs by 10.7% or 2.4% depending on the assumptions made about physical activity. While meat made the strongest contribution to GHGEs, the impact of different meat reduction scenarios was modest. In particular, when fruit and vegetables were isocalorically substituted for meat, either null or positive diet-associated GHGE variations were observed because of the need for large amounts of fruit and vegetables to maintain the energy content of the diet.[29] A further study by this research group classified diets into four categories according to their nutritional quality. On evaluating the environmental impact, they found that high nutritional quality diets had a higher GHG impact than poorer diets. However, the differences in the nutritional quality of the diets had little to do with the meat content but rather in the quantities of fruit and vegetables and sweets and snacks. Better diets tend to be richer in fruit and vegetables which are substituted by sweets and snacks in poorer diets. Since sugary and carbohydrate-containing snacks have a lower GHG footprint, this explains the difference. Further research by this French group suggests that a reduction in diet-related GHGE by 20% while maintaining high nutritional quality seems realistic. This goal could be achieved at no extra cost by reducing energy intake and energy density and by increasing the share of plant-based products.[194]

A Mediterranean-type diet (low in meat, rich in fresh fruit and vegetables, low in salty and sugary snacks, dietary fat obtained from plant-based oil) is linked with low environmental impact in several studies,[199, 203–206] reducing GHG emissions, land use and, when measured, water use compared with the usual dietary pattern. A regional Nordic diet, mimicking the Mediterranean diet but with regional foods produced in Northern Europe (high in locally grown vegetables, including legumes, roots, fish, whole-grain products, nuts, and fruit and berries in season, and 35% less meat than the average Danish diet), found that reducing the meat content of the diet and excluding most long-distance imports was of substantial environmental advantage compared with the average Danish diet, but including large amounts of organic produce was a disadvantage because of the lower productivity of organic agriculture.[207, 208]

## Conclusions

The food system is a key element in the world's environmental challenge. From a consideration of the environment alone, can we really continue to eat what we like? Europe and North America consume resources as if they inhabit multiple planets and food is a key factor in this picture. The food system contributes 20–30% of anthropogenic GHG emissions and is the leading cause of deforestation, land-use change, water use and loss of biodiversity. Although the entire food system from agriculture through to distribution, manufacturing, cooking and waste disposal contributes to these problems, agriculture has the biggest impact. Both livestock and crop production contribute to these problems but it is clear that the rearing of livestock for meat, milk and eggs are significant sources of the environmental problems in the food system.

This problem can be conceptualised as a production challenge, the solution to which is to change how food is produced by improving the efficiency of food production; a consumption challenge, which requires changes to the dietary drivers that determine food production; and a socio-economic challenge, which requires changes in how the food system is governed.[45] The idea that technological efficiency alone can avert environmental problems in the food system is widely held, and clearly there is much that can be done to improve environmental efficiency throughout the food system. But we cannot ignore the need to tackle consumption and how to normalise the consumption of a low environmental impact diet. Eating less meat and other animal food is a first step towards a sustainable diet but, as we showed for the issue of biodiversity, simply to reduce meat does not necessarily improve dietary diversity. A consumer can derive diversity from the supermarket shelf which has come from monocropping and biodiversity-destroying agricultural practices. Truly sustainable diets must build quite a few environmental metrics into daily life, much as healthy lifestyles need to build physical activity and healthier diets into daily life. Reducing energy intake where necessary to maintain a healthy body weight and reducing waste throughout the food system would also make a significant contribution to reducing environmental impact. These dietary changes would also reduce health risks (see Chapter 3).

## References

1  Tukker A, Huppes G, Guinée J, et al. *Environmental Impact of Products (EIPRO): Analysis of the Life Cycle Environmental Impacts Related to the Final Consumption of the EU-25.* Seville, Spain: European Commission Joint Research Centre, 2006

2  FAOSTAT. *Agri-environmental Indicators: Land.* Available at: http://faostat3.fao.org/search/*/E (accessed March 12, 2016). Rome: Food and Agricultural Organization of the United Nations, 2016

3 Garnett T. Where are the best opportunities for reducing greenhouse gas emissions in the food system (including the food chain)? *Food Policy*, 2011; 36: S23–S32, doi: 10.1016/j.foodpol.2010.10.010

4 Foley JA, Ramankutty N, Brauman KA, *et al.* Solutions for a cultivated planet. *Nature*, 2011; 478(7369): 337–42

5 Hoekstra AY, Mekonnen MM. The water footprint of humanity. *Proceedings of the National Academy of Sciences*, 2012; 109(9): 3232–7

6 Foley JA, DeFries R, Asner GP, *et al.* Global consequences of land use. *Science*, 2005; 309(5734): 570–4

7 Lang T, Barling D. Nutrition and sustainability: an emerging food policy discourse. *Proceedings of the Nutrition Society*, 2013; 72(01): 1–12

8 Rockström J, Steffen W, Noone K, *et al.* A safe operating space for humanity. *Nature*, 2009; 461(7263): 472–5

9 Jackson T. *Prosperity without Growth? The Transition to a Sustainable Economy.* Available at: www.sd-commission.org.uk (accessed January 15, 2015). London: Sustainable Development Commission, 2009

10 Daly HE, Farley JC. *Ecological Economics: Principles and Applications.* Washington, DC; London: Island Press, 2004

11 Stocker T, Qin D, Plattner G, *et al.*, IPCC. *Climate Change 2013: The Physical Science Basis.* Contribution of Working Group I to the Fifth Assessment Report of the Intergovernmental Panel on Climate Change. Geneva: Intergovernmental Panel on Climate Change, 2013

12 Pachauri RK. *Climate Change 2007: Synthesis Report.* Contribution of Working Groups I, II and III to the Fourth Assessment Report. Geneva: Intergovernmental Panel on Climate Change, 2008

13 European Commission. *Limiting Global Climate Change to 2 Degrees Celsius: The Way Ahead for 2020 and Beyond.* Communication from the Commission to the Council, the European Parliament, the European Economic and Social Committee and the Committee of the Regions. Available at: http://eur-lex.europa.eu/legal-content/EN/TXT/?uri=URISERV%3Al28188 (accessed March 12, 2016). Brussels: EUR-Lex, 2007

14 UNEP. *The Emissions Gap Report 2013.* Available at: www.unep.org/pdf/UNEPEmissionsGapReport2013.pdf (accessed March 12, 2015). Nairobi: United Nations Environment Programme, 2013

15 Garnett T. *Cooking Up a Storm: Food, Greenhouse Gas Emissions and Our Changing Climate.* Guildford, University of Surrey: Food and Climate Research Network Centre for Environmental Strategy, 2008

16 Ripple WJ, Smith P, Haberl H, *et al.* Ruminants, climate change and climate policy. *Nature Climate Change*, 2014; 4(1): 2–5

17 Metz B, Davidson OR. *Climate Change 2007: Mitigation.* Contribution of Working Group III to the Fourth Assessment Report of the Intergovernmental Panel on Climate Change. Geneva: Intergovernmental Panel on Climate Change, 2007

18 Vermeulen SJ, Campbell BM, Ingram JS. Climate change and food systems. *Annual Review of Environment and Resources*, 2012; 37(1): 195

19 Audsley E, Brander M, Chatterton J, *et al.* How Low Can We Go? An Assessment of Greenhouse Gas Emissions from the UK Food System and the Scope to Reduce Them by 2050. Woking, Surrey: WWF-UK, 2009

20 Bellarby J, Foereid B, Hastings A, *et al. Cool Farming: Climate Impacts of Agriculture and Mitigation Potential.* Amsterdam: Greenpeace International, 2008

21 Audsley E, Chatterton J, Graves A, *et al*. *Food, Land and Greenhouse Gases: The Effect of Changes in UK Food Consumption on Land Requirements and Greenhouse Gas Emissions*. London: The Committee on Climate Change, 2010

22 House of Commons Energy and Climate Change Committee. *Consumption-Based Emissions Reporting: Twelfth Report of Session 2010–12*. Available at: www.publications.parliament.uk/pa/cm201012/cmselect/cmenergy/1646/1646.pdf (accessed March 16, 2013). London: The Stationery Office, 2012

23 de Ruiter H, Macdiarmid JI, Matthews RB, *et al*. Global cropland and greenhouse gas impacts of UK food supply are increasingly located overseas. *Journal of The Royal Society Interface*, 2016; 13(114): 20151001

24 Committee on Climate Change. *Reducing the UK's Carbon Footprint and Managing Competitiveness Risks*. Available at: www.theccc.org.uk/publication/carbon-footprint-and-competitiveness/ (accessed June 10, 2016), 2013

25 Pendolovska V, Fernandez R, Mandl N, *et al*. Annual European Union Greenhouse Gas Inventory 1990–2011 and Inventory Report. Available at: www.eea.europa.eu/publications/european-union-greenhouse-gas-inventory-2013 (accessed July 30, 2016). Brussels: European Environment Agency, 2013

26 FAOSTAT. *FAOSTAT Emissions: Agriculture*. Available at: http://faostat3.fao.org/browse/G1/*/E (accessed July 27, 2016). Rome: Food and Agricultural Organization of the United Nations, 2015

27 Carlsson-Kanyama A, Gonzalez AD. Potential contributions of food consumption patterns to climate change. *The American Journal of Clinical Nutrition*, 2009; 89(5): 1704S–09S, doi: 10.3945/ajcn.2009.26736AA

28 Nilsson K, Sund V, Florén B. *The Environmental Impact of the Consumption of Sweets, Crisps and Soft Drinks*. Available at: www.diva-portal.org/smash/get/diva2:702819/FULLTEXT01.pdf (accessed July 31, 2016). Copenhagen: Nordic Council of Ministers, 2011

29 Vieux F, Darmon N, Touazi D, *et al*. Greenhouse gas emissions of self-selected individual diets in France: changing the diet structure or consuming less? *Ecological Economics*, 2012; 75(0): 91–101

30 Gerber P, Steinfeld H, Henderson B, *et al*. Tackling climate change through livestock: a global assessment of emissions and mitigation opportunities. Available at: www.fao.org/3/i3437e.pdf (accessed March 3, 2014). Rome: Food and Agricultural Organization, 2013

31 Steinfeld H, Gerber P, Wassenaar T, *et al*. *Livestock's Long Shadow: Environmental Issues and Options*. Rome: Food and Agricultural Organization, 2006

32 Lake I, Abdelhamid A, Hooper L, *et al*. *Food and Climate Change: A Review of the Effects of Climate Change on Food Within the Remit of the Food Standards Agency*. London: Food Standards Agency, 2010

33 Carlsson-Kanyama A, Ekström MP, Shanahan H. Food and life cycle energy inputs: consequences of diet and ways to increase efficiency. *Ecological Economics*, 2003; 44(2): 293–307

34 Kramer KJ, Moll HC, Nonhebel S, *et al*. Greenhouse gas emissions related to Dutch food consumption. *Energy Policy*, 1999; 27(4): 203–16

35 Westhoek H, Rood G, Berg M, *et al*. The protein puzzle: the consumption and production of meat, dairy and fish in the European Union. *European Journal of Food Research & Review*, 2011; 1(3): 123–44

36 Nijdam D, Rood T, Westhoek H. The price of protein: review of land use and carbon footprints from life cycle assessments of animal food products and their substitutes. *Food Policy*, 2012; 37(6): 760–70

37 Smil V. *Should We Eat Meat?* Chichester, UK: Wiley-Blackwell, 2013, 140–1

38 Williams A, Chatterton J, Daccache A. *Are Potatoes a Low-Impact Food for GB Consumers Compared with Rice and Pasta?* A report for the Potato Council. Milton Keynes, UK: Cranfield University, 2013

39 Health Council of the Netherlands. *Guidelines for a Healthy Diet: The Ecological Perspective*, publication no.2011/08E. The Hague: Health Council of the Netherlands, 2011

40 Barrett J, Vallack H, Jones A, *et al.* *A Material Flow Analysis and Ecological Footprint of York.* Stockholm: Stockholm Environment Institute, 2002

41 Wallén A, Brandt N, Wennersten R. Does the Swedish consumer's choice of food influence greenhouse gas emissions? *Environmental Science & Policy*, 2004; 7(6): 525–35, doi: 10.1016/j.envsci.2004.08.004

42 World Bank. *World Development Report 2010: Development and Climate Change.* Available at: https://openknowledge.worldbank.org/handle/10986/4387 (accessed March 23, 2015). Washington, DC: World Bank, 2010

43 Myers S, Zanobetti A, Kloog I, *et al.* Increasing CO2 threatens human nutrition. *Nature*, 2014, Jun 5; 510(7503): 139–42

44 Smith P, Gregory PJ. Climate change and sustainable food production. *Proceedings of the Nutrition Society*, 2013; 1(1): 1–8

45 Garnett T. Food sustainability: problems, perspectives and solutions. *Proceedings of the Nutrition Society*, 2013; 72(01): 29–39

46 Dickie A, Streck C, Roe S, *et al.* *Strategies for Mitigating Climate Change in Agriculture: Abridged Report.* Climate Focus and California Environmental Associates, prepared with the support of the Climate and Land Use Alliance. Available at: www.agriculturalmitigation.org (accessed October 19, 2014). San Francisco: Climate Focus and California Environmental Associates, 2014

47 UNCTAD. *Trade and Environment Review 2013. Wake Up Before It Is Too Late: Make Agriculture Truly Sustainable Now for Food Security in a Changing Climate.* Available at: http://unctad.org/en/pages/PublicationWebflyer.aspx?publicationid=666 (accessed February 10, 2015). Geneva: United Nations Conference on Trade and Development, 2013

48 Popp A, Lotze-Campen H, Bodirsky B. Food consumption, diet shifts and associated non-CO$_2$ greenhouse gases from agricultural production. *Global Environmental Change*, 2010; 20(3): 451–62

49 Ray DK, Mueller ND, West PC, *et al.* Yield trends are insufficient to double global crop production by 2050. *PLoS ONE*, 2013; 8(6): e66428

50 Hedenus F, Wirsenius S, Johansson DJ. The importance of reduced meat and dairy consumption for meeting stringent climate change targets. *Climatic Change*, 2014: 1–13

51 Garnett T. Livestock-related greenhouse gas emissions: impacts and options for policy makers. *Environmental Science & Policy*, 2009; 12(4): 491–503, doi: 10.1016/j. envsci.2009.01.006

52 Garnett T, Appleby M, Balmford A, *et al.* Sustainable intensification in agriculture: premises and policies. *Science*, 2013; 341(6141): 33–4

53  Eshel G, Shepon A, Makov T, *et al.* Land, irrigation water, greenhouse gas, and reactive nitrogen burdens of meat, eggs, and dairy production in the United States. *Proceedings of the National Academy of Sciences*, 2014; 111(33): 11996–12001

54  Fairlie S. *Meat: A Benign Extravagance*. East Meon, Hampshire: Permanent Publications, 2010

55  Woods J, Williams A, Hughes JK, *et al.* Energy and the food system. *Philosophical Transactions of the Royal Society B: Biological Sciences*, 2010; 365(1554): 2991–3006, doi: 10.1098/rstb.2010.0172

56  FAO. *Energy Smart Food for People and Climate*. Available at: www.fao.org/docrep/014/i2454e/i2454e00.pdf (accessed May 15, 2014). Rome: Food and Agricultural Organization, 2011

57  Pimentel D. Reducing energy inputs in the agricultural production system. *Monthly Review*, 2009; 61(03): 1–11

58  Canning P. *Energy Use in the US Food System*. Collingdale, PA: Diane Publishing, 2010

59  Cuéllar AD, Webber ME. Wasted food, wasted energy: the embedded energy in food waste in the United States. *Environmental Science & Technology*, 2010; 44(16): 6464–9

60  Mrema GC, Baker D, Kahan D. *Agricultural Mechanization in Sub-Saharan Africa: Time for a New Look*. Agricultural Management, Marketing and Finance Occasional Paper (FAO). Rome: Food and Agriculture Organization of the United Nations, 2008

61  Dawson C, Hilton J. Fertiliser availability in a resource-limited world: production and recycling of nitrogen and phosphorus. *Food Policy*, 2011; 36: S14–S22

62  Safa M, Samarasinghe S, Mohssen M. A field study of energy consumption in wheat production in Canterbury, New Zealand. *Energy Conversion and Management*, 2011; 52(7): 2526–32

63  Tenkorang F, Lowenberg-DeBoer J. Forecasting long-term global fertilizer demand. *Nutrient Cycling in Agroecosystems*, 2009; 83(3): 233–47

64  Carlsson-Kanyama A, Faist M. *Energy Use in the Food Sector: A Data Survey*. Stockholm: Swedish Environmental Protection Agency, 2000

65  Pimentel D, Pimentel M. Sustainability of meat-based and plant-based diets and the environment. *The American Journal of Clinical Nutrition*, 2003; 78(3): 660S–3S

66  Jägerskog A, Jønch Clausen T. *Feeding a Thirsty World: Challenges and Opportunities for a Water and Food Secure Future: Report*. Stockholm: Stockholm International Water Institute, 2012

67  Mekonnen MM, Hoekstra AY. *National Water Footprint Accounts: The Green, Blue and Grey Water Footprint of Production and Consumption*, Value of Water Research Report Series No. 50, UNESCO-IHE. Delft, the Netherlands: UNESCO-IHE, 2011

68  Fox T, Fimeche C. *Global Food: Waste Not, Want Not*. London: Institute of Mechanical Engineers, 2013

69  Hoekstra AY, Chapagain AK, Aldaya MM, *et al.* *The Water Footprint Assessment Manual: Setting the Global Standard*. London: Earthscan, 2011

70  Arjen YH, Mesfin MM. Imported water risk: the case of the UK. *Environmental Research Letters*, 2016; 11(5): 055002

71  UN Water. *Coping with Water Scarcity: Challenge of the Twenty-First Century, 2007*. Available at: www.fao.org/nr/water/docs/escarcity.pdf (accessed March 25, 2014). Geneva: United Nations Water, 2007

72  Mekonnen MM, Hoekstra AY. A global assessment of the water footprint of farm animal products. *Ecosystems*, 2012; 15(3): 401–15

73 Gerbens-Leenes PW, Mekonnen MM, Hoekstra AY. The water footprint of poultry, pork and beef: a comparative study in different countries and production systems. *Water Resources and Industry*, 2013; 1–2: 25–36, doi: 10.1016/j.wri.2013.03.001

74 Chapagain AK, Hoekstra AY. *Water Footprints of Nations*. Delft, The Netherlands: UNESCO-IHE, 2004

75 Williams ED, Ayres RU, Heller M. The 1.7 kilogram microchip: energy and material use in the production of semiconductor devices. *Environmental Science & Technology*, 2002; 36(24): 5504–10

76 Hoekstra AY. The water footprint of animal products, in: J D'Silva and J Webster (Eds). *The Meat Crisis: Developing More Sustainable Production and Consumption*. London, UK: Earthscan, 2010, 22–33

77 Vanham D, Mekonnen MM, Hoekstra AY. The water footprint of the EU for different diets. *Ecological Indicators*, 2013; 32: 1–8, doi: 10.1016/j.ecolind.2013.02.020

78 Gibbs HK, Rausch L, Munger J, et al. Brazil's soy moratorium: supply chain governance is needed to avoid deforestation. *Science*, 2015; 347(6220): 377–8

79 Lam H-M, Remais J, Fung M-C, et al. Food supply and food safety issues in China. *The Lancet*, 2013; 381(9882): 2044–53

80 Kastner T, Rivas MJI, Koch W, et al. Global changes in diets and the consequences for land requirements for food. *Proceedings of the National Academy of Sciences*, 2012; 109(18): 6868–72

81 Gerbens-Leenes P, Nonhebel S. Consumption patterns and their effects on land required for food. *Ecological Economics*, 2002; 42(1): 185–99

82 Gerbens-Leenes W, Nonhebel S. Food and land use: the influence of consumption patterns on the use of agricultural resources. *Appetite*, 2005; 45(1): 24–31, doi: 10.1016/j.appet.2005.01.011

83 Elferink EV, Nonhebel S. Variations in land requirements for meat production. *Journal of Cleaner Production*, 2007; 15(18): 1778–86, doi: 10.1016/j.jclepro.2006.04.003

84 Wirsenius S, Azar C, Berndes G. How much land is needed for global food production under scenarios of dietary changes and livestock productivity increases in 2030? *Agricultural Systems*, 2010; 103(9): 621–38

85 Wilkins JL, Peters C, Hamm MW, et al. Increasing acres to decrease inches: comparing the agricultural land requirements of a low-carbohydrate, high-protein diet with a MyPyramid Diet. *Journal of Hunger & Environmental Nutrition*, 2008; 3(1): 3–16, doi: 10.1080/19320240802163480

86 Temme EH, van der Voet H, Thissen JT, et al. Replacement of meat and dairy by plant-derived foods: estimated effects on land use, iron and SFA intakes in young Dutch adult females. *Public Health Nutrition*, 2013; 16(10): 1900–7, doi: 10.1017/S1368980013000232

87 Peters CJ, Wilkins JL, Fick GW. Testing a complete-diet model for estimating the land resource requirements of food consumption and agricultural carrying capacity: the New York State example. *Renewable Agriculture and Food Systems*, 2007; 22(02): 145–53

88 Meier T, Christen O, Semler E, et al. Balancing virtual land imports by a shift in the diet: using a land balance approach to assess the sustainability of food consumption. Germany as an example. *Appetite*, 2014; 74(0): 20–34

89 Howard SA. *An Agricultural Testament*. Oxford: Oxford University Press, 1940

90 Hyams E. *Soil and Civilization*. London: Thames and Hudson, 1952

91 Tansey G, Worsley T. *The Food System: A Guide*. London: Earthscan Publications Ltd, 1995

92  GEF-IFAD Partnership. *Tackling Land Degradation and Desertification*. Available at: www.ifad.org/events/wssd/gef/gef_ifad.htm (accessed March 25, 2015). Washington, DC: Global Environmental Fund and International Fund for Agricultural Development, 2002, 2

93  Pimentel D. Soil erosion: a food and environmental threat. *Environment, Development and Sustainability*, 2006; 8(1): 119–37

94  Metson GS, Bennett EM, Elser JJ. The role of diet in phosphorus demand. *Environmental Research Letters*, 2012; 7(4): 044043, doi: 10.1088/1748-9326/7/4/044043

95  Heywood V. Overview of agricultural biodiversity and its contribution to nutrition and health, in: J Fanzo, D Hunter, T Borelli and F Mattei (Eds) *Diversifying Food and Diets, Using Agricultural Biodiversity to Improve Nutrition and Health*. Abingdon, UK: Earthscan from Routledge, 2013, 35–67

96  TEEB. *The Economics of Ecosystems and Biodiversity (TEEB) for Agriculture & Food: An Interim Report*. Geneva: United Nations Environment Programme, 2015, 124

97  Berti P, Jones A. Biodiversity's contribution to dietary diversity, in: J Fanzo, D Hunter, T Borelli and F Mattei (Eds) *Diversifying Food and Diets, Using Agricultural Biodiversity to Improve Nutrition and Health*. Abingdon, Oxon: Earthscan from Routledge, 2013, 186–206

98  Johns T, Sthapit BR. Biocultural diversity in the sustainability of developing-country food systems. *Food and Nutrition Bulletin*, 2004; 25(2): 143–55

99  Shimbo S, Kimura K, Imai Y, *et al*. Number of food items as an indicator of nutrient intake. *Ecology of Food and Nutrition*, 1994; 32(3): 197–206

100  FAO. *Key Recommendations for Improving Nutrition through Agriculture and Food Systems*. Rome: Food and Agriculture Organization, 2015

101  Bellon MR, Ntandou-Bouzitou GD, Caracciolo F. On-farm diversity and market participation are positively associated with dietary diversity of rural mothers in Southern Benin, West Africa. *PLoS ONE*, 2016; 11(9): e0162535

102  Remans R, Wood SA, Saha N, *et al*. Measuring nutritional diversity of national food supplies. *Global Food Security*, 2014; 3(3–4): 174–82, doi: 10.1016/j. gfs.2014.07.001

103  Khoury CK, Bjorkman AD, Dempewolf H, *et al*. Increasing homogeneity in global food supplies and the implications for food security. *Proceedings of the National Academy of Sciences*, 2014; 111(11): 4001–6, doi: 10.1073/pnas.1313490111

104  Jones AD, Ejeta G. A new global agenda for nutrition and health: the importance of agriculture and food systems. *Bulletin of the World Health Organisation*, 2015; 94(228–229), doi: 10.2471/BLT.15.164509

105  Jones AD, Hoey L, Blesh J, *et al*. A systematic review of the measurement of sustainable diets. *Advances in Nutrition: An International Review Journal*, 2016; 7(4): 641–64

106  Jones AD, Shrinivas A, Bezner-Kerr R. Farm production diversity is associated with greater household dietary diversity in Malawi: findings from nationally representative data. *Food Policy*, 2014; 46: 1–12

107  La Vecchia C, Muñoz SE, Braga C, *et al*. Diet diversity and gastric cancer. *International Journal of Cancer*, 1997; 72(2): 255–7, doi: 10.1002/(SICI)1097-0215(19970717)72:2<255::AID-IJC9>3.0.CO;2-Q

108  Garavello W, Giordano L, Bosetti C, *et al*. Diet diversity and the risk of oral and pharyngeal cancer. *European Journal of Nutrition*, 2008; 47(5): 280–4, doi: 10.1007/s00394-008-0722-y

109 Isa F, Xie LP, Hu Z, *et al.* Dietary consumption and diet diversity and risk of developing bladder cancer: results from the South and East China case-control study. *Cancer Causes & Control*, 2013; 24(5): 885–95. doi: 10.1007/s10552-013-0165-5

110 Kant AK, Schatzkin A, Harris TB, *et al.* Dietary diversity and subsequent mortality in the first National Health and Nutrition Examination Survey Epidemiologic Follow-up Study. *The American Journal of Clinical Nutrition*, 1993; 57(3): 434–40

111 Marshall TA, Stumbo PJ, Warren JJ, *et al.* Inadequate nutrient intakes are common and are associated with low diet variety in rural, community-dwelling elderly. *The Journal of Nutrition*, 2001; 131(8): 2192–6

112 Ruel MT. Operationalizing dietary diversity: a review of measurement issues and research priorities. *The Journal of Nutrition*, 2003; 133(11): 3911S–26S

113 Fitzherbert EB, Struebig MJ, Morel A, *et al.* How will oil palm expansion affect biodiversity? *Trends in Ecology & Evolution*, 2008; 23(10): 538–45

114 Koh LP, Wilcove DS. Is oil palm agriculture really destroying tropical biodiversity? *Conservation Letters*, 2008; 1(2): 60–4

115 Geiger F, Bengtsson J, Berendse F, *et al.* Persistent negative effects of pesticides on biodiversity and biological control potential on European farmland. *Basic and Applied Ecology*, 2010; 11(2): 97–105

116 FAO. *Biodiversity*. Available at: www.fao.org/biodiversity/en/ (accessed May 6, 2014). Rome: Food and Agricultural Organization, 2014

117 Kuhnlein HV, Erasmus B, Spigelski D (Eds). *Indigenous Peoples' Food Systems: The Many Dimensions of Culture, Diversity and Environment for Nutrition and Health.* Rome: Food and Agriculture Organization and Centre for Indigenous Peoples' Nutrition and Environment (CINE), 2009

118 Kuhnlein HV, Receveur O. Dietary change and traditional food systems of indigenous peoples. *Annual Review of Nutrition*, 1996; 16: 417–42, doi: 10.1146/annurev. nu.16.070196.002221

119 Kuhnlein HV, Erasmus B, Spigelski D, *et al.* (Eds). *Indigenous Peoples' Food Systems and Well-Being: Interventions and Policies for Healthy Communities.* Rome: Food and Agricultural Organization and Centre for Indigenous Peoples' Nutrition and Environment (CINE), 2013

120 Damman S, Wenche BE, Kuhnlein HV. Indigenous peoples' nutrition transition in a right to food perspective. *Food Policy*, 2008; 33(2): 135–55

121 Lang T, Heasman M. *Food Wars: The Global Battle for Mouths, Minds and Markets* (2nd Ed.). Abingdon: Routledge Earthscan, 2015

122 Burlingame B, Dernini S. *Sustainable Diets and Biodiversity: Directions and Solutions for Policy, Research and Action.* Rome: Food and Agriculture Organization of the United Nations, 2010

123 Wahlqvist ML, Specht RL. Food variety and biodiversity: econutrition. *Asia Pacific Journal of Clinical Nutrition*, 1998; 7(3 & 4): 314–19

124 UNESCO. *Facts and Figures on Marine Biodiversity*. Available at: www.unesco. org/new/en/natural-sciences/ioc-oceans/focus-areas/rio-20-ocean/blueprint-for-the-future-we-want/marine-biodiversity/facts-and-figures-on-marine-biodiversity/ (accessed May 4, 2015). Paris: United Nations Educational Scientific and Cultural Organisation, 2015

125 Pitcher TJ, Cheung WWL. Fisheries: hope or despair? *Marine Pollution Bulletin*, 2013; 74(2): 506–16

126 FAO. The State of World Fisheries and Aquaculture Opportunities and Challenges. Available at: www.fao.org/3/a-i3720e.pdf (accessed June 16, 2016). Rome: Food and Agricultural Organization of the United Nations, 2014

127 Bijma J, Pörtner H-O, Yesson C, et al. Climate change and the oceans: what does the future hold? Marine Pollution Bulletin, 2013; 74(2): 495–505

128 Cheung WW, Lam VW, Sarmiento JL, et al. Projecting global marine biodiversity impacts under climate change scenarios. Fish and Fisheries, 2009; 10(3): 235–51

129 Lam VW, Cheung WW, Swartz W, et al. Climate change impacts on fisheries in West Africa: implications for economic, food and nutritional security. African Journal of Marine Science, 2012; 34(1): 103–17

130 Rogers AD, Laffoley D. Introduction to the special issue: the global state of the ocean; interactions between stresses, impacts and some potential solutions. Synthesis papers from the International Programme on the State of the Ocean 2011 and 2012 workshops. Marine Pollution Bulletin, 2013; 74(2): 491–4

131 FAO. The State of the World's Fisheries and Aquaculture. Available at: www.fao.org/docrep/016/i2727e/i2727e.pdf (accessed June 16, 2016). Rome: Food and Agricultural Organization of the United Nations, 2016

132 Cole DW, Cole R, Gaydos SJ, et al. Aquaculture: environmental, toxicological, and health issues. International Journal of Hygiene and Environmental Health, 2009; 212(4): 369–77

133 Costello MJ. Ecology of sea lice parasitic on farmed and wild fish. Trends in Parasitology, 2006; 22(10): 475–83

134 Cabello FC. Heavy use of prophylactic antibiotics in aquaculture: a growing problem for human and animal health and for the environment. Environmental Microbiology, 2006; 8(7): 1137–44, doi: 10.1111/j.1462-2920.2006.01054.x

135 Brunner EJ, Jones PJ, Friel S, et al. Fish, human health and marine ecosystem health: policies in collision. International Journal of Epidemiology, 2009; 38(1): 93–100, doi: 10.1093/ije/dyn157

136 Esteban A, Crilly R. Fish Dependence – 2012 Update: The Increasing Reliance of the EU on Fish from Elsewhere. OCEAN2012/New Economics Foundation (NEF), 2012

137 Edwards-Jones G, Milà i Canals L, Hounsome N, et al. Testing the assertion that 'local food is best': the challenges of an evidence-based approach. Trends in Food Science & Technology, 2008; 19(5): 265–74

138 Williams A, Pell E, Webb J, et al. Final Report for Defra Project FO0103. Comparative Life Cycle Assessment of Food Commodities Procured for UK Consumption through a Diversity of Supply Chains. Available at: http://randd.defra.gov.uk/Default.aspx?Module=More&Location=None&ProjectID=15001 (accessed May 18, 2015). London: Department for Environment, Food and Rural Affairs, 2008

139 Hospido A, Milà i Canals L, McLaren S, et al. The role of seasonality in lettuce consumption: a case study of environmental and social aspects. The International Journal of Life Cycle Assessment, 2009; 14: 381–91

140 Webb J, Williams AG, Hope E, et al. Do foods imported into the UK have a greater environmental impact than the same foods produced within the UK? The International Journal of Life Cycle Assessment, 2013; 18(7): 1325–43

141 Foster C, Guében C, Holmes M, et al. The environmental effects of seasonal food purchase: a raspberry case study. Journal of Cleaner Production, 2014; 73: 269–74

142 Mila i Canals L, Cowell SJ, Sim S, et al. Comparing domestic versus imported apples: a focus on energy use. Environmental Science and Pollution Research International, 2007; 14(5): 338–44

143  Edwards-Jones G. Does eating local food reduce the environmental impact of food production and enhance consumer health? *Proceedings of the Nutrition Society*, 2010; 69(04): 582–91, doi: 10.1017/S0029665110002004

144  Defra. *Food Transport Indicators to 2010*. Available at: www.gov.uk/government/publications/food-transport-indicators (accessed May 9, 2014). London: Department for Environment, Food and Rural Affairs, 2012

145  Smith A, Watkiss P, Tweddle G, et al. *The Validity of Food Miles as an Indicator of Sustainable Development, Final Report: Report ED50254*. London: Department for Environment, Food and Rural Affairs, 2005

146  Coley D, Howard M, Winter M. Local food, food miles and carbon emissions: a comparison of farm shop and mass distribution approaches. *Food Policy*, 2009; 34(2): 150–5, doi: 10.1016/j.foodpol.2008.11.001

147  Edwards-Jones G, Plassmann K, York E, et al. Vulnerability of exporting nations to the development of a carbon label in the United Kingdom. *Environmental Science & Policy*, 2009; 12(4): 479–90

148  Plassmann K, Edwards-Jones G. Carbon footprinting and carbon labelling of food products, in: U Sonesson, J Berlin and F Ziegler (Eds) *Environmental Assessment and Management in the Food Industry*. Cambridge, UK: Woodhead Publishing Ltd, 2010, 272–94

149  Garnett T. What Is a Sustainable Healthy Diet? A Discussion Paper. Available at: www.fcrn.org.uk/sites/default/files/fcrn_what_is_a_sustainable_healthy_diet_final. pdf (accessed May 2, 2014). Oxford: Food and Climate Research Network, 2014

150  Stoessel F, Juraske R, Pfister S, et al. Life cycle inventory and carbon and water food-print of fruits and vegetables: application to a Swiss retailer. *Environmental Science & Technology*, 2012; 46(6): 3253–62

151  Jungbluth N, Itten R, Schori S. *Environmental Impacts of Food Consumption and Its Reduction Potentials*. Eighth International Conference on Life Cycle Assessment in the Agri-Food Sector: LCA Food 2012. Rennes, 2012

152  Mondelaers K, Aertsens J, Van Huylenbroeck G. A meta-analysis of the differences in environmental impacts between organic and conventional farming. *British Food Journal*, 2009; 111(10): 1098–119

153  Pimentel D, Hepperly P, Hanson J, et al. Environmental, energetic, and economic comparisons of organic and conventional farming systems. *BioScience*, 2005; 55(7): 573–82

154  Alliance to Save Our Antibiotics. *The Campaign*. Bristol: Soil Association, 2013

155  Yussefi M. *The World of Organic Agriculture: Statistics and Emerging Trends 2009*. London: Earthscan, 2009

156  Nemecek T, Dubois D, Huguenin-Elie O, et al. Life cycle assessment of Swiss farming systems: I. Integrated and organic farming. *Agricultural Systems*, 2011; 104(3): 217–32

157  Tuomisto H, Hodge I, Riordan P, et al. Does organic farming reduce environmental impacts? A meta-analysis of European research. *Journal of Environmental Management*, 2012; 112: 309–20

158  Williams A, Audsley E, Sandars D. *Determining the Environmental Burdens and Resource Use in the Production of Agricultural and Horticultural Commodities*. Main Report, Defra Research Project IS0205. London: Department for Environment, Food and Rural Affairs, 2006

159  Seufert V, Ramankutty N, Foley JA. Comparing the yields of organic and conventional agriculture. *Nature*, 2012; 485(7397): 229–32, doi: 10.1038/nature11069

160  Bengtsson J, Ahnström J, Weibull AC. The effects of organic agriculture on biodiversity and abundance: a meta-analysis. *Journal of Applied Ecology*, 2005; 42(2): 261–9

161  Gabriel D, Sait SM, Hodgson JA, *et al.* Scale matters: the impact of organic farming on biodiversity at different spatial scales. *Ecology Letters*, 2010; 13(7): 858–69

162  Tuck SL, Winqvist C, Mota F, *et al.* Land-use intensity and the effects of organic farming on biodiversity: a hierarchical meta-analysis. *Journal of Applied Ecology*, 2014; 51(3): 746–55, doi: 10.1111/1365-2664.12219

163  Gustavsson J, Cederberg C, Sonesson U, *et al. Global Food Losses and Food Waste*. Rome: Food and Agriculture Organization of the United Nations, 2011

164  Quested T, Ingle R, Parry A. *Household Food and Drink Waste in the United Kingdom 2012.* Available at: www.wrap.org.uk/content/household-food-and-drink-waste-uk-2012 (accessed February 10, 2015). Banbury: Waste Resources Action Programme (UK), 2013

165  Quested TE, Parry AD, Easteal S, *et al.* Food and drink waste from households in the UK. *Nutrition Bulletin*, 2011; 36(4): 460–7

166  FAO. *Food Wastage Footprint Impacts on Natural Resources*. Technical Report. Available at: www.fao.org/docrep/018/i3347e/i3347e.pdf (accessed May 6, 2014). Rome: Food and Agricultural Organization, 2013

167  Rutten M, Nowicki P, Bogaardt M-J, *et al. Reducing Food Waste by Households and by Retail in the EU: a Prioritisation using Economic, Land Use and Food Security Impacts.* Available at: www.wageningenur.nl/upload_mm/b/c/8/27078547-595c-48c2-a016-d9ad8b8b3164_2013-035%20Rutten_DEF_WEB%205-11_Totaal. pdf (accessed February 19, 2014). Wageningen, Netherlands: LEI, Wageningen University and Research Centre, 2014

168  Kummu M, de Moel H, Porkka M, *et al.* Lost food, wasted resources: global food supply chain losses and their impacts on freshwater, cropland, and fertiliser use. *Science of The Total Environment*, 2012; 438(0): 477–89

169  ReFood. *Vision 2020: UK Road Map to Zero Food Waste to Landfill*. www.saria.co.uk/pdfs/vision2020_roadmap.pdf (accessed June 16, 2016), 2013

170  Regmi A, Gehlhar M. *New Directions in Global Food Markets: Agriculture Information Bulletin Number 794*. Washington, DC: United States Department of Agriculture/Economic Research Service, 2005

171  Gustavsson J, Cederberg C, Sonnesson U, *et al. Global Food Losses and Food Waste: Extent, Causes and Prevention*. Rome: Food and Agriculture Organization, 2011

172  Worldwatch Institute. *Global Plastic Production Rises, Recycling Lag*. Available at: www.worldwatch.org/global-plastic-production-rises-recycling-lags-0 (accessed August 10, 2016). Washington, DC: Worldwatch Institute, 2015

173  Claudio L. Our food: packaging and public health. *Environmental Health Perspectives*, 2012; 120(6): a232–7

174  Muncke J, Myers JP, Scheringer M, *et al.* Food packaging and migration of food contact materials: will epidemiologists rise to the neotoxic challenge? *Journal of Epidemiology and Community Health*, 2014; 68: 592–4, doi: 10.1136/jech-2013-202593

175  Ellen MacArthur Foundation. *The New Plastics Economy: Rethinking the Future of Plastic*. Ellen MacArthur Foundation, World Economic Forum and McKinsey & Company, 2016

176  Jungbluth N, Tietje O, Scholz RW. Food purchases: impacts from the consumers' point of view investigated with a modular LCA. *International Journal of Life Cycle Assessment*, 2000; 5: 134–42

177  Gussow JD. *The Feeding Web*. Palo Alto, CA: Bull Publishing Company, 1978

178 Gussow JD. Ecology and vegetarian considerations: does environmental responsibility demand the elimination of livestock? *The American Journal of Clinical Nutrition*, 1994; 59(5): 1110S–16S

179 Leitzmann C. Nutrition ecology: the contribution of vegetarian diets. *The American Journal of Clinical Nutrition*, 2003; 78(3): 657S–9S

180 Baroni L, Cenci L, Tettamanti M, et al. Evaluating the environmental impact of various dietary patterns combined with different food production systems. *European Journal of Clinical Nutrition*, 2007; 61(2): 279–86, doi: 10.1038/sj.ejcn.1602522

181 Reijnders L, Soret S. Quantification of the environmental impact of different dietary protein choices. *The American Journal of Clinical Nutrition*, 2003; 78(3 Suppl): 664S–8S

182 Stehfest E, Bouwman L, Vuuren DP, et al. Climate benefits of changing diet. *Climatic Change*, 2009; 95(1–2): 83–102, doi: 10.1007/s10584-008-9534-6

183 Berners-Lee M, Hoolohan C, Cammack H, et al. The relative greenhouse gas impacts of realistic dietary choices. *Energy Policy*, 2012; 43: 184–90, doi: 10.1016/j.enpol.2011.12.054

184 Macdiarmid JI, Kyle J, Horgan GW, et al. Sustainable diets for the future: can we contribute to reducing greenhouse gas emissions by eating a healthy diet? *The American Journal of Clinical Nutrition*, 2012; 96(3): 632–9, doi: 10.3945/ajcn.112.038729

185 Scarborough P, Allender S, Clarke D, et al. Modelling the health impact of environmentally sustainable dietary scenarios in the UK. *European Journal of Clinical Nutrition*, 2012; 66(6): 710–15

186 Meier T, Christen O. Environmental impacts of dietary recommendations and dietary styles: Germany as an example. *Environmental Science & Technology*, 2013; 47(2): 877–88, doi: 10.1021/es302152v

187 Biesbroek S, Bueno-de-Mesquita HB, Peeters PH, et al. Reducing our environmental footprint and improving our health: greenhouse gas emission and land use of usual diet and mortality in EPIC-NL – a prospective cohort study. *Environmental Health*, 2014; 13(1): 27

188 Westhoek H, Lesschen JP, Rood T, et al. Food choices, health and environment: effects of cutting Europe's meat and dairy intake. *Global Environmental Change*, 2014; 26: 196–205

189 Davis J, Sonesson U, Baumgartner DU, et al. Environmental impact of four meals with different protein sources: case studies in Spain and Sweden. *Food Research International*, 2010; 43(7): 1874–84, doi: 10.1016/j.foodres.2009.08.017

190 Tukker A, Goldbohm RA, De Koning A, et al. Environmental impacts of changes to healthier diets in Europe. *Ecological Economics*, 2011; 70(10): 1776–88

191 Cassidy ES. *Quantifying Environmental Impacts of Diets*. Available at: www.slideshare.net/EmilyCassidy/cassidy-emily-quantifying (accessed August 1, 2016). Minneapolis, MN: Institute for the Environment, University of Minnesota, 2013

192 Aston LM, Smith JN, Powles JW. Impact of a reduced red and processed meat dietary pattern on disease risks and greenhouse gas emissions in the UK: a modelling study. *BMJ Open*, 2012; 2(5): e001072

193 Hendrie GA, Ridoutt BG, Wiedmann TO, et al. Greenhouse gas emissions and the Australian diet: comparing dietary recommendations with average intakes. *Nutrients*, 2014; 6(1): 289–303

194  Masset G, Vieux F, Verger EO, *et al*. Reducing energy intake and energy density for a sustainable diet: a study based on self-selected diets in French adults. *The American Journal of Clinical Nutrition*, 2014; doi: 10.3945/ajcn.113.077958

195  Van Kernebeek H, Oosting S, Feskens E, *et al*. The effect of nutritional quality on comparing environmental impacts of human diets. *Journal of Cleaner Production*, 2013; 73: 88–99

196  Cassidy ES, West PC, Gerber JS, *et al*. Redefining agricultural yields: from tonnes to people nourished per hectare. *Environmental Research Letters*, 2013; 8(3): 034015

197  Vanham D, Hoekstra A, Bidoglio G. Potential water saving through changes in European diets. *Environment International*, 2013; 61: 45–56

198  Peters CJ, Picardy J, Darrouzet-Nardi AF, *et al*. Carrying capacity of U.S. agricultural land: ten diet scenarios. *Elementa*, 2016; 4: doi: 10.12952/journal.elementa.000116

199  Van Dooren C, Marinussen M, Blonk H, *et al*. Exploring dietary guidelines based on ecological and nutritional values: a comparison of six dietary patterns. *Food Policy*, 2014; 44: 36–46

200  Gerber PJ, Steinfeld H, Henderson B, *et al*. *Tackling Climate Change Through Livestock: A Global Assessment of Emissions and Mitigation Opportunities*. Rome: Food and Agriculture Organization of the United Nations, 2013

201  Carbon Trust. *The Eatwell Guide: A More Sustainable Diet*. Available at: www.carbontrust.com/resources/reports/advice/sustainable-diets/ (accessed June 9, 2016). London: Carbon Trust, 2016

202  Carbon Trust. *The Case for Protein Diversity*. Available at: www.carbontrust.com/resources/reports/advice/the-case-for-protein-diversity/ (accessed June 9, 2016), 2016

203  Duchin F. Sustainable consumption of food: a framework for analyzing scenarios about changes in diets. *Journal of Industrial Ecology*, 2005; 9(1–2): 99–114

204  Saez-Almendros S, Obrador B, Bach-Faig A, *et al*. Environmental footprints of Mediterranean versus Western dietary patterns: beyond the health benefits of the Mediterranean diet. *Environmental Health: A Global Access Science Source*, 2013; 12: 118, doi: 10.1186/1476-069X-12-118

205  De Marco A, Velardi M, Camporeale C, *et al*. The adherence of the diet to Mediterranean principle and its impacts on human and environmental health. *International Journal of Environmental Protection and Policy*, 2014; 2(2): 64–75

206  Pairotti MB, Cerutti AK, Martini F, *et al*. Energy consumption and GHG emission of the Mediterranean diet: a systemic assessment using a hybrid LCA-IO method. *Journal of Cleaner Production*, 2015, 103: 507–16

207  Saxe H. The New Nordic Diet is an effective tool in environmental protection: it reduces the associated socioeconomic cost of diets. *The American Journal of Clinical Nutrition*, 2014; 99(5): 1117–25, doi: 10.3945/ajcn.113.066746

208  Saxe H, Larsen TM, Mogensen L. The global warming potential of two healthy Nordic diets compared with the average Danish diet. *Climatic Change*, 2013; 116: 249–62

# Chapter 5

# Culture and society
## The social conditions shaping eating patterns

## Contents

## Core arguments

Food means much more than just nutrients. It is imbued with social, emotional and cultural meaning. It is associated with pleasure and identity but can and does bring pain and social dislocation. Choice of food is determined by many factors. Food preferences are themselves determined by income and/or birth circumstances. Access to land to produce food is a key factor in rural areas but less so in urban ones. Citizen skills in sourcing and preparing food, the influence of marketing and consumerism, information and labelling, socio-cultural norms and, increasingly, ethics, be they issues of animal welfare or fairness in trade, are all important social factors that have entered the debates about sustainability of food and diet.

This chapter discusses how this complex mix of social and cultural factors feeds into the concept of sustainable diets. Social determinants range from socio-economic status to culture, from family upbringing to aspirations, from gender to generational differences. These are the focus of lively debates about the politics of equality and justice through food. In an ideal world a sustainable diet should not only be healthy for people and the planet, but should be culturally appropriate and accessible to everyone. Reality is different. The links between society and diet go in both directions: the food system both shapes and reflects society. These societal elements are or ought to be central to any notion of sustainable diets but, so far, debate has tended to focus more on either environment or health, yet social meanings imbue what people eat and their notions of good diet and food. The concept of cultural appropriateness is delicate but essential in this debate.

The chapter suggests that sustainable diets require a population approach that goes beyond single-issue diet 'solutions'. No matter how good a diet is for health and the environment, if it is not available to everyone in a form that is culturally appropriate such a diet cannot be judged sustainable. This social dimension already has a presence in the debate, but it is set to matter even more in the twenty-first century as tensions emerge over resources and societal progress. The role of social movements such as those for fair trade, animal welfare and eco-friendly foods suggests the importance of civil society in civilising the food system. They often champion the 'social' when pursuing better food supply and diets. In an era of weak governance and strong corporate messaging about food, the social element of sustainable diets is highly contested. There is no dominant social or moral compass shaping the sustainability of diets.

## Food is social

This chapter explores the relevance of the combination of factors that shape how humans experience their food and diets as social beings. The 'social' elements of diets have been highlighted from years of findings, mostly from social scientists, about the importance of issues such as: food access; the social context of eating; the effects of culture, class, family, gender, ethnicity, education, skills, time, knowledge, attitudes and beliefs. This complex mix of social elements means that yet more meanings and factors have to be included in what is meant by sustainable diet. The transition to sustainable diets must take account of social factors underpinning eating patterns. How well this is done could make or mar the transition. The importance of the socio-cultural dimension was recognised by Johnston and colleagues in a review of the determinants and processes influencing sustain-ability of diets that singled out the importance of social norms, seasonality, family dynamics, gender, knowledge, religion and income inequalities.[1]

Food is a source of social pleasure and identity, not just something only con-sumed and experienced as 'fuel' consumed on one's own. Modern diets across the world, or anywhere where people live at above subsistence level, are partly affected by consumerism. Indeed, they are outcomes of consumerism. A world that over-produces and mal-distributes food – FAO figures suggest there is not too little food but almost too much at present – has an imperative to keep us eating, snacking and drinking value-added drinks all the time. The social function of eating has thus been transformed from a need to a want in the twentieth century on an unprecedented scale. Marketing funded by corporations committed to processed diets attempts to shape what people eat. In 2015, an estimated US$30.7 billion was spent on global food advertising. Food is the second highest advertised segment after automobiles.[2] It targets us everywhere, and is particularly sensitive in relation to children.[3]

By starting young, advertising and marketing exploit what might be called the mass psychology of diet. This is not just seeking behaviour change, as current policy makers like to use the term, but is the systematic setting of norms at the societal and supra-individual level. In theory, better food labelling, education and information give consumers some countervailing power – some tools with which they can reassert consumer power. But these are comparatively weak ways of injecting societal responsibilities into food systems. The terms of reference have already been set. There is a lock-in to the obesogenic food system; there is an assumption that food progress is packaged, and meals come from takea-ways or supermarkets, and that cooking is increasingly what happens in factories. Meanwhile, there is a mirror-image lock-in to the hunger sphere of the food sys-tem. Over-eating sits alongside under- and mal-eating. Each sphere can eye the other but not easily meet. A divided culture remains.

Many social factors determine people's food and nutrition intake. 'Soft' cul-tural factors such as the norms, meanings and assumptions that imbue food in everyday life mix with 'harder' socio-economic factors such as income, social class, status and geo-politics. These are overlaid onto biological factors such as hunger, appetite, taste and palatability; and psychological factors such as mood, pleasure/pain, disgust/like and stress. It is no wonder, given this immense range of factors, that some academics have preferred to subscribe to simpler theories and models of how food behaviour develops and changes. One of the most cited is Fishbein and Ajzen's 'Knowledge-Behaviour-Action' model, the Theory of Reasoned Action (TRA). This posited that, to predict behaviour, one primar-ily needs to know a person's beliefs, attitudes and intentions.[4, 5] Outsiders can try to alter attitudes, but the relationship between the major factors are hard to alter. The TRA model has been criticised for being over-simple and reduction-ist, so this chapter explores the case for a more complex understanding. Our argument is that diet invokes broader social and cultural meanings than simply reason or genetics, for that matter. If the notion of sustainable diets is to be of societal value, it must be translated into population and national/global norms and habits. The re-setting of these is what matters. Societal change is more than the aggregation of individual actions.

This is anathema to neoliberals, who argue that society is best left to individual choice. Indeed, the 'social' can be painted as a top-down force emerging like the giant foot from the sky to squash the viewer at the start of each episode of *Monty Python's Flying Circus*. Social control, in that top-down sense, does happen under dictatorships, or in what the Canadian sociologist Erving Goffman called 'total institutions' such as prisons; caged places where inmates have limited autonomy.[6] Yet studies of even these stark circumstances have shown that there is room for agency;[7] the life of Nelson Mandela in prison is a celebrated example.[8] Sociologists have argued for over a century about the social tensions between top-down control and democratic pressures for more fluidity. Most now agree that modern societies exhibit a mix of order and agency. They have structures and institutions – the family, work, education, political forms – but these are malleable and subject to change. Taking this lead, we see the social elements of diet as not just controlled or shaped by social context but as features that can also be altered. Societies can and do redesign what a normal diet is. This process of change may be rapid – for example, in times of war and rationing – or may slow.[9, 10] It may be shaped by commerce or by campaigns or religions and will certainly be by climate change.[9]

To the social scientist, inequality is probably one of the most important social factors shaping current diets.[11–13] After the Great Recession (2007–10), it troubled even the World Bank and International Monetary Fund.[14] Open debate resumed about the case for reducing the gap across society as a whole.[15] Policies and politics can and do make a difference. *The World Happiness Report* produced by the Sustainable Development Solutions Network based at Columbia University, USA shows that more equal societies tend to be happier, but that in recent years most of the 156 societies studied have become both less equal and less contented.[16] This suggests the need to rebuild the long traditions of work by nutritionists on social divisions in food availability in developing and developed countries.[17]

Inequalities raise a moral dimension in the sustainable diet debate. In an individualised world, volition is everything. A world where humans have to choose the 'right thing' means they cannot be just passive recipients of what is presented.[18] Ethical and social values matter for food and diet. Religious and other moral 'rules' operationalise choice. They set norms and reflexes of likes and dislikes. Campaigners for animal welfare or fairer trade or improvements in food working conditions are, in effect, trying to recalibrate those norms. They enter a multi-layered mix of tensions: dietary choice vs little dietary choice; inherited food rules vs created food rules; individualisation of food systems vs sharing as a principle; fair distribution between the sexes and age groups vs unequal distribution; commercialised information flows vs educated information; and so on. But if consumers in an affluent society can affect the lives of farm labourers far away, as the fair trade movement suggests they can,[19] how could social factors be addressed to underpin sustainable diets?

## Seeking the social determinants of dietary change

The 1987 Brundtland report's approach to sustainability was to see it as the overlap of economy, environment and society. In fact, few food sustainability analysts gave much attention to the societal element of diet until comparatively recently. It was left to civil society movements such as trades unions or campaigners for animal welfare to flesh out exactly what this can mean in practice. Organisations with their own social indicators emerged, such as the Ethical Trade Initiative and the movement for minimum wages.[20] That is how fair trade campaigners, arguing for more of the money consumers pay for foods (coffee, sugar, chocolate) to get down to primary workers, paradoxically ended up supporting commodities not known for their high health attributes. The campaigns put priority on the social needs of small farmers above more affluent far-away consumers. From a sustainable diet perspective, the fair trade sugar might be bad for you but it's helping the grower live.

Anthropologists were arguably among the first social researchers to begin to dissect the dynamics and meaning of food cultures in the nineteenth century. Critics sometimes depict this as part of the Western imperial attempt to understand their subjects in order to control them.[21] Certainly, there was an element of desire for control that informed studies of how very different peoples ate what (to Westerners) were strange diets.[22] But there has also been a profoundly sympathetic and liberal element to this academic inquiry, through which the 'plasticity' of food cultures became clear.[23] The diversity of diets on the planet showed dietary choice is not fixed. They reflect context, time, geography, trade opportunities and more. Diet and food are prisms through which the structures and dynamics of societies could be viewed and compared. Women are key actors in food culture; they are primary food managers, mediating the needs of children and men.[24, 25]

Today, there is more comprehensive recognition of the subtlety yet diversity of diets, beliefs about food and social assumptions about what a good diet is. There is more humility, too, about how important the social aspects of food are, and how societies vary in what they consider good.[26] Diets have been shown to change remarkably fast. British children's favourite foods include pizza and burgers. *Buzzfeed*, the list-obsessed web-based news source, can offer guidance for 'healthy' versions of US children's favourite foods: lasagne, nuggets, pasta, fries, and so on![27] More worryingly, food's social meanings and 'rules' have been actively subverted in the name of the promoters of more processed foods. Why else are $, € and £ trillions used to market, position and brand foods? Indeed, there is an interesting *folie à deux* between researchers on modern food trends and sections of the food industry desperately trying to keep 'hip' or to look for new niche markets which they might grow into vast new brands. Smoothies came from seemingly nowhere; fusion foods, too. The search for new products, new tastes is ceaseless. But only in the over-consuming world. This fissured reality to dietary choice is perhaps the indicator of a food cultural neophiliac tendency: the cult of the new. Meanwhile hundreds of millions of people in Asia or Africa live on restricted diets beyond the realm of choice culture.

Critics seeking more sustainable diets have sometimes appealed to tradition and historic authenticity as a motive for change. The Swedish government did this in its 2008 environmentally effective food choice guidance, and Michael Pollan, too, in his often-quoted appeal not to eat what your grandmother would not recognise.[28, 29] 'Real food' is pitched as something from the past. While one can understand this logic, surely part of the social challenge of sustainable diets must be to explore the social meaning of diet in order to hone more diverse messaging appropriate for many different contexts. An argument or a set of determinants in one context might be completely irrelevant in another. Possibly more than for any other topic or chapter in this book, the 'social' element in diet will inevitably retain this 'plastic', malleable, loose characteristic. The policy task is to negotiate how to unpick the range of barriers on dietary change and in order to reframe social norms.

The sustainable diet challenge means searching for new food literacies in the age of climate change and obesity.[30, 31] The notion of food literacy can be invoked to highlight the existence (and malleability) of public modes of understanding about diet and food. Sustainable diets must be underpinned by the 'everyday rules' people apply to food, without necessarily thinking too hard about it. A plethora of rules are applied in the eating process: choice of foods, the mode of sitting or standing, the use of hands or utensils, the pace of eating, the time of day, occasions when not to eat, whether to eat outside (if so how) or inside only, and so on. Historically and still today, religions have been important in framing this architecture of food culture. While religions are still immensely powerful, they cannot compete with the new commercial forces who now shape social and cultural mores. The commercial vies with the historically inherited, the simple with the complex, the pre-processed versus the home-cooked, and so on. Why bother to make a burger or custard when you can buy it ready-made so cheaply?

It can be hard to disentangle all the reasons why people eat what they do, yet it is now possible to conceptualise a multi-factoral model, which goes beyond the psychological reductionism of Fishbein and Ajzen's TRA outlined earlier. Figure 5.1 (which has been used in some form in the UK over several decades) maps out at the household level the important socio-economic determinants of food access and intake, together with some of the broad national and local policies that have an impact. There are now many such schema. One that focuses on family dynamics is given in Figure 5.2. Our concern here is that people's diet – whether sustainable or unsustainable – sits in a web of interactions and social forces. These are interpreted and modelled differently by the various social science disciplines. Any transition to a more sustainable diet must therefore engage with these insights or risk being undermined by counter-forces. We now address some of these social factors in more detail, highlighting their significance for sustainable diets. Other chapters add further detail (see Chapters 7 and 8 for more on culture and food labour, for example).

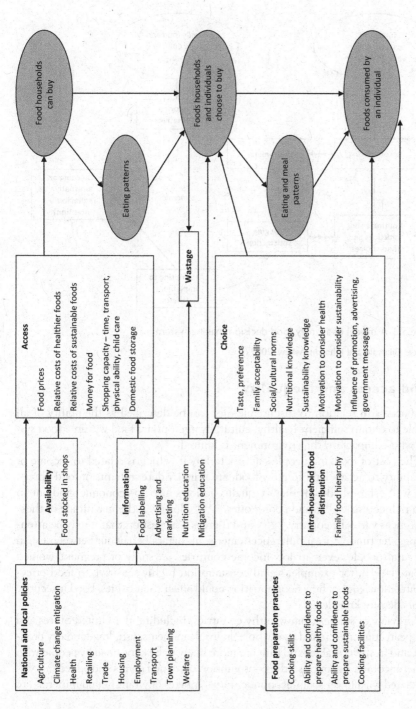

*Figure 5.1* Determinants of food and nutrition intake in the UK

Source: Dowler et al., 2007.[32]

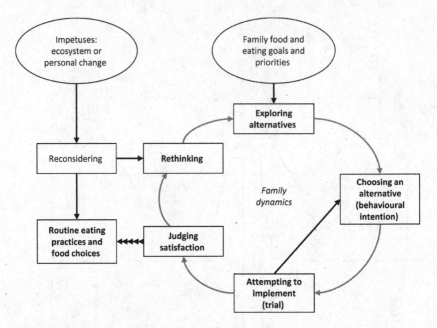

*Figure 5.2* A model of a family food decision-making system

Source: Gillespie and Johnson-Askew, 2009.[33]

## Food access and inequality

Food access in relation to sustainable diet can be described as the ability of all people to obtain sufficient healthy, culturally appropriate food within a food system whose impact on the environment is limited.

The cost of food and people's ability to buy it, which is related to income or the ability to access land to grow food, are primary determinants of food access. It is well established that dietary quality follows a socio-economic gradient in both rich countries,[34–42] and poorer ones.[36, 43–46] However, the magnitude of these differences varies by country,[36, 47, 48] and there is a suggestion that it may be attenuating over time.[49] Great differences emerge in dietary behaviour between urban and rural people, even in low-income countries. A study of pregnant women in Bangladesh, for example, found consumption highly sensitive to food prices despite knowledge of how poor nutrition could affect their babies. Food insecurity occurs despite knowledge.[50]

A review of studies from wealthy countries, including the United States and European countries, found that whole grains, lean meats, fish, low-fat dairy products, and fresh vegetables and fruit are more likely to be consumed by people with higher incomes. In contrast, the consumption of refined grains and added fats was associated with lower socio-economic status. Intakes of vitamins and minerals are also lower in people with limited incomes but there is little evidence to indicate that socio-economic status affects either total energy intakes or the macronutrient (fat and carbohydrate) composition of the diet.[34]

In the UK, differences in household or individual dietary patterns, nutrient intakes and blood levels have been observed in national surveys of people on low incomes compared with the rest of the population. The Low Income Diet and Nutrition Survey (LIDNS) found that people on low incomes were less likely to eat whole grains and fruit and vegetables and to consume more fat spreads, soft drinks, beef, pork, lamb and veal dishes, pizza, processed meat, whole milk and table sugar.[51] Energy intakes and vitamin and mineral intakes were similar across socio-economic groups. In the USA, people on low incomes have been found to have lower intakes of calcium, vitamin D and fibre.[52] In the UK LIDNS, higher proportions of people on low incomes had haemoglobin levels below the threshold for anaemia and vitamin D blood levels below the cut-off point for low vitamin D status.

A study of the Scottish diet indicated that, while energy density was highest in the most deprived population groups, there was no difference in total fat intake.[53] Cheese, butter and cream contributed more fat in the least deprived versus the most deprived groups. Sugar intake was highest in the most deprived groups, but saturated fat and fibre intake was highest in the least deprived groups. In this survey there was no difference in overall red meat intake by socio-economic group, but meat product consumption was higher in the most deprived groups. While there was no difference in confectionery consumption between the most and least deprived groups, consumption of cakes, biscuits and pastries was highest in the least deprived groups.

In poorer countries the picture is different. A systematic review of 33 studies from 17 low- and middle-income countries (5 low-income countries and 12 middle-income countries; 31 cross-sectional and 2 longitudinal studies) indicated that a higher socio-economic group or living in an urban area was associated with higher intakes of calories, protein, total fat, polyunsaturated, saturated and monounsaturated fatty acids, iron and vitamins A and C, and with lower intakes of carbohydrates and fibre. Being in a high socio-economic group was also associated with higher fruit and/or vegetable consumption, diet quality and diversity. Although few studies in this review were performed in low-income countries, similar patterns were generally observed in both low- and middle-income countries except for fruit intake, which was lower in urban than in rural areas in low-income countries.[43] In China, where incomes have increased very rapidly, for some people dietary quality is mixed in that people in higher socio-economic groups have been associated with raised fast-food intake (hamburgers, soft drinks),[54, 55] and also higher fruit intake.[55] In health terms, one step forward, one – or is it two? – back. If life expectancy rises with income, will the acculturation of US-style fast food undermine the positive cultural elements of 'traditional' Chinese diets?

As is well known, obesity is increasingly prevalent throughout the world, but the incidence of obesity actually varies with socio-economic status, although the patterns of obesity differ between countries. A seminal piece of research in 1989 studied the relationship between obesity and socio-economic group in both richer and poorer countries.[56] Primary findings included the observation of a consistently inverse association for women in richer countries, with a higher likelihood of obesity among women in lower socio-economic groups, but the relation for men and children was inconsistent. By contrast, in poorer countries, a strong direct relation was observed for women, men and children, with a higher likelihood of obesity among persons in higher socio-economic groups. An update of this review published in 2007 identified an overall pattern, for both men and women, of an increased likelihood of obesity in rich compared with poor countries.[57] In richer countries there was a lower likelihood of obesity among women with more education and higher-paid occupations, while in low- and middle-income countries obesity increased in women with income and material possessions, but these differences were less striking than those observed in the earlier review.

Obesity in poorer countries is increasingly no longer solely a disease of richer people,[58] although the burden of overweight remains concentrated among wealthier people in both low- and middle-income countries.[59, 60] More affluent people in the lowest-income countries are at the greatest risk of obesity,[61, 62] while in middle-income countries the association becomes largely mixed for men and mainly negative for women.[61] In upper-middle-income countries, higher socio-economic status confers protection against obesity.[62] The burden of obesity in each developing country tends to shift towards the groups with lower socio-economic status as the country's gross national product (GNP) increases. The shift of obesity towards women with low socio-economic status apparently occurs at an earlier stage of economic development than it does for men.[58]

## Causes of dietary inequalities

The links between poor diet and socio-economic status are important but complex. In rich countries there is a long history of health professionals and other scientists describing the diets of people on low incomes as unhealthy because of ignorance. Deficiencies of skills in relation to shopping, budgeting and cooking have been posited as leading to undesirable dietary habits.[32] Actually, it is far harder to disentangle the reasons why people eat what they do than it might appear. This is partly because socio-economic status represents a variety of indices, including household income, receipt of benefits, education and employment, that are not necessarily interchangeable in terms of their relationship with food purchasing patterns and nutritional outcomes. However, differences in dietary quality between people who are richer compared with those who are poorer are particularly observed when comparison is by household income, economic activity (employed versus unemployed or in receipt of welfare benefits) or household composition.[63] In short, differences are more marked if indicators of material well-being are used rather than differences based on occupation or educational level, which are proxy indicators for wealth, cultural and social capital.

The meaning and practice of cooking, for example, changes with time, food retail markets and the status of women.[64-68] Since the 1970s the food system has been subject to major changes, including accelerated globalisation of tastes and market concentration. Supermarketisation has increased around the world, spreading the availability of highly processed food and ready-prepared meals into culinary cultures where they were sparse. Commercial spending on marketing, particularly to children and young people, has grown at a time of pressures on state welfare.[69, 70] In this shifting cultural context, the effects of social class and ethnic or cultural identity in food purchasing and intake is itself altered. Traditional patterns of food use can be quickly altered in the nutrition transition. Some have argued that diets (and societies) become more homogenous in this process – seeing the emergence of a 'globo-diet' and what is called in the literature 'dietary convergence' – but the evidence suggests that considerable differences remain; there is uneven dietary development.[71-73] A study comparing approaches to cooking even in two rich societies, the UK and France, found major historical differences remained in the time spent cooking, how people ate and the meaning of food.[68] The differences between rich and poor societies are even more marked. While affluent people eat out more, poorer people are most likely to buy familiar foods and meals. Tight budgets are a barrier to trying new dishes and leave little financial room for experimentation, failure or a meal being thrown away by a family member. Pleasing the household and being able to prepare and eat a meal quickly are also likely to be more important than health outcomes such as reducing environmental damage from dietary choices or the risk of future cardiovascular disease and diabetes. Income and status shape people's mental 'space' and culinary room for manoeuvre.

The list of social factors that determine diet and its (un)sustainability is potentially huge. Like other accounts, we can therefore only summarise. What matters is how the various factors interact and mix, and which has salience under this or that circumstance. The cost of food and its relation to income are particularly important for a sustainable diet almost everywhere. They can restrict preparedness to change. How much money people have, what food is available and at what cost in the shops people use, as well as food skills, taste and cultural aspects, play significant roles. Beliefs and attitudes about food also have significant roles in food choice. For instance, religious views affect methods of rearing and slaughtering animals. They provide historically derived norms and cultural rules about what is good or bad, clean or dirty, pleasurable or disgusting. They provide guidance, which becomes routine in how people live and work. Physical factors such as the availability of food and type or location of shops and markets provide the conditions under which cultural norms can be activated.

### The social dynamics of food prices

Food prices are widely accepted to provide a key linkage between socio-economic disparities and diet intake and quality. Cost and income are key dietary gatekeepers.

A systematic review and meta-analysis of 151 studies found that foods of lower nutritional value and lower-quality diets generally cost less per calorie and tended to be selected by groups of lower socio-economic status,[74] while diets of higher nutritional value tend to cost more.[37] A study in the Australian city of Adelaide found that households on low incomes would have to spend approximately 30% of household income on eating healthily, whereas high-income households needed to spend about 10%.[75] A study in West Sydney, Australia, found that households in the lowest income quintile would have to spend up to 48% of their weekly income to buy a healthy food basket while households in the highest income quintile had to spend only 9% of their income.[76] The cost of the healthy food basket also varied by neighbourhood, with people in the most deprived neighbourhood having to spend proportionately more for the same basket of healthy food.[76]

A concern is that the cost of healthy food appears to have risen more than that of less healthy options. A 2015 report by the UK Overseas Development Institute (ODI) concluded that this has been the case in rich countries over the past 30 years, but that the same may also apply in emerging economies such as Brazil, China, Korea and Mexico where incomes have risen very rapidly during the last 20 years.[77] A 2014 UK study found a 35% rise in the price of both more and healthy food between 2002 and 2012 from £3.87 per 1,000 kcal to £5.21 per 1,000 kcal.[78] Price per 1,000 kcal was always highest for fruit and vegetables, lowest for starchy foods (bread, rice, potatoes and pasta), and second lowest for foods and drinks high in fat and/or sugar. The price of starchy foods per 1,000 kcal stayed roughly the same between 2002 and 2012, while the other groups showed price rises. Each of the food categories, with the exception of fruit and vegetables, contained both foods classified as more healthy and some as less healthy. Healthier foods increased in price per 1,000 kcal more rapidly than less healthy foods. Healthier foods increased in price by an average of 17 pence per 1,000 kcal per year while less healthy foods rose seven pence per 1,000 kcal per year. In 2012 the average price of more healthy foods was about three times higher – £7.49 for 1,000 kcal compared with £2.50 for 1,000 kcal of less healthy foods.

The high cost of healthy foods leaves households on low incomes vulnerable to diet-related health problems because they may have to rely on cheaper foods that are high in fat, sugar and salt. Households on low incomes often face a very difficult financial struggle to afford healthy food and, when food costs are considered, families on low incomes often face circumstances of poverty. Food poverty is an indicator of overall poverty as it is strongly linked to household income.[63] Where basic expenditure on rent, fuel and water constitute a high proportion of outgoings, and this has risen in relation to income, including that from benefits and pensions, the cost of food can be critical in determining food-purchasing decisions. Households may have little flexibility in how they prioritise expenditures, which may include compulsory deductions of rent arrears, loan repayments and fines, such that food is the only flexible part of the budget. People then economise by buying cheaper or different items, fewer vegetables, no fruit, cheap processed foods, filling comfort foods or sometimes omitting meals altogether.

Within the household, historically, it has been usual for women/mothers to act as gatekeepers of food allocation in the home.[79, 80] They tend to prioritise children first, husband/partners next and themselves last. Even when men participate more in provisioning of food, this female role emerges as significant for resource allocation. Roles and power relations are different when eating out of the home and, as the world urbanises, family patterns alter and challenge these roles.[81] These changes suggest that, if there is to be a shift towards sustainable diets, women and mothers are likely to be highly significant leaders. The appeal to responsibility for young people's dietary future may be contested.[82] Proponents of sustainable diets will almost certainly have either to subvert or counteract the power of marketing, which tries to use children and young people as pressures on parents to buy particular, mostly unhealthy, foods.

### Physical and social environment

Research into the immediate environmental (i.e., locational) influences on diet has been primarily concerned with physical access to, and availability of, food and drink. This relates to the physical location of food outlets, including their relative accessibility by public transport or on foot. It also relates to whether outlets that are physically accessible provide a range of healthy and affordable foods. Work is now needed to test availability of sustainable diets. Meanwhile, studies from the USA,[83] Canada and Australia[76] have shown that in many poorer neighbourhoods healthy food is either not available, unacceptable, inaccessible or unaffordable; but this has not been conclusively shown in the UK and New Zealand.[84, 85] In relation to accessibility, two 'natural experiments' evaluating the impact of new large food retail stores in low-income communities have had differing results. One study found positive changes in fruit and vegetable consumption and the other did not.[86, 87] Two further studies conducted in major urban centres in the UK found no independent association between the food environment (in terms of availability), individual diet and fruit and vegetable consumption.[88, 89] The evidence supporting a relationship between area deprivation and diet is also mixed. For example, one large-scale, cross-sectional, population-based study has shown that residential area deprivation predicts fruit and vegetable consumption independently of individual educational level and occupational social class.[90] However, other evidence indicates a more complex picture. A 2013 qualitative study suggests that the relationship between area deprivation, food environment and dietary intake at an individual level is inconsistent and is influenced by multiple interrelated social, economic and cultural factors.[91]

### Hunger amid affluence

While the vast majority of serious malnutrition occurs in low-income countries, there is a persistent problem of poor diets among people on low incomes in affluent societies.[92] There has been a growth of food welfare systems of the type that post-Second World War policy makers hoped would be banished by economic growth: charity food banks, soup kitchens, hand-outs. Food welfare schemes have proliferated, encouraged by attacks on 'state hand-outs' and the denigration of welfare. Long policy traditions of distinguishing between the worthy and unworthy recipients of welfare have been reinvented, as have old policy arguments about whether it is more 'efficient' to give food welfare as 'cash or in kind' (i.e., as food itself).[93, 94] While food charity serves as a moral safety valve, allowing us to feel good about what we do, it leaves unaddressed the systemic causes of lack of access to a good diet – low wages, inadequate benefits and unfair income distribution.

Austerity cuts have led to the proliferation of food banks in the United States and Canada and, more recently, in other rich countries including the UK. Food banks have become institutionalised in the USA where public assistance programmes as a response to poverty have been historically preferred to income transfers as in Europe. Some countries see food poverty as the primary responsibility of charity and not the moral, legal and political obligation of the state. Surplus food within Western supply chains is creating new markets for manufacturing and retail actors to direct surplus food to food banks (and sometimes win tax credits when doing so). There are moral questions here. If people's incomes are too low to access a good diet, is it right that they edge towards the humiliation and stigma of hand-outs?[95] The counter-argument is that it is also immoral to perpetuate waste in the food so why not redirect surpluses or food approaching 'sell by' dates to the poor? This rise of food banks and food distribution schemes enables government to downplay its responsibilities for income poverty and the right to food.[94, 96] A 2015 Fabian Society report recommended British food banks and other forms of food charity, which rose rapidly in the Great Recession, should be phased out by 2020, and that the real goal ought to be for all citizens to have access to healthy sustainable food they can afford.[97] That and other reports reiterate an older analysis that decent work is the best way of achieving food security and that welfare should aim to be a last resort and short in duration.[98–100]

## Human right to food: could sustainable diets fit in?

Food has been recognised as a basic human need since the 1948 Universal Declaration of Human Rights,[101] and as a fundamental human right and a legal entitlement.[95] It is a core element of the International Covenant on Economic, Social and Cultural Rights,[102] ratified by some governments but not the USA. Government is the primary duty bearer for realising the right to food and, under international law, is accountable for achieving national food security – for ensuring not only a nation's food supply but access to it, especially for at-risk social groups. Though food is produced and distributed as a market commodity, some argue that it is a 'public good' to which all have a rightful claim. In 1999 the United Nations Committee on Economic, Social and Cultural Rights stated that the right to food is fully realised only when all have physical and economic access at all times to adequate food or the means for its procurement.[103, 104]

The 'right to food' continues to be fought over in law and in politics.[95] Could sustainable diets be incorporated into this debate? Might it be a UN-recognised social right that ideal diets are low carbon and socially appropriate as well as affordable? If it was, it would obligate governments and other actors to respect, protect and fulfil the right to a sustainable diet, and for the social dimension to have this legal basis. This might seem ambitious but so, too, were the aspirations of the UN Declaration.

## Cultural appropriateness

What is deemed a culturally appropriate diet will vary in detail and meaning, if not in overall principle, across different cultures. Cultural appropriateness lies not simply in the meal or an item of food but an amalgamation of all the rules, habits, meanings, rituals and practices in their production and consumption.[105] Context can be key; the same food, eaten with different people, in a different place and a different time, may hold an entirely different cultural meaning and connotation. Culturally appropriate food is not only a matter of what we eat but about how and with whom we eat. In addition, culturally appropriate food is not simply about eating the foods traditionally consumed in one's country of origin; it is a meaningful experience that cannot be easily replicated or articulated artificially. Food that is understood as nutritious for one group may be inappropriate or taboo for others. For example, insects are eaten across many cultures of the world but Westernised urban populations generally do not eat them, although there is a view that insects may become more common fare in the future and are already being industrialised in Europe for animal feed.[106] Culture, in general, is complex and fluid; culturally appropriate foods are continuously changing based on context and understanding.

Like everything discussed in this chapter, notions of cultural appropriateness are in flux. Simple diets have become more complex; everyday assumptions of what is desirable can change. Meals eaten in the home are replaced by eating more frequently out of the home and on the street. Markets are replaced by supermarkets and, instead of walking to shop, food purchasing is a car trip to the store. Food and eating have shifted from a shared (if domestically unequal) experience of eating to an individual act of market consumption; the food becomes an object not just an experience.[105] Its authenticity changes. 'Heritage' brands can be manufactured by clever marketing in years rather than centuries.[107] Regardless of this commodification, people still look for authenticity.

## Pleasure: the subversive element of sustainable diets

It seems obvious that, in an ideal world, food should be a source of pleasure and a delightful part of life, yet sustainable diets can easily tap into motives that could be interpreted as anti-pleasure – a hair-shirt tendency.[108] Certainly, the rise of phobias, fads and anxieties associated with food suggests a worrying cultural fragmentation, as do movements for 'clean eating', mass fears about allergies, neuroses about body shape, bulimia and self-disgust at not looking like celebrity superstars. These are signs of food cultures not at ease with themselves. It would be wrong, as well as counter-productive, to dismiss this as the concerns of the 'worried well'. But care needs to be taken about what these phenomena mean and what causes them. These are more than simply ethical concerns about food production, safety, provenance, quality and security.[109] It can be argued that the pleasure of food has been problematised for centuries.[110] In ancient Greece, for example, the teachings of Epicurus advocated that pleasure is the greatest good, but this was not understood in the modern sense of hedonistic excess, or even guilty pleasure, but rather that the way to attain pleasure was to live modestly and limit one's desires. By Roman times the emphasis had shifted to the role that food played in the care of the individual and how, through fasting and austerity, pleasure could be enhanced, a concept different from the contemporary understanding of moderation that suggests the limitation of pleasure. In Christian times food and appetite became linked with lust and illness with disease, which were considered to be manifestations of evil and sin.[110] Pleasure was to be eliminated altogether and the civilising of appetite emerged as a concern only in the Middle Ages.[111] The current concern about obesity coincided with growing concerns about slimming, the fear of fatness, dietary restraint and the emergence of eating disorders.[109] This is, perhaps, a dichotomised food cultural legacy. Despite, or perhaps because of, these concerns, an appeal to food's sensual pleasure has re-emerged during recent years. Some television cooks and food writers have re-popularised the sensual and even sexual dimension of cooking and eating.[112, 113] This has added an extra complication to culinary skills and the function of TV chefs and the mass-processing of foods.[114, 115]

To the industrial food scientist, the sensory engagement with food's organoleptic properties is seen as an end in itself, be this concerned with the taste, flavour, smell or texture of food. While feeding a household or family is considered to have an oppressive dimension in some feminist narratives,[116, 117] there is also acknowledgement of the pleasure to be gained from feeding others, including cooking for friends. Sharing food either cooked at home or eaten out can produce high social rewards.

A strong social movement championing pleasure through food and tradition emerged with the rise of the Slow Food movement, an antidote to globalisation and culinary homogenisation.[118, 119] However, beyond its alternative political narrative, the Slow Food movement champions the cultural base of the pleasure associated with food. Indeed the key principle of Slow Food is the pleasure to be found in flavours, cuisines and practices of local sustainable food. Pleasure in food and eating is partly derived from a consciousness of the lives and locality from which food comes. Critics counter that high quality sustainably produced food is not distributed equitably and is impossible for mass urban societies. In Italy, where the Slow Food movement originated as an antidote to the rise of 'fast food', it was intended to be an inclusive movement in which people across all social groups would participate.

## Identity

Food makes a significant contribution to both individual and collective identity and can signify national, regional, class, ethnic or religious grouping.[120] First-generation migrants living in a new land often display strong inertia in food habits even when the ingredients for their traditional type of cookery may be difficult to obtain. Second and third generations find assimilation unavoidable but some dishes survive as a link with the past, and opening cafés and restaurants is often the migrant's route to autonomous economic activity. Their food culture is the route to employment. In North America, for example, not only specific foods such as Cornish pasties but, in some cases, whole cuisines, including Italian, Jewish and Mexican, have survived as a source of pride.[121] They are part of the US cultural assimilation through retention of identity. It can also become a parody: the English on holiday seeking fish and chips, Australians hunting for Vegemite on toast in Asia and North Americans searching for burgers. Sometimes, too, migration is an opportunity to shed culinary characteristics perceived as negative; not all identity foods are positive. Crawfish in the US Cajun community, for example, has been a source of shame, a link with poverty.[122]

Nevertheless, since the 1960s, consciousness about the importance of ethnicity in relation to food has grown. Ethnic minorities see and use culinary roots to celebrate their existence and develop a strong economic presence.[122] Curry, for example, has become one of the UK's favourite dishes.[123]

One of the most striking expressions of identity through food is the love of the Japanese people for rice. Although rice is less dominant in the Japanese diet than it was half a century ago, Japan has held strongly to the view that it remains central to the country's identity. Rice farmers were until recently heavily subsidised and grains from elsewhere excluded by import tariffs. This was not just for economic protection but because the highly urbanised Japanese people value their links with the countryside and the rural way of life is still seen as central to their culture.[122] Rice also has spiritual meaning and is believed to be a medium between earthly and godly realms.

At an individual level, food can be a powerful symbol of who we are.[121] To set yourself apart from others by what you will and will not eat sends powerful social signals.[124] As something that all humans share, food can also be a vehicle for social differentiation. Vegetarian parents, for example, will be familiar with the child who declares that he or she is going to eat meat or vice versa. You identify with others by eating the same things in the same way as they do. To achieve such identification, people will struggle to eat things they loath and avoid perfectly tasty food that is on the forbidden list. In the process of social climbing, for example, people have to learn to like high status foods such as caviar, artichokes, snails and asparagus, and to scorn dumplings, fish and chips and meat and potato pie because they are tainted with lower-class associations. Such status associations will affect the sustainable diet transition. At the same time, the permeability of social and status associations gives grounds for optimism.[122]

## Marketing

Marketing has captured a significant place in both understanding and defining social values on food; it is a major shaper of the social environment of food and diet. US young children see 10–12 food advertisements each day.[125] Coca-Cola, the world's largest brand by value and by sales, is reported as having spent $4 bn on advertising in 2015.[126] This was the same as the WHO's entire two-year budget for 2014–15, and much more than its budget for non-communicable diseases ($0.32 bn) or for promoting health through the life-course ($0.39 bn).[127] Historically, 98% of such advertisements in the USA promoted foods high in salt, fat and sugar.[128] A meta-analysis concluded that food advertising targeted at children does affect their dietary choices.[129] In this respect alone, today's food environment is quite different from that experienced by previous generations. Globally, an extensive variety of food and drink products are now available in most markets, offering palatability, convenience and novelty. In the rich world, but increasingly in poorer countries too, there are too many calories seeking consumers' mouths. One study has suggested that soft drink (cola) companies now target developing country markets where pressures to contain or refute marketing are weaker.[130] 'Buy me, eat me' messages are everywhere in the competition for sales. The 'consciousness industries' compound this by their large investment in marketing, branding and now the virtual media, distorting government health messages and health-related behaviour among citizens.

The food industry's advertising budget is enormous compared to the budgets of government departments. A 2003 report *Broadcasting Bad Health* by the International Association of Consumer Food Organizations (IACFO), a campaign group, found that the food industry's global advertising budget was $40 bn, larger than the gross domestic product (GDP) of 70% of the world's nations.[131] For every dollar spent by the World Health Organization (WHO) on preventing the diseases caused by Western-style diets, more than $500 is spent by the food industry promoting these diets. The US fast-food industry spent more than $4.6 bn in 2012 on TV advertising, radio, magazines, newspapers, outdoor advertising and other media.[132] While TV, magazine and newspaper advertising remains important for the food industry, it worries that consumers are paying less attention to it as it interrupts their lives and as internet advertising grows in importance. In the UK, total advertising expenditure across media was forecast to be £18,517 m in 2014 (up from £17,510 m in 2013), with internet advertising spending amounting to 38.5% of the total and TV advertising 26.8%.[133]

The wide availability and heavy marketing of many food products, and especially those with a high content of fat, sugar and/or salt, challenge efforts to eat healthily and maintain a healthy weight, particularly in children. Public education, for example in schools and on a variety of information channels, cannot effectively or sufficiently alter the mismatch between the food supply, the marketing environment and public health.

Advertising and other forms of food and beverage marketing to children are extensive and excessively associated with high fat, sugar or salt products.[134–137] A 2015 report from the University of Connecticut's Rudd Center for Food Policy and Obesity[138] found that food companies have been increasing their advertising to children for chips and unhealthy snack foods, while marketing of healthier snacks such as yogurt has not kept pace. The majority of snack adverts that pre-school children, school-age children and teenagers saw were for sweet snacks and savoury snacks, and only about a quarter of these snacks were considered healthy by the US Department of Agriculture (USDA) Smart Snacks standards.[139] These standards are based on levels of calories, sodium, fats and sugar in the snack and determine which snacks can be sold in schools. For some of the age groups, advertising of unhealthy snacks increased from 2010 to 2014: marketing of savoury snacks to children increased by 23% and advertising of sweet snacks to youngsters in their teens increased by 17%. Meanwhile, from 2010 to 2014, exposure to advertising of yogurt products, nearly all of which are considered healthy based on the USDA Smart Snacks standards, did not change. The number of adverts for fruits increased between 3.5 and 6 times to the different age groups and the number of adverts for nuts nearly doubled. But even after the increase, marketing for fruits and nuts represented only about 5% of all snack adverts.

Why, if evidence shows that television advertising influences children's food preferences, purchase requests and consumption patterns, is this systematic moulding of food consciousness legal when its effects are so costly?[135, 140] Even a 30-second exposure to an advertisement can significantly influence the food preferences of a young child, even though they may not be able to recognise an advert, particularly in the newer media.[134] Children in the developing world may be particularly vulnerable to food promotion because they are less familiar with advertising. These children are considered to be key entry points for new food products by Western food manufacturers as they are more responsive than their parents and they continue to associate Western brands with desirable lifestyles. A wide range of techniques are used to market products, reaching children in schools, nurseries and supermarkets. The many routes through which messages can be conveyed include: television and the internet using interactive games, blogs, free downloads, SMS texting to children's mobile phones, brand advertising in educational materials.

There is a huge disparity between the proportion of advertisements promoting foods high in fats, sugars and salt and the space these nutrients ought to take if our diets were healthy. Televised food adverts, which encourage viewers to eat the foods promoted for sale, constitute a *de facto* set of dietary endorsements. A US study that compared the nutritional content of food choices endorsed on television during four hours of prime-time viewing in autumn 2004 found that a diet consisting of observed food items would provide 2,560% of the recommended daily servings of sugars, 2,080% of the recommended daily servings for fat, 40% of the recommended daily servings for vegetables, 32% of the recommended daily servings for dairy and 27% of the recommended daily servings for fruits. The same diet would substantially oversupply protein, total fat, saturated fat, cholesterol and sodium, while substantially undersupplying carbohydrates, fibre, vitamins A, E and D, pantothenic acid, iron, phosphorus, calcium, magnesium, copper and potassium. Overall, the food choices endorsed on television failed to meet US nutrition guidelines and would encourage nutritional imbalance.[141] A 2013 review indicated that little progress had been made towards rebalancing the food marketing landscape between 2003 and 2012.[136]

In response to the increasing evidence that advertising of foods and beverages affects children's food choices and food intake, several national governments and many of the world's larger food and beverage manufacturers have acted to restrict the marketing of their products to children or to advertise only 'better for you' products or 'healthier dietary choices' to children. Independent assessment of the impact of these pledges has been difficult due to the different criteria being used in regulatory and self-regulatory regimes. A 2013 systematic review examined the data available on levels of exposure of children to the advertising of less-healthy foods since the introduction of the statutory and voluntary codes. The results indicated a sharp division in the evidence, with scientific, peer-reviewed papers showing that high levels of such advertising of less-healthy foods continue to be found in several different countries worldwide. In contrast, the evidence provided in industry-sponsored reports indicated a remarkably high adherence to voluntary codes.[142] These findings suggest that adherence to voluntary codes may not sufficiently reduce the advertising of foods that undermine healthy diets, or reduce children's exposure to this advertising.

## Labelling, education and information

In theory, in consumer societies, informed choices are and can be made by educated consumers armed with full knowledge of what they buy. This is the market theory. So could sustainable diets be aided simply by better labels and consumer information? Is information deficit and distortion part of the lock-in to unsustainable diets?

Pre-packed foods carry a range of information from lists of ingredients, including allergens, best-before and use-by dates, to nutrition information and health claims. The information that appears on the label depends on a mixture of national food-labelling regulations and voluntary activities. Food labelling, education and information are not politically neutral. In North America, Europe, Australia, New Zealand and increasingly in other countries, debates about the content of food labels in terms of nutritional content, country of origin, fair trade, animal welfare, expiry dates and the presence of allergens and genetically modified ingredients go to the heart of what is meant by a good diet.[143]

Food labelling is not new, of course. In the late nineteenth century, food manufacturers introduced labels on packaged foods to make claims about the qualities of their products, and labels subsequently came under policy scrutiny. Indeed, labels can be thought of as a battle zone in which the concerns, claims and counterclaims of regulators, the food industry, activists and consumers are expressed and contested.[144] In the USA the 1906 Pure Food and Drug Act prohibited food labels from bearing statements that were 'false or misleading in any particular', an injunction that remains central to labelling guidelines round the world as, for example, in the EU regulations on health claims and in the UN's Codex Alimentarius Commission's setting of standards.

There are many types of food labels, from simple symbols to complex ingredient lists, each with differing aims, audiences and histories. They can be positive, as in the case of health claims, or negative as with warning labels. For regulators and consumer groups, labels are seen as a means of increasing transparency, opening up the contexts of food production or the constituents of foods to scrutiny, but the ability of industry actors to adapt labelling systems to their own ends can distort this transparency. Thus, labels have been denounced as misleading, opaque and inadequate.[145] Food industry bodies tend to see labelling regulations as restrictive or burdensome.

Some labelling is mandatory and some voluntary. International non-binding Codex Alimentarius standards suggest eight mandatory labels: the name of the food, the list of ingredients, net contents and drained weight, the name and address of the producer or distributor, the country of origin, lot identification, date marking, storage instructions and instructions for use. As the case of expiry-date labelling illustrates, even mandatory labelling can be the subject of heated debate. When date labels were first introduced, they supported clearly defined lines of traceability and safety devices such as HACCP (Hazard Analysis and Critical Control Point) plans. More recently, however, date labels have become the focus of criticisms about food safety and waste, which have transformed labels from tools of consumer protection to instruments of consumer discipline and criticism.[143] For example, consumers are regularly accused of mistaking 'best before' labels (intended as a marker of food quality) for 'use by' labels (intended as a marker of food safety), and there is further confusion about 'display until' labels (intended for use by retail managers rather than consumers themselves).

Significant variation in labelling systems exists round the world. The form labelling takes reflects the political economy, culture and, often, the ability of powerful interests to adapt labelling systems for their ends. In the EU and the United States, and a number of other countries, basic nutritional back-of-pack (BOP) labels are mandatory, generally in the form of a standardised nutrition box. There has been a rapid spread of mandatory, as opposed to voluntary, nutrition labelling across the world, as consumer and health agencies push for this reform. Figure 5.3 shows the change between 2007 and 2015 in countries where BOP labels were mandatory or voluntary.

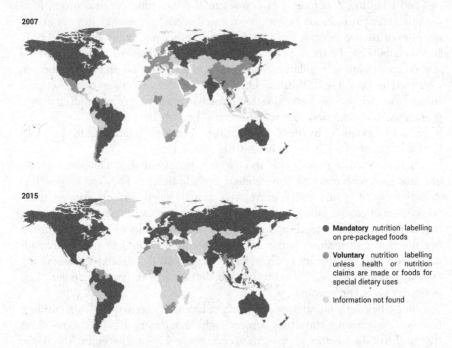

2007

2015

Mandatory nutrition labelling on pre-packaged foods

Voluntary nutrition labelling unless health or nutrition claims are made or foods for special dietary uses

Information not found

*Figure 5.3* The spread of mandatory nutrition labelling, 2007–15

Source: EUFIC.[146]

With rising obesity, however, there are doubts about the ability of labels to communicate sufficient information about food with regard to sustainability. Decades have passed in trying to get effective health labelling. Can climate change or biodiversity loss wait that long? Health campaigners point to the slow advance to achieve front-of-pack (FOP) labelling, presenting consumers with key nutritional features. For example, in 2012 Norway, Sweden and Denmark agreed to use the 20-year-old Swedish keyhole symbol, a logo from a trusted governmental health agency, to encourage healthy choices.[147] In 2006, the UK FSA adopted a colour-based traffic-light system, which highlights total fat, saturated fat, sugar and salt content on the front of the food packages. Similar systems have been proposed in Australia and New Zealand and, in 2010, the US FDA launched a consultation on rationalising FOP labelling. The initial reporting of the FDA consultation supported the UK FSA's argument for the introduction of single standards for labelling. However, in both Europe and the USA, such labelling schemes remain voluntary and their format remains open. In May 2011, Thailand became the first country to introduce mandatory FOP nutrition labels, while South Korea was the first country in Asia to press ahead with voluntary traffic-light labels on children's food.

Recognising that food labelling policy is highly complex, in 2013 the Australian Government Department of Health introduced a conceptual framework to provide a principles-based approach for decision-making regarding food labelling regulation.[148] The framework is underpinned by a risk-based issues hierarchy that is to be applied in the development of food-labelling policy. Within this framework (see Figure 5.4) food-labelling policy is to be guided by a three-tier issues hierarchy in descending order of food safety, preventative health and consumer values issues, including animal welfare, GM, fair trade, and so on, all of which can change with time. Food safety would include direct, acute, immediate threats to health. It particularly relates to poisoning and communicable diseases. Labelling in relation to food safety should primarily be initiated by government. Preventative health includes the indirect, long-term impacts on health and particularly includes chronic disease. Labelling in relation to preventative health may be initiated by government, or in tandem with stakeholders, including industry. The suggestion is that the level of intervention will be informed by governments' health priorities, public health research and the effectiveness or otherwise of co-regulatory measures. Consumer values reflect consumer perceptions and ethical values. Labelling in relation to consumer values should, according to this Australian framework, generally be initiated by industry in response to consumer demand, with the possibility of some specific methods or processes of production being referenced in regulation, where this is justified.

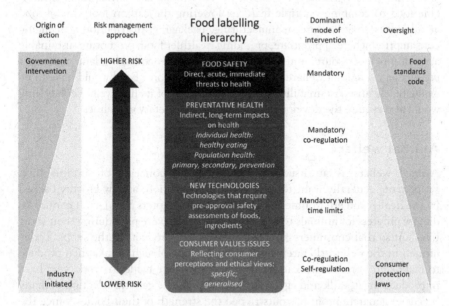

*Figure 5.4* Food labelling policy conceptual framework and issues hierarchy

Source: Blewett, 2011.[149]

With regard to sustainable diets, there is international experience, if not of fully formed multi-criteria sustainable diet labels, then of at least some constituent elements. The German Council of Sustainable Development, for example, encourages consumers to use logo and assurance schemes to favour organic produce or sustainably sourced seafood (see Chapter 8). There is a range of such voluntary labels related to various ethical, environmental and quality issues around food, responding to different pressures: fair trade, animal welfare, organics and marine conservation. These reflect the effectiveness of alternative food movements, and enable market differentiation. But full sustainable diet labelling requires more information and more institutional backing.

One possibility is to carbon label foods. This approach received some attention in the late 2000s. The UK Government-backed Carbon Trust, for example, helped industry develop carbon footprint labels. The British retailer Tesco stated that it would eventually put carbon labels on all of its 70,000 products but, by 2012, it dropped its pledge, citing the amount of work and the fact that other retailers were not following its lead.[150]

The viability of food eco-labelling has been explored across Europe at various levels, including the industry-led EU Sustainable Consumption and Production Food Round Table[151] and through the EU Ecolabel,[152] which does not, at the time of writing, cover food. Research from the Vermont School of Law in the USA has also considered the merits of developing a national ecolabel.[153] An ecolabel would go beyond, for example, existing organic, carbon footprint and country of origin labelling, and embrace the broader principles of sustainable food to combine multiple features: lowering the carbon footprint of food at all stages – agriculture, manufacturing, packaging, distribution – reducing consumption where appropriate, providing healthier food, promoting sustainable agriculture (less resource intensive, less polluting), encouraging land and water use efficiency, animal welfare and fair labour conditions. Food would have to be evaluated against sustainability criteria at all stages of its life-cycle. Ecolabelling would also require the development of sustainable dietary guidelines.

## Animal welfare

Animal welfare is an issue often included in concepts of sustainability. Proponents generally want to see less meat production, a view broadly backed by the health and environmental evidence (see Chapters 3 and 4). It cannot be dietary progress for animals to suffer discomfort or severe pain during their short lives just so that consumers can buy cheap animal products in the shops. Today farmers in the rich world rarely use oxen to pull the plough or take their produce to market in horse-drawn carts, but farm animals are made to 'work' very hard to produce meat, milk and eggs, not least because the genetic selection of many breeds to generate profit has outstripped the strength of their bodies. Since the 1950s, animal farming in the European Union and North America has been affected by intensive livestock production, a system of rearing animals that uses intensive production-line methods that aim to maximise the amount of meat, milk and eggs while minimising costs; this method of animal farming is becoming increasingly widespread in developing countries too.

Increasing output is a way to increase farming income or, more accurately, to try to maintain farmer income. Actually farm incomes are squeezed. In the UK the productivity of dairy cows multiplied by two and a half, from an average of 2,800 litres in 1950 to 7,000 litres in 2010.[154] The number of dairy cattle per farm has also risen from 17 to 125 over the same period and dairy farms are producing 18 times as much milk as they were in the 1950s. Selective breeding has contributed, as has the feeding of concentrates and, in some countries, the injection of bovine somatotropin (BST). However, the animal's body may be reaching the end of its biological capacity, beyond which its welfare could be threatened. Increased risk of disease such as mastitis, anaemia and lameness, where the animal's hind legs cannot bear the pressure of the enlarged udder, is a problem.[122] While the natural lifespan of a cow is about 20 years, it is today quite common for them to be sent to slaughter at six or seven years, either because their yield is no longer adequate or they are worn out. Similarly with broiler (purpose-grown meat) chickens: in the EU the industry produces approximately 6 bn broilers each year, of which approximately 890 m are produced in the UK.[155] In the UK, the bulk of the chicken-meat production comes from flocks of more than 100,000 birds that are kept in large dimly lit sheds and are fed and watered automatically. The broiler has been specially bred to put on weight quickly. What used to take 60 days in the 1960s for a bird to reach market weight now takes about 34 days.[156] This places great strain on the birds' legs, and during the last one to two weeks of the fattening period the birds may have bone deformities that hamper their ability to walk and cause chronic pain. Turkeys are subject to the same deformities if intensively farmed. This may affect the quality of the meat for the consumer and certainly can cause suffering for the birds (see below).

In some countries campaigns against such methods have influenced public opinion and government agencies. Animal welfare may be considered according to the framework of the so-called 'Five Freedoms', i.e., freedom from hunger, thirst and malnutrition; freedom from discomfort; freedom from pain, injury and disease; freedom to express normal behaviour; freedom from fear and distress (see Chapter 2).[157] The EU banned battery cages for egg-laying hens from 2012.[158] Battery production continues in the USA where improvements in animal welfare have appeared more slowly. In Australia, too, the majority of egg-laying hens are intensively reared, and each hen may be allocated space less than the size of an A4/foolscap-sized sheet of paper, which is insufficient room to act on natural instincts such as dust bathing, foraging and wing flapping.[159] Similarly with pigs, the average intensively reared sow produced 23 weaned piglets a year, a considerable strain for some animals.[122] Sows are tethered in stalls such that they cannot turn round. The UK was the first nation to ban tethering and sow stalls in 1999 while, in the EU, tethering has been banned since 2006 and sow stalls since 2013.[160] Cruelty is also alleged in relation to how animals are slaughtered.

This is socially delicate as some religions have clear rules about methods. The profitability of abattoirs is, to a certain extent, a function of the speed of killing and corners on animal welfare may be cut.

Intensive farming may also be harmful to human health. Animals in cramped conditions easily catch and transmit diseases, which may then be passed to humans. Dirty conditions of production can lead to the infection of eggs with salmonella. Farmers routinely using antibiotics in animals may be contributing to antibiotic resistance in humans (see Chapter 3). The usual argument for the continuation of intensive livestock farming is that these methods of production are the only means of ensuring cheap animal food. However, the 'true cost' of the meat in terms of animal disease and human health is not paid by the consumer at the till but elsewhere. Environmental costs are also high; industrial farming units are heavy polluters and can make massive demands on land and water (see Chapter 4). In addition, increasing production beyond demand, which is the current case with milk on the world market, may maintain cheap prices for consumers but depresses prices for producers, such that the livelihoods of small-scale farmers in particular are undermined as they are unable to benefit from the economies of scale derived by the larger intensive farm units. Moreover, the conversion of crops into animal food, meat in particular, is a nutritionally inefficient (see Chapter 3) and costly way of feeding rapidly increasing populations when a proportion of the grain, legumes and oil seed could be fed directly to humans. For people in rich countries, as well as wealthy people in poorer countries who are increasing meat consumption, the best way of helping to improve animal welfare may be to reduce the numbers of farm livestock, farm less intensively and for the consumer to eat less meat of higher quality.

## Fair trade

All diets should be 'fair' in terms of accessibility and affordability for everyone while providing fair prices to food producers. Food producers in poor rural economies, which are found mainly in poor countries but also in richer countries, are often jeopardised by constraints on the opportunity to produce through restricted access to the resources – such as land and capital – needed to farm, and on the opportunity to sell, through restricted access to local and global markets, so they need support to be able to produce and sell their produce.

Fair trade provides one model for providing this support; giving producers a fairer return, investing in community development and enhancing environmental integrity. The fair trade mark is specific to commodities traded internationally, such as coffee, tea, chocolate and cotton. Fair trade fosters the re-embedding of international commodity production and distribution in 'equitable social relations', with the aim of developing a more stable and advantageous system of trade for agricultural and non-agriculture goods produced under more favourable social conditions.[161] The overall goal of fair trade and other alternative trade initiatives is to question and counter the organisation of trade around abstract market principles that devalue and exploit poor people, particularly in poorer regions of the global south.

Fair trade is not without its challenges. A review of research into the impact of fair trade found strong evidence of positive empowerment effects, including improved self-confidence and self-esteem, greater access to training and improved market and export knowledge – in addition to positive effects such as increased democracy and levels of participation.[162] However, a study of Kenyan fair trade tea production, reported in a 2014 Food Ethics Council report, found that, while some producers did experience empowerment effects through fair trade, the exclusion that some groups had experienced prior to the introduction of fair trade certification persisted. Women were under-represented on fair trade-related boards and committees, and voting for the Social Premium Committee was restricted to registered farmers, fewer than 20% of whom are women. This restriction also meant that landless people continued to be excluded from decision-making.[163] A 2014 report by the UK School of Oriental and African Studies (SOAS) that looked at fair trade production in Ethiopia and Uganda found no difference in working conditions between fair trade and non-fair trade producers and no improvement in wages for waged workers.[164] The SOAS report made various recommendations, suggesting that fair trade could be improved by, for example, the promotion of independent trade unions and the reduction in gender-based wage discrimination.

## Conclusions

The chapter has suggested the complex ways in which there are social and cultural threads running through the search for sustainable diets. As with other chapters, we find that the 'social' is in fact a complex bundle of factors, but it is possible to identify and clarify them. The chapter has shown that the social dimension to sustainable diets is important. A culturally appropriate diet must be available and accessible to everyone. Everyone needs access to a decent living and/or land to produce acceptable food. Social movements such as for fair trade, animal welfare and workers' rights are refining what the 'social' element in diet is. The distortion of knowledge about production processes and the limits of information transfer to consumers undermines the neoliberal belief that markets are driven by 'informed consumers'. Serious inequalities in society shape what and how people eat. If there are limits to how much we really choose our diets, this chapter reinforces again a central message of the book that we need to think more seriously about how to engineer systemic change, and not leave the transition to sustainable diets to individual choice. Consumers need help in this cultural transition.

## References

1 Johnston JL, Fanzo JC, Cogill B. Understanding sustainable diets: a descriptive analysis of the determinants and processes that influence diets and their impact on health, food security, and environmental sustainability. *Advances in Nutrition*, 2014; 5: 418–29

2 Maddox K. Global ad spending will be up an average 4.2% next year – automotive, food and wireless will be top spenders, Schonfeld reports. *AdvertisingAge*. Available at: http://adage.com/article/btob/global-ad-spending-average-4-2-year/298980/ (accessed August 10, 2016), 2015

3 Bernhardt AM, Wilking C, Adachi-Mejia AM, *et al.* How television fast food marketing aimed at children compares with adult advertisements. *PLoS ONE*, 2013; 8(8): e7247

4 Fishbein M, Ajzen I. *Belief, Attitude, Intention, and Behavior: An Introduction to Theory and Research*. Reading, MA: Addison-Wesley, 1975

5 Ajzen I, Fishbein M. *Understanding Attitudes and Predicting Social Behavior*. Englewood Cliffs, NJ: Prentice-Hall, 1980

6 Goffman E. The characteristics of total institutions. Paper to Symposium on Preventive and Social Psychiatry, 15–17 April 1957, Walter Reed Army Institute of Research, Washington, DC, in: E Goffman, *Asylums: Essays on the Social Situation of Mental Patients and Other Inmates*. New York: Anchor Books, 1961

7 Taylor I, Walton P, Young J. *The New Criminology*. London: Routledge, 1973

8 Mandela N. *Long Walk to Freedom: The Autobiography of Nelson Mandela*. London: Little, Brown and Company, 1995

9 Cohen MJ. Is the UK preparing for 'war'? Military metaphors, personal carbon allowances, and consumption rationing in historical perspective. *Climatic Change*, 2011; 104(2): 199–222

10 Minns R. *Bombers and Mash: The Domestic Front 1939–1945*. London: Virago, 1980

11 Fabian Commission on Food and Poverty. *A Recipe for Inequality: Why Our Food System Is Leaving Low-Income Households Behind*. London: Fabian Society, 2015

12 Alesina A, Di Tella R, MacCulloch R. Inequality and happiness: are Europeans and Americans different? *Journal of Public Economics*, 2004; 88(9–10): 2009–42

13 Belfield C, Cribb J, Hood A, *et al. Living Standards, Poverty and Inequality in the UK: 2015*. London: Institute of Fiscal Studies, 2015

14 Ostry JD, Berg A, Tsangarides CG. *Redistribution, Inequality, and Growth*. Washington, DC: International Monetary Fund, 2014

15 Wilkinson RG, Pickett K. *The Spirit Level: Why More Equal Societies Almost Always Do Better*. London: Allen Lane, 2009

16 Helliwell J, Layard R, Sachs J. *World Happiness Report 2016 (Update, Volume 1)*. New York: Sustainable Development Solutions Network, 2016

17 Dowler E. Food poverty and food policy. *IDS Bulletin: Poverty and Social Exclusion in North and South*, 1998; 29(1): 58–65

18 Shaw D, Carrington M, Chatzidakis A (Eds). *Ethics and Morality in Consumption: Interdisciplinary Perspectives*. Abingdon: Routledge Studies in Business Ethics, 2016

19 Lamb H. *Fighting the Banana Wars and Other Fairtrade Battles*. London: Rider/Ebury, 2008

20 ETI. *Ethical Trade Initiative: About Us*. Available at: www.ethicaltrade.org/ (accessed August 30, 2015). London: Ethical Trade Initiative, 2015

21 Gough K. New proposals for anthropologists. *Current Anthropology*, 1968; 9(5): 403–7

22 Evans-Pritchard EE. *The Nuer: A Description of the Modes of Livelihood and Political Institutions of a Nilotic People*. Oxford: Clarendon Press, 1940

23 Douglas M. Deciphering a meal. *Daedalus*, 1972; 101: 61–82

24 Charles N, Kerr M. *Women, Food and Families*. Manchester: Manchester University Press, 1988

25 Mennell S, Murcott A, Otterloo AHv, *et al. The Sociology of Food: Eating, Diet and Culture*. London: Sage, 1992

26 Mintz SW, Du Bois CM. The anthropology of food and eating. *Annual Review of Anthropology*, 2002; 31: 99–119

27 Shanker D. 27 healthy versions of your kids' favorite foods. *Buzzfeed*. Available at: www.buzzfeed.com/deenashanker/healthy-versions-of-foods-your-kids-love?utm_term=.ikd0PRx4W#.esMeQPEAz (accessed August 10, 2016), 2014

28 Pollan M. *Food Rules: An Eater's Manual*. London: Penguin, 2010

29 National Food Administration, Environment Agency. *Environmentally Effective Food Choices: Proposal Notified to the EU*. Stockholm: National Food Administration, 2008

30 Pennell M. Community food literacies: an introduction. *Community Literacy Journal*, 2015; 10(1): 1–3

31 Vidgen H (Ed.). *Food Literacy: Key Concepts for Health and Education*. Abingdon: Routledge, 2016

32 Dowler E, Caraher M, Lincoln P. Inequalities in food and nutrition: challenging 'lifestyle', in: E Dowler and N Spence (Eds) *Challenging Health Inequalities: From 'Acheson' to Choosing Health*. Bristol, UK: Policy Press, 127–57, 2007

33 Gillespie AMH, Johnson-Askew WL. Changing family food and eating practices: the family food decision-making system. *Annals of Behavioral Medicine*, 2009; 38(Supplement 1): S31–6

34 Darmon N, Drewnowski A. Does social class predict diet quality? *The American Journal of Clinical Nutrition*, 2008; 87(5): 1107–17

35 Lallukka T, Laaksonen M, Rahkonen O, et al. Multiple socio-economic circumstances and healthy food habits. *European Journal of Clinical Nutrition*, 2007; 61(6): 701–10

36 Boylan S, Lallukka T, Lahelma E, et al. Socio-economic circumstances and food habits in Eastern, Central and Western European populations. *Public Health Nutrition*, 2011; 14(4): 678–87

37 Monsivais P, Aggarwal A, Drewnowski A. Are socio-economic disparities in diet quality explained by diet cost? *Journal of Epidemiology and Community Health*, 2012; 66(6): 530–5

38 Maguire ER, Monsivais P. Socio-economic dietary inequalities in UK adults: an updated picture of key food groups and nutrients from national surveillance data. *The British Journal of Nutrition*, 2014; 113(1): 1–9

39 Barton KL, Wrieden WL, Sherriff A, et al. Trends in socio-economic inequalities in the Scottish diet: 2001–2009. *Public Health Nutrition*, 2015; 18(16): 2970–80

40 van Lenthe FJ, Jansen T, Kamphuis CB. Understanding socio-economic inequalities in food choice behaviour: can Maslow's pyramid help? *The British Journal of Nutrition*, 2015; 113(7): 1139–47

41 Niven P, Scully M, Morley B, et al. Socio-economic disparities in Australian adolescents' eating behaviours. *Public Health Nutrition*, 2014; 17(12): 2753–8

42 Ward PR, Verity F, Carter P, et al. Food stress in Adelaide: the relationship between low income and the affordability of healthy food. *Journal of Environmental and Public Health*, 2013; (1): 1–10, 968078

43 Mayen AL, Marques-Vidal P, Paccaud F, et al. Socioeconomic determinants of dietary patterns in low- and middle-income countries: a systematic review. *The American Journal of Clinical Nutrition*, 2014; 100(6): 1520–31

44 Hong R, Banta JE, Betancourt JA. Relationship between household wealth inequality and chronic childhood under-nutrition in Bangladesh. *International Journal for Equity in Health*, 2006; 5: 15

45 Hong R, Mishra V. Effect of wealth inequality on chronic under-nutrition in Cambodian children. *Journal of Health, Population, and Nutrition*, 2006; 24(1): 89–99

46 Hong R. Effect of economic inequality on chronic childhood undernutrition in Ghana. *Public Health Nutrition*, 2007; 10(4): 371–8

47 Roos G, Johansson L, Kasmel A, *et al.* Disparities in vegetable and fruit consumption: European cases from the north to the south. *Public Health Nutrition*, 2001; 4(1): 35–43

48 Dowler E. Inequalities in diet and physical activity in Europe. *Public Health Nutrition*, 2001; 4(2b): 701–9

49 Crotty P, Germov J. Food and class, in: J Germov and I Williams (Eds) *A Sociology of Food and Nutrition: The Social Appetite* (2nd Ed.). Victoria: Oxford University Press, 241–62, 2004

50 Levay AV, Mumtaz Z, Rashid SF, *et al.* Influence of gender roles and rising food prices on poor, pregnant women's eating and food provisioning practices in Dhaka, Bangladesh. *Reproductive Health*, 2013; 10(53)

51 Nelson M, Ehrens B, Bates B, *et al. Low Income Diet and Nutrition Survey: Key Findings.* A survey carried out on behalf of the Food Standards Agency. Available at: http://tna.europarchive.org/20110116113217/http://www.food.gov.uk/multimedia/pdfs/lidnssummary.pdf (accessed August 6, 2015). London: The Stationery Office, 2007

52 Dietary Guidelines Advisory Committee. *Scientific Report of the 2015 Dietary Guidelines Advisory Committee.* Washington, DC: USDA and US Department of Health and Human Services, 2015

53 Wrieden W. *Is the Scotish Diet Getting Any Better?* Presentation at ESRC Seminar Series, The Politics of Food and Nutrition: Resilience, Security and Justice in a Global Context, Edinburgh, 4th February. Available at: http://foodresearch.org.uk/the-politics-of-food-and-nutrition/#wendy-wrieden-human-nutrition-research-centre-newcastle-university (accessed August 6, 2015). London: Food Research Collaboration, 2015

54 Du S, Mroz TA, Zhai F, *et al.* Rapid income growth adversely affects diet quality in China – particularly for the poor! *Social Science & Medicine*, (1982) 2004; 59(7): 1505–15

55 Shi Z, Lien N, Kumar BN, *et al.* Socio-demographic differences in food habits and preferences of school adolescents in Jiangsu Province, China. *European Journal of Clinical Nutrition*, 2005; 59(12): 1439–48

56 Sobal J, Stunkard AJ. Socioeconomic status and obesity: a review of the literature. *Psychological Bulletin*, 1989; 105(2): 260–75

57 McLaren L. Socioeconomic status and obesity. *Epidemiologic Reviews*, 2007; 29: 29–48

58 Monteiro CA, Moura EC, Conde WL, *et al.* Socioeconomic status and obesity in adult populations of developing countries: a review. *Bulletin of the World Health Organization*, 2004; 82(12): 940–6

59 Neuman M, Finlay JE, Davey Smith G, *et al.* The poor stay thinner: stable socioeconomic gradients in BMI among women in lower- and middle-income countries. *The American Journal of Clinical Nutrition*, 2011; 94(5): 1348–57

60 Subramanian SV, Perkins JM, Ozaltin E, *et al.* Weight of nations: a socioeconomic analysis of women in low- to middle-income countries. *The American Journal of Clinical Nutrition*, 2011; 93(2): 413–21

61 Dinsa GD, Goryakin Y, Fumagalli E, *et al.* Obesity and socioeconomic status in developing countries: a systematic review. *Obesity Reviews*, 2012; 13(11): 1067–79

62 Monteiro CA, Conde WL, Lu B, *et al.* Obesity and inequities in health in the developing world. *International Journal of Obesity and Related Metabolic Disorders*, 2004; 28(9): 1181–6

63 Caraher M, Dowler E. Food for poorer people: conventional and 'alternative' transgressions, in: MK Goodman, C Sage *Food Transgressions: Making Sense of Food Politics*. Abingdon, UK: Ashgate (Routledge), 2014, 228–46

64 Caraher M. *Food Poverty and Inequality: The Growth of Hunger in the UK*. Available at: www.city.ac.uk/events/2010/may/food-poverty-and-inequality-the-growth-of-hunger-in-the-uk-a-lecture-by-martin-caraher (accessed January 19, 2012). London: City University, 2010

65 Caraher M, Baker H, Burns M. Children's views of cooking and food preparation. *British Food Journal*, 2004; 106(4): 255–73

66 Lang T, Caraher M. Is there a culinary skills transition? Data and debate from the UK about changes in cooking culture. *Journal of the Home Economics*, Institute of Australia, 2001; 8(2): 2–14

67 Short F. *Kitchen Secrets: The Meaning of Cooking in Everyday Life*. Oxford: Berg, 2006

68 Gatley A, Caraher M, Lang T. A qualitative, cross cultural examination of attitudes and behaviour in relation to cooking habits in France and Britain. *Appetite*, 2014; 75: 71–81

69 Lang T, Heasman M. *Food Wars: The Global Battle for Mouths, Minds and Markets*, (2nd Ed.). Abingdon: Routledge Earthscan, 2015

70 Lang T, Dowler E, Hunter DJ. *Review of the Scottish Diet Action Plan: Progress and Impacts 1996–2005*. Edinburgh: NHS Health Scotland, 2006

71 Hawkes C. Uneven dietary development: linking the policies and processes of globalization with the nutrition transition, obesity and diet-related chronic diseases. *Globalization and Health*, 2006; 2(4), doi:10.1186/744-8603-2-4

72 Pinstrup-Andersen P, Cheng F. *Case Studies in Food Policy for Developing Countries: Domestic Policies for Production, Markets, and Environment*. Ithaca, NY: Cornell University Press, 2009

73 Fanzo J, Hunter D, Borelli T, *et al.* (Eds). *Diversifying Food and Diets: Using Agricultural Biodiversity to Improve Nutrition and Health*. Abingdon: Routledge/Earthscan, 2013

74 Darmon N, Drewnowski A. Contribution of food prices and diet cost to socio-economic disparities in diet quality and health: a systematic review and analysis. *Nutrition Reviews*, 2015; 73(10): 643–60

75 Ward PR, Verity F, Carter P, *et al.* Food stress in Adelaide: the relationship between low income and the affordability of healthy food. *Journal of Environmental and Public Health*, 2013; 2013: 10

76 Barosh L, Friel S, Engelhardt K, *et al.* The cost of a healthy and sustainable diet – who can afford it? *Australian and New Zealand Journal of Public Health*, 2014; 38(1): 7–12

77 Wiggins S, Keats S, Shimokawa S, *et al.* *The Rising Cost of a Healthy Diet*. Available at: www.odi.org/rising-cost-healthy-diet (accessed October 19, 2015). London: The Overseas Development Institute, 2015

78 Jones NRV, Conklin AI, Suhrcke M, *et al.* The growing price gap between more and less healthy foods: analysis of a novel longitudinal UK dataset. *PLoS ONE*, 2014; 9(10): e109343

79 Savage JS, Fisher JO, Birch LL. Parental influence on eating behavior: conception to adolescence. *Journal of Law, Medicine & Ethics*, 2007; 35(1): 22–34

80  WHO. *Health Nutrition: The Role of Women.* Report of a WHO meeting, Murmansk, June 14–15. Copenhagen: World Health Organization Regional Office for Europe, 2000

81  Wang MC, Naidoo N, Ferzacca S, *et al.* The role of women in food provision and food choice decision-making in Singapore: a case study. *Ecology of Food and Nutrition,* 2014; 53(6): 658–77

82  Lindsay J, Maher J. *Consuming Families: Buying, Making, Producing Family Life in the 21st Century.* Abingdon: Routledge, 2013

83  Walker RE, Keane CR, Burke JG. Disparities and access to healthy food in the United States: a review of food deserts literature. *Health & Place,* 2010; 16(5): 876–84

84  Caspi CE, Sorensen G, Subramanian SV, *et al.* The local food environment and diet: a systematic review. *Health & Place,* 2012; 18(5): 1172–87

85  Cummins S, Macintyre S. 'Food deserts' – evidence and assumption in health policy making. *BMJ (Clinical Research Ed.),* 2002; 325(7361): 436–8

86  Wrigley N, Warm D, Margetts B. Deprivation, diet, and food-retail access: findings from the Leeds 'food deserts' study. *Environment and Planning A,* 2003; 35(1): 151–88

87  Cummins S, Petticrew M, Higgins C, *et al.* Large scale food retailing as an intervention for diet and health: quasi-experimental evaluation of a natural experiment. *Journal of Epidemiology and Community Health,* 2005; 59(12): 1035–40

88  White M, Bunting J, Williams L, *et al. Do Food Deserts Exist? A Multi-level, Geographical Analysis of the Relationship Between Retail Food Access, Socio-economic Position and Dietary Intake.* London: Food Standards Authority, 2004

89  Pearson T, Russell J, Campbell MJ, *et al.* Do 'food deserts' influence fruit and vegetable consumption? A cross-sectional study. *Appetite,* 2005; 45(2): 195–7

90  Shohaimi S, Welch A, Bingham S, *et al.* Residential area deprivation predicts fruit and vegetable consumption independently of individual educational level and occupational social class: a cross sectional population study in the Norfolk cohort of the European Prospective Investigation into Cancer (EPIC-Norfolk). *Journal of Epidemiology and Community Health,* 2004; 58(8): 686–91

91  Thompson C, Cummins S, Brown T, *et al.* Understanding interactions with the food environment: an exploration of supermarket food shopping routines in deprived neighbourhoods. *Health & Place,* 2013; 19: 116–23

92  Riches G, Silvasti T. *First World Hunger Revisited: Food Charity or the Right to Food?* London: Palgrave Macmillan, 2014

93  Caraher M and Coveney J (Eds) *Food Poverty and Insecurity: International Food Inequalities.* Cham, Switzerland: Springer, 2015

94  Poppendieck J. *Sweet Charity? Emergency Food and the End of Entitlement.* London: Penguin, 1999

95  Riches G. Surplus food or the right to food. Available at: http://thirdforcenews.org.uk/blogs/surplus-food-or-the-right-to-food (accessed October 21, 2015). *Third Force News,* 2015

96  MacLeod M. *Making the Connections: A Study of Emergency Food Aid in Scotland.* Glasgow: Poverty Alliance, 2015

97  Tait C. *Hungry for Change.* The final report of the Fabian Commission on Food and Poverty. Available at: www.fabians.org.uk/publications/hungry-for-change/ (accessed November 2, 2015). London: Fabian Society, 2015

98  Freudenberg N, Silver M. *Jobs for a Healthier Diet and a Stronger Economy. Opportunities for Creating New Good Food Jobs in New York City.* New York: Food Policy Center Hunter College and City University of New York School of Public Health, 2013: 49

99 Titmuss RM. *Commitment to Welfare*. London: Unwin University Books, 1968

100 Boyd Orr SJ. *Food and the People. Target for Tomorrow No 3*. London: Pilot Press, 1943

101 UN. *Universal Declaration of Human Rights*. Adopted and proclaimed by General Assembly resolution 217 A (III) of 10 December. Geneva: United Nations, 1948

102 United Nations Human Rights Office of the High Commissioner. *International Covenant on Economic, Social and Cultural Rights, 1966*. Available at: www.ohchr.org/EN/ProfessionalInterest/Pages/CESCR.aspx (accessed November 18, 2015), 1966

103 UN Commission on Human Rights. *The Realization of Economic, Social and Cultural Rights: Report Updating the Study on the Right to Food*, prepared by Mr. Asbjørn Eide, Commission on Human Rights Sub-Commission on Prevention of Discrimination and Protection of Minorities, fiftieth session, item 4 of the provisional agenda, E/CN.4/Sub.2/1998/9, 29 June. New York: UN Commission on Human Rights Sub-Commission on Prevention of Discrimination and Protection of Minorities, 1998

104 UN Economic and Social Council. *General Comment No. 12: The Right to Adequate Food* (Art. 11 of the Covenant), 12 May. Available at: www.refworld.org/docid/4538838c11.html (accessed October 21, 2015). Geneva: UN Committee on Economic, Social and Cultural Rights (CESCR), 1999

105 Aronson R. *Eating in Crisis: Culturally Appropriate Food and the Local Food Movement in the Lives of Domestic Violence Survivors*. UVM Honors College Senior Theses. Paper 21. University of Vermont ScholarWorks @ UVM, 2014

106 van Huis A, Van Itterbeeck J, Klunder H, *et al*. *Edible Insects: Future Prospects for Food and Feed Security*. FAO Forestry Paper 71. Available at: www.faoorg/docrep/018/i3253e/i3253e00htm (accessed October 13, 2015). Rome: Food and Agricultural Organization, 2013

107 Cavanaugh JR, Shankar S. Producing authenticity in global capitalism: language, materiality, and value. *American Anthropologist*, 2014; 116(1): 51–64

108 Lang T. Sustainable diets: hairshirts or a better food future? *Development*, 2014; 57(4): 240–56

109 Griffiths S, Wallace J. *Consuming Passions: Cooking and Eating in the Age of Anxiety*. Manchester: Manchester University Press, 1998

110 Coveney J. *Food, Morals and Meaning*. Abingdon, Oxon: Routledge, 2000

111 Mennel S, Murcott A, van Otterloo A. *The Sociology of Food, Eating, Diet and Culture* (2nd Ed.). London: Sage, 1992

112 Lawson N. *Feast: Food that Celebrates Life*. London: Chatto and Windus, 2004

113 Lawson N. *How To Eat: The Pleasures and Principles of Good Food*. London: Chatto and Windus, 2014

114 Oliver J. *The Ministry of Food* (TV series and book). London: Channel 4 TV, 2008

115 Oliver J. *Cutting Food Waste: Reclaiming Wonky Veg*. Available at: www.jamieoliver.com/news-and-features/features/reclaiming-wonky-veg/#SiOQ8PtZYCVUpU06.97 (accessed July 30, 2016). London: Jamie Oliver Organisation, 2016

116 Julier A, Lindenfeld L. Mapping men onto the menu: masculinities and food. *Food and Foodways*, 2005; 13(1–2): 1–16

117 Murcott A, Gamarnikow E. 'It's a Pleasure to Cook for Him': *Food, Mealtimes and Gender in Some South Wales Households*. London: Heinemann, 1983

118 Bossy S. Slow food movement. *The Wiley-Blackwell Encyclopedia of Social and Political Movements*. Chichester, UK: Wiley-Blackwell, 2013

119 Andrews G. *The Slow Food Story: Politics and Pleasure*. London: Pluto Press, 2008

120 Caplan P. *Food, Health and Identity*. London: Routledge, 2013

121   Gabaccia DR, Gabaccia DR. *We Are What We Eat: Ethnic Food and the Making of Americans*. Cambridge, MA: Harvard University Press, 2009

122   Atkins P, Bowler I. *Food in Society: Economy, Culture, Geography*. London: Arnold, Hodder Headline Group, 2001

123   Basu S. *Curry: The Story of Britain's Favourite Dish*. Kolkata, India: Rupa Publications, 2011

124   Cooks L. You are what you (don't) eat? Food, identity, and resistance. *Text and Performance Quarterly*, 2009; 29(1): 94–110

125   Powell LM, Schermbeck RM, Szczypka G, *et al*. Trends in the nutritional content of television food advertisements seen by children in the United States: analyses by age, food categories, and companies. *Archives of Pediatric and Adolescent Medicine*, 2011; 165(12): 1078–86

126   The Grocer. World's biggest brand: in 'Grocery's Gold Winner' (annual review). *The Grocer*, 2016: 24–9

127   World Health Organization. *WHO Programme Budget 2014–2015*. Available at: www.who.int/about/resources_planning/PB14-15_en.pdf?ua=1 (accessed August 12, 2016). Geneva: World Health Organization, 2014

128   Powell LM, Szczypka G, Chaloupka FJ, *et al*. Nutritional content of television food advertisements seen by children and adolescents in the United States. *Pediatrics*, 2007; 120(3): 576–83

129   Boyland EJ, Nolan S, Kelly B, *et al*. Advertising as a cue to consume: a systematic review and meta-analysis of the effects of acute exposure to unhealthy food and non-alcoholic beverage advertising on intake in children and adults. *The American Journal of Clinical Nutrition*, 2016; 103(2): 519–33

130   Taylor AL, Jacobson MF. *Carbonating the World: The Marketing and Health Impact of Sugar Drinks in Low- and Middle-Income Countries*. Washington, DC: Center for Science in the Public Interest, 2016

131   Dalmeny K, Hanna E, Lobstein T. *Broadcasting Bad Health: Why Food Marketing to Children Needs to be Controlled*. London: The International Association of Consumer Food Organizations, 2003

132   Rudd Center for Food Policy and Obesity. *Fast Food Marketing Ranking Tables*. Available at: www.fastfoodmarketing.org/media/FastFoodFACTS_Marketing Rankings.pdf (accessed October 21, 2015). Connecticut: Rudd Centre for Food Policy and Obesity, 2014

133   AA/Warc. *Advertising Association Downgrades Forecast and Economic Caution*, 13 January. London: Advertising Association and Warc, 2015

134   Mason P. Marketing to children: implications for obesity. *Nutrition Bulletin*, 2012; 37(1): 86–91

135   Halford JC, Boyland EJ, Hughes G, *et al*. Beyond-brand effect of television (TV) food advertisements/commercials on caloric intake and food choice of 5–7-year-old children. *Appetite*, 2007; 49(1): 263–7

136   Cairns G, Angus K, Hastings G, *et al*. Systematic reviews of the evidence on the nature, extent and effects of food marketing to children: a retrospective summary. *Appetite*, 2013; 62: 209–15

137   Zimmerman FJ, Shimoga SV. The effects of food advertising and cognitive load on food choices. *BMC Public Health*, 2014; 14: 342

138   Harris J, Schwarz M, Sheehan C. Snack FACTS 2015. *Evaluating Snack Food Nutrition and Marketing to Youth*. UConn Rudd Center for Food Policy & Obesity. Available at:

www.uconnruddcenter.org/files/Pdfs/SnackFACTS_2015_Fulldraft02.pdf (accessed November 7, 2015), 2015

139  USDA. *Agriculture Secretary Vilsack Highlights New 'Smart Snacks in School' Standards; Will Ensure School Vending Machines, Snack Bars Include Healthy Choices.* Available at: www.fns.usda.gov/pressrelease/2013/013413 (accessed November 7, 2015). Washington, DC: United States Department of Agriculture, 2013

140  Boyland EJ, Halford JC. Television advertising and branding. Effects on eating behaviour and food preferences in children. *Appetite*, 2013; 62: 236–41

141  Mink M, Evans A, Moore CG, *et al.* Nutritional imbalance endorsed by televised food advertisements. *Journal of the American Dietetic Association*, 2010; 110(6): 904–10

142  Galbraith-Emami S, Lobstein T. The impact of initiatives to limit the advertising of food and beverage products to children: a systematic review. *Obesity Reviews*, 2013; 14(12): 960–74

143  Milne R. Labelling, in: P Jackson and CONANX Group, *Food Words: Essays in Culinary Culture*. London: Bloomsbury, 2013

144  Lang T, Heasman M. *Food Wars: The Global Battle for Mouths, Minds and Markets* (2nd Ed.). Abingdon, Oxon: Earthscan, 2015

145  Lawrence F. *Not on the Label: What Really Goes into the Food on Your Plate*. London: Penguin UK, 2004

146  EUFIC. *Global Update on Nutrition Labelling Executive Summary*. Available at: www.eufic.org/upl/1/default/doc/ExecutiveSummary.pdf (accessed June 20, 2016). Brussels: European Food Information Council, 2016

147  Nordic Council of Ministers. Nordic Nutrition Recommendations: Keyhole Nutrition Label. Available at: www.norden.org/en/theme/nordic-nutrition-recommendation/keyhole-nutrition-label (accessed June 17, 2016). Copenhagen: The Nordic Council, 2012

148  Australian Government Department of Health. *Overarching Strategic Statement for the Food Regulatory System*. Available at: www.health.gov.au/internet/main/publishing.nsf/Content/foodsecretariat-stategic-statement (accessed November 7, 2015), 2013

149  Blewett N. *Labelling Logic: Review of Food Labelling Law and Policy*. London: Department of Health and Ageing, 2011

150  Vaughan A. Tesco drops carbon-label pledge. Available at: www.theguardian.com/environment/2012/jan/30/tesco-drops-carbon-labelling (accessed June 10, 2016). London: *The Guardian*, 2012

151  European Food SCP Round Table. *European Food SCP Round Table*. Available at: www.food-scp.eu/ (accessed June 10, 2016). Brussels: European Food Sustainable Consumption and Production Round Table, 2016

152  European Commission. *The EU Ecolabel*. Available at: http://ec.europa.eu/environment/ecolabel/ (accessed June 10, 2016). Brussels: European Commission, 2016

153  Czarnezki JJ. The future of food eco-labeling: organic, carbon footprint, and environmental life-cycle analysis. *Stanford Environmental Law Journal*, 2011; 30(3). Available at: http://digitalcommons.pace.edu/lawfaculty/914/ (accessed 7 August 2016)

154  Fairlie S. Dairy miles. *The Land*, Winter 2012–13; 13: 48–57

155  Compassion in World Farming. *Statistics: Broiler Chickens*. Available at: www.ciwf.org.uk/media/5235303/Statistics-Broiler-chickens.pdf (accessed June 6, 2016), 2013

156  FAWC. *Opinion on the Welfare Implications of Breeding and Breeding Technologies in Commercial Livestock Agriculture*. Available at: www.gov.uk/government/uploads/system/uploads/attachment_data/file/324658/FAWC_opinion_on_the_welfare_implications_of_

breeding_and_breeding_technologies_in_commercial_livestock_agriculture.pdf (accessed June 10, 2016). London: Farm Animal Welfare Committee, 2012

157  FAWC. *Farm Animal Welfare in Great Britain: Past, Present and Future.* London: Farm Animal Welfare Council, 2009

158  Andrews J. European Union bans battery cages for egg-laying hens. *Food Safety News,* January 19, 2012. Available at: www.foodsafetynews.com/2012/01/european-union-bans-battery-cages-for-egg-laying-hens/#.V2MZYOYrJuU (accessed June 10, 2016), 2012

159  Voiceless. *Battery Hens.* Available at: www.voiceless.org.au/the-issues/battery-hens (accessed June 10, 2016). Paddington, Australia: Voiceless, 2016

160  Stevenson P. *European Union Legislation on the Welfare of Farm Animals.* Available at: www.ciwf.org.uk/research/policy-economics/the-european-union-legislation-of-farmed-animals/ (accessed June 10, 2016). Godalming: Compassion in World Farming, 2012

161  Raynolds LT. Re-embedding global agriculture: the international organic and fair trade movements. *Agriculture and Human Values,* 2000; 17(3): 297–309

162  Nelson V, Pound B. *The Last Ten Years: A Comprehensive Review of the Literature on the Impact of Fairtrade.* Natural Resources Institute, 2009: 1–48

163  Food Ethics Council. *Food Justice: The Report of the Food and Fairness Inquiry.* London: Food Ethics Council, 2014.

164  Cramer C, Johnston D, Oya C, *et al. Fairtrade, Employment and Poverty Reduction in Ethiopia and Uganda,* Final Report to the DFID, April 2014. London: Department for International Development, 2014

# Chapter 6

# Food quality
## Everyone likes their own food

## Core arguments

In this chapter we look at the concept of food quality and acceptability, which we consider to be an essential component of a sustainable diet, for reasons we began to explore in Chapter 5. Food quality is sometimes said to be hard to define as it means different things to different people, but within the notion of quality there are some characteristics that cross cultural and geographical boundaries. Everyone aspires to have access to food of a quality they like and would choose if it is available and affordable. In this chapter we discuss the various attributes of food quality and what they might mean for the debate about sustainable diets. Attributes of food quality cut across many aspects of sustainable diets, including the environment, health and nutrition, social and economic factors and governance. We also consider how quality is decided upon and established, including the use of quality standards. Who decides them, on whose behalf and through which institutions are matters of considerable importance in shaping what is meant by quality. Food history suggests that quality is a moveable but contested policy terrain.

## What is food quality?

Food quality is a multi-faceted concept, which one might initially think is too woolly to include under sustainable diets. It can appear to be tricky to define because it suggests a subjective element although, as we show in this chapter, it is possible to nail down some clear features. Whole journals are in fact dedicated to sharing specialist knowledge on quality, with titles such as *Food Quality and Preference* and *Food Control*. Clarification of 'quality' is helped by considering its reverse: adulteration. *The Lancet*, a respected medical journal, made its reputation in a celebrated battle between science, government and the food industry over adulteration in the mid-nineteenth century.[1, 2]

The notion of food quality has a variety of meanings depending on who is attempting to define it, whether the person is a food researcher, a food producer, a food manufacturer or retailer, and so on. Quality is a matter of perspective, literally a matter of where one stands. The literature on food quality has many studies of binary options: perception vs. reality of quality; consumer vs. supply approaches to quality; pre- and post-purchase experience of quality; short- versus long-term judgements of quality; willingness to pay vs. actual purchasing behaviour; and so on.[3] Economists and psychologists have combined to create conceptual models of how decisions about food quality might be made. Figure 6.1 gives one of these – the Total Food Quality Model developed by Grunert and colleagues.[3, 4] This suggests that what one could have dismissed as purely intuitive or subjective verdicts on food quality can be broken down into a decision-tree type format.

The Total Food Quality Model, like all models, carries assumptions. It breaks down the pursuit of quality into computer-like decisions in a series of on/off switches. Gestalt psychology sees consumers as approaching choice with predilections to choose through overviews rather than attention to minutiae, while other psychologists stress the learned nature of taste.[5] The relative appeals of sweetness and sourness are learned.[6] Taste buds are trained and therefore can be retrained at a population level.[7] Habits are the operationalisation of experienced quality in that they are repeated behaviours that reinforce themselves. Learning what is 'nice' to eat is a habituation process, the bedding down of norms in culturally meaningful ways at the personal level. The notion of habits used to be central in early twentieth-century social psychology (for example, in the work of MacDougall who talked of 'semi-mechanical' behaviour,[8] or that of William

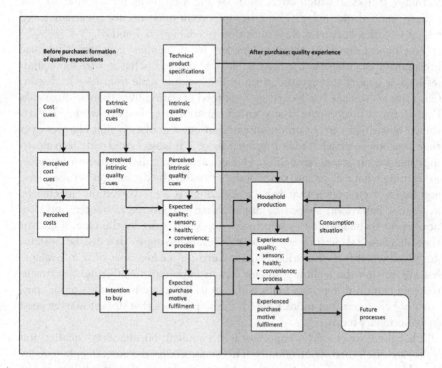

*Figure 6.1* Total Food Quality Model
Source: Grunert.[3]

James, brother of novelist Henry James[9]) but this was pushed aside by the search of Freudian psychoanalysis for deep meanings. It has returned with the realisation of the case for tackling undesirable behaviour. Alan Warde, a sociologist, has recently suggested it warrants a central place in a modern understanding of eating.[10]

Debates about the differences between models of learned behaviour need not divert us too much here, fascinating though they are. What matters for sustainable diets is that academics have created a useful pool of insights and studies of processes on what is meant by quality. Notions of quality are an essential element in the clarification of whether and how a transition to sustainable diets is conceivable and deliverable, and these do need to be invoked in how that transition is managed. Currently, the model favoured in the West is what is now called behavioural economics, a marriage of economics and behavioural psychology.[11, 12] This has emerged as policy makers come to realise the enormity of various societal challenges such as climate change or obesity. This questions the consumerist model in which market sovereignty lies with the purchaser. Change may be needed for 'their own good'. The fashionable association for this is 'nudge' thinking, which offers methods and a rationale for attempts to shift culture 'beneath the radar'. This raises important questions for governance and who is in control of any dietary transition (see Chapters 7 and 8).

For the consumer, at the very simplest level, 'quality' may stand for basic acceptance, i.e. whether the food is liked or disliked. That is why some studies look at quality through the prism of the hedonic scale from love to disgust. Gastronomic science has looked more at food or eating likes than at disgust, as Paul Rozin, a psychologist, has pointed out in a large body of work.[13] He has shown how disgust is not an on/off emotion but a gradation that changes over time as people learn what to be disgusted about.[14] It is associated with deep meanings about what enters our bodies. This is learned in childhood as, for instance, in learning what can go into our mouths – notably the distinction between food and faeces.[13] He argues that behaviour change is more powerfully affected by avoidance behaviour, shaped by disgust, than by positive attributes, and does not appear to be affected by personality type, but more by the type of elicitor (how disgusting something is perceived to be). Rozin argues that disgust taps into deep feelings of fear of death.[15] Valerie Curtis, a medical specialist in hygiene, has argued that the feeling of disgust has an important health role. It warns us to avoid certain things, and helps build (or to habituate in Warde's terms) patterns of behaviour that protect health.[16] She proposes that disgust may be good in evolutionary terms.

That the taste of food is important is self-evident, but the terms 'quality' and 'taste' are often used synonymously. This is not always the case. People may say they like the taste of a particular product even though they think it is of low quality. A beef burger bought from a fast-food restaurant may be judged to be of lower quality than a burger from a farmers' market. But on what basis is such a judgement made? Blind testing often confounds prejudice. A well-made hand-baked loaf of bread may be judged to be of higher quality than a mass-produced sliced loaf from a mass food retailer. However, some people may prefer the taste of a food they judge to be of lower quality. It is what they are used to. Psychologists see this as fear of the unknown or unfamiliar. For example, some children who are used to vegetables from a large retailer may find the taste of vegetables from a farmers' market or community growing project less to their liking until they get used to the different taste. The definition of, and the criteria for, the quality of an item sold in a fast-food restaurant may differ from the criteria for the same food sold at a farmer's market or a supermarket. In the search for convenience, the consumer may be happy to eat food of a different quality than they would, say, if they were cooking a meal from scratch at home. Perception of quality is thus a function of experience.

Although everyone has an internal barometer of quality, they may not be able to define what they mean by quality or what aspects make up quality. It may therefore be impossible to define food quality in a rigid fashion given the influence of these individual differences and the effects of context. To some extent, the advent of postmodernism has made it even more difficult to define quality as it has challenged the traditional cultural hierarchy whereby the food preferences of rich and powerful people were canonised as 'good quality' and 'good taste'. Sociologists such as Bourdieu have described taste (in both culinary and domestic meanings) as a function of socio-economic status.[17]

Although meat-eating consumers might agree that a lean, tender steak in a fine restaurant is of higher quality than a hot dog bought at a street vendor, it is no longer so easy to accept older conceptions of 'good quality' and 'good taste' that often went unquestioned and were embodied by those who somehow inherited impeccable judgement and whose judgements were neither scrutinised nor challenged. Indeed, the fashion for and importance of 'street food' suggests that fast food has won quality adherents. However, the desire to use food to maintain cultural and social distinction still remains, as Bourdieu sketched. Food perceived to be of high quality, for example, artisan food, often hand-made to a traditional recipe or traditional production process, may be purchased as a means of distinguishing oneself from others who, if such food is perceived to be or genuinely is, more expensive than its mass-produced equivalents, will not be able or may not want to buy it. Food perceived as 'posh' may be rejected by some people who may also want to distinguish themselves from others by not eating such food. Tastes change, while class distinction may remain. One moment the affluent favour fitted kitchens; the next they prefer the unstructured look. Thus, as the sociologists have noted, taste becomes a motor force for consumerism; it oils the wheels of commerce.

So is the issue of quality a culinary or social game of cat and mouse? Academics think not. Nor does the food industry, which knows only too well how sensitive consumers are to perceived quality. This is why such vast sums are spent by marketers when launching new food products. Tens of thousands of new food products are launched annually, but the attrition rate of failures is high.

### Why food quality matters: adulteration and trust

The notion of quality itself changes, and is subject to long-term tussles between science and technology, on the one hand, and 'ordinary' consumer culture, on the other. The emergence of food chemistry in the eighteenth century became highly political when a new generation of chemists started exposing the adulterated state of food. Frederick Accum produced his *Treatise on Adulteration* in 1820,[18] in which he outlined the frauds and dangers in British food that he had subjected to analytic techniques. He thought – naively as it turned out – that his published results would lead to a clean-up and that he would be seen to have done a public service. In fact, his career was quickly broken and for a variety of reasons he fled the country. It was not until others took up the anti-adulteration cause in the 1850s that controls began to be put into place.[1] Even so, sections of the food industry fought back, and it was not until the late nineteenth century that the UK's food adulteration laws were broadly fixed.[19] Other countries had not dissimilar experiences, notably the USA regarding its meat quality controls. It took a major scandal in 1906 – Upton

Sinclair exposing that the Chicago meat packing factories had not halted production when a worker fell in the cauldrons[20] – to get President Theodore Roosevelt
and Congress to institute tough new food laws and create an institution to monitor them. Tough, focused inspection was essential to ensure food quality, argued
Sinclair in an exchange of letters with the President.[20]

So is food quality simply a matter of politics? Yes and no. Yes, to some extent,
in that political considerations undoubtedly frame how and whether food quality is brought into the sphere of governance. The long struggle to clean up food
shows that.[2, 21] But no, in that this does not mean that food quality is too vague to
be made sense of. The science of food chemistry has certainly prospered since its
nineteenth-century trials over levels of adulteration.[22] Indeed, critics might even
suggest that food chemistry, once seen as the foe of the mainstream food industry
in the early nineteenth century, has become one of its key agents in the twentieth
and twenty-first. Food technologists and chemists have become key agents of
new product development, mainly working for food companies and contributing
to the production of ultra-processed foods and the spread of the nutrition transition. The nineteenth-century argument articulated by Hassall and others was
that food chemistry should help hold the food industry to account, and that is
why independent government offices of inspection should be funded. The process
of inspection and auditing would maintain quality and consumer trust.

In this chapter we take a broad view of quality. It matters for the discourse on
sustainable diets because the last century of research into consumer preferences
shows how sensitive public understanding is. The notion of quality goes to the
heart of what it is to be a consumer. One review of what is meant by quality in
food suggested that quality can be broken down to the following features.[23]

- Organoleptic and sensory attributes: colour, appearance, texture, juiciness,
  taste, astringency and aroma.
- Safety: contaminants, mycotoxins and pathogens.
- Nutritional value: bioavailable nutrients such as proteins, essential amino
  acids, vitamins and minerals.
- Functionality: use-value for food processing.
- Service and stability: resistance to rapid deterioration.
- Healthiness: value for consumer health.
- Psychological factors: convenience, price, ease of use, novelty, etc.

Beyond simple acceptance of a food and its taste, there may be other expectations
about the quality of a food such as its nutritional value, ingredients, storage ability
and shelf life, safety in terms of microbiological and toxicological contaminants,
the presence of genetically modified organisms and additives, labelling and packaging. Quality is also at the heart of many of the contemporary discussions about
changing food systems; towards increasing industrialisation on the one hand and
'alternative' food systems on the other. New conceptualisations of food quality
have emerged within alternative food networks; from the expansion of local and

organic food to a focus on animal welfare, eating food in season, artisanal or ethical production and heritage, tradition, traceability and authenticity, all of which can be included in a description of food quality. In this context, food quality can carry 'ethical' connotations, telling consumers about production methods and a product's relationship to animal welfare and the environment.[24] It can also refer to geographical origin.

The definition of quality therefore encompasses several different attributes and combines objective features dealt with, in the case of industrialised food, by food technologists, engineers and nutritionists, with the subjective needs of consumers. The presence of quality is often a key message in food marketing. There has been a growth of messages conveyed to the consumer in the form of 'quality marks' such as the UK's Red Tractor farm assurance scheme,[25] or the many half-way house approaches between agrichemical-based farming and organics such as the USA's Integrated Pest Management Institute of North America,[26] or the UK's LEAF (Linking Environment and Farming) Marque.[27] Throughout the world, retailers now have own-labels pronouncing high-quality products by labelling them as 'finest' or 'award winning' or 'better for you'. In the case of small producers, the notion of quality is often about the food being locally produced, from an identifiable source and involving face-to-face contact between producer or retailer and consumer. The producer will often have a 'story' to tell about how they produce their food and where they get their ingredients. In this context, quality is understood less in terms of global standards but within alternative food networks; there is often an insistence that quality exists only at the margins of globalised and industrialised food networks.

## Taste

Taste has both physical and social meanings. All palates are attuned to distinguish between bitter, sour, salty and sweet tastes and to identify common flavours. Universal standards around which foods are pleasant to taste are difficult to identify. While it is possible to distinguish between a food that tastes bitter or sweet, it is impossible to provide a universally valid verdict on whether any particular bitterness or sweetness is pleasant. The taste of food can be influenced by many aspects of the eating experience including the use (or not) of cutlery and plates, the colour of the plates and the shape of the glasses, the names used to describe the dishes and the choice of background music and, if eating out, the behaviour of the people serving the food.

Although humans are omnivorous, they are not necessarily attracted or able to eat everything that may be edible. Understandably, people are suspicious of certain foods because of possible poisoning or risk of infection or other disease, but they also have food preferences or avoidances that are culturally and socially derived. In Britain and the United States, for example, horsemeat is regarded with some distaste, while in Germany, Switzerland and China it is consumed without a second thought. However, horsemeat did become a scandal in Europe when, in 2013, it was found to be being sold as beef by many reputable retailers.[28, 29] Commercial assurance schemes were seen to be thin. Also, despite the demise of older conceptions of 'good taste' in food, distinctions between social groups and classes in their preferences for food remain important, and tastes in food certainly become a badge of identity, a means of social orientation and a sense of place in society. Food sends signals. The question is: how could sustainable diets be seen as desirable?

Taste in food can evolve through changing circumstances of supply and demand. The spread of 'exotic', 'ethnic' and processed foods may become acceptable to new consumers who enjoy novelty, as is the case with tropical fruits and vegetables that have become a feature of modern diets in rich countries. These can be cheaper and easier to prepare, as has been the case with wheat food aid in Africa, which has become more popular than locally grown grains and root crops, or they can be heavily promoted in the medias, for example, with soft drinks and ready to eat 'fast foods'. The globalisation process – the loosening of food borders between nations – has entered the frame in this respect, because tastes in heavily processed foods or soft drinks have spread.[30, 31] Although one line of criticism has feared an increasing culinary homogenisation in this process, the reality is still fairly regionalised eating patterns.

The sheer diversity of food on offer in contemporary urban settings is enormous. That said, companies seeking global markets for their products do aim for consistency of appeal and product. A burger and fries from one fast-food chain will taste very much the same whether bought in Beijing, Moscow, Washington or London. Commercially, a food world is emerging of 'diminishing contrasts' alongside 'increasing variety': diminishing contrasts in terms of the quantities of processed food based on a small number of ingredients such as white flour, sugar, soya and corn oil, but increasing variety in terms of the tens of thousands of food products vying for our attention and money in the supermarkets. While trends in eating styles leap across borders – affected by tourism, too – there are some mega-trends that dwarf others. The rise of over-processed foods is one and the spread of soft drinks is another.[6, 30, 32] The marketing push of soft drinks into developing countries is particularly insidious for health, a sign of corporates seeking growth in low-income countries now that their own home markets are saturated and under scrutiny for causing ill-health.[33] Much of the food in the contemporary food market is high in sugar and fat, which appeals to the human taste for sweet, energy dense foods and therefore helps to grow food company profits. The counter trend here is the increasing popularity of localised food, partly as a statement of identity and partly resulting from the rediscovery of distinctive, 'traditional' and supposedly authentic foods, recipes and tastes promoted by alternative food networks.[34, 35, 36]

Another issue related to taste is the criticism that fresh food bought from large retailers may lack distinctive taste. If it is mass-produced, how can it be special? For example, fruits and vegetables purchased from supermarkets can taste bland, as they are cultivated for length of shelf life (durability), low waste, uniformity of colour, shape and consistency. For just-in-time supply chains, the harvesting of an entire crop at the same time makes sense. The retailer/ distributor has the power. Such crops must also be easily transportable, sometimes over long distances, without spoilage.[37, 38] However, local and seasonal fruit and vegetables are often described as tastier, fresher and better quality than the equivalent imported produce or those produced out of season.[39] Fruit and vegetables of better taste and quality may increase the likelihood of increased consumption of these healthy foods.

### Fresh

Fresh is a generally positive term for food and particularly a desirable feature in produce such as fruit and vegetables. However, what is often sold as fresh may depend on a whole series of technological innovations such as refrigeration, sprout suppression and even airfreight. Part of the motivation may be positive: to reduce spoilage and ensure quality is maintained to the point of purchase. But this may not be liked or understood by the consumer. Who knows that the 'fresh' citrus fruit is waxed with an anti-fungicide? Or that the ready-washed mixed leaf salad has been washed in chlorine?[40] Until recently, access to fresh foods such as vegetables, fruit, meat and fish could be regarded as a luxury for the elite few as the perishability of these foodstuffs limited their availability and increased their value.[41] Seasonality ruled availability. The food technologist was seen as a liberator, widening the seasons and making a bigger range of foods more available to more people.[42, 43]

The demand for freshness can have hidden environmental costs. While freshness is now being deployed as a term in food marketing as part of a return to nature, the demand for year-round supplies of fresh produce such as soft fruit and exotic vegetables has led to the widespread use of hot houses in cold climates and increasing reliance on total quality control – management by temperature control, use of pesticides and computer/satellite-based logistics. The demand for freshness has also contributed to concerns about food wastage. Use of 'best before', 'sell by' and 'eat by' labels has legitimised institutional waste. Campaigners have exposed the scandal of over-production and waste.[44] Tristram Stuart, one of the global band of anti-waste campaigners, argues that, with freshly made sandwiches, over-ordering is standard practice across the retail sector to avoid the appearance of empty shelf space, leading to high volumes of waste when supply regularly exceeds demand.

Definitions of freshness are complex and contested. Suzanne Freidberg has shown how, according to the US Food and Drug Administration (FDA), for example, the use of the label 'fresh' is not permitted on frozen, heat-treated or chemically preserved foods with the exception of pasteurised milk.[45] Strict adherence to the rules has, however, led to the emergence of categories such as 'fresh-frozen' and to the advertising of irradiated salads as fresh. The picture the social scientists paint of the notion of 'fresh' is that it has become plastic and malleable.[46] The FDA may have its 2009 *FDA Food Code* and the European Commission may have its product labelling directive, but such regulations can be stretched by reality, hence the need for constant review and inspection (as Upton Sinclair recognised over a century ago).

A 2008 report from the UK FSA stated that the term 'fresh' is helpful where it differentiates produce that is sold within a short time after production or harvesting.[47] However, modern distribution and storage methods can significantly increase the time period before there is loss of quality for a product, and it has become increasingly difficult to decide when the term 'fresh' is being used legitimately. For example, foods that have been vacuum packed to retain their freshness have not necessarily been recently harvested. Chill temperatures and other controlled atmospheres are used in the food production chain for the delayed ripening and/or extended storage of fruit and vegetables. In the UK, the term 'fresh' when applied to fruit and vegetables generally indicates that they are not processed (for example, canned, pickled, preserved or frozen), rather than that they have been recently harvested. However, use of the term 'fresh' to imply that only a short period after harvesting or preparation has elapsed before sale may be misleading.

Milk and meat represent particularly interesting cases for the quality of freshness. The production of fresh milk on an industrial scale involves all kinds of interventions in the food chain from the domestication of cattle to the use of artificial growth hormone such as bovine somatotropin (now banned in many countries). As societies urbanised, milk travelled further to market, increasing the dangers of spoilage and infection associated with diseases such as diphtheria, scarlet fever and tuberculosis. The mass consumption of milk depends on the elimination of bacteria through heat treatment and pasteurisation to ensure its safety. For meat, the term 'fresh' is traditionally used to differentiate raw meat from that which has been (chemically) preserved. Virtually all carcass meat is chilled following slaughter for hygiene reasons. The best quality beef will be carefully aged and not fresh in the way the term is routinely defined. Good quality cheese is painstakingly matured. However, use of the term 'fresh' in these cases is acceptable.

### Cosmetic (appearance)

Cosmetic appearance of food (usually fruit and vegetables) refers to external attributes that do not necessarily affect taste, yield or nutritional value. These attributes include shape, colour, size or other aesthetic properties. Buyers for large retailers and other middle-men in the food system can reject perfectly edible food because it does not meet their requirements in terms of cosmetic appearance (or other standards). For example, up to 30% of the UK's vegetable crop never reaches the marketplace, primarily the supermarket, as a result of trimming, quality selection and failure to conform to purely cosmetic criteria. This can include such reasons as the packaging is slightly dented, one piece of fruit is bad in an otherwise perfectly good bag of fruit, or it is thrown out in the warehouse because it had ripened too soon.[48, 49] In this way the global food industry produces large amounts of food waste, with retailers generating 1.6 million tonnes of food waste per year.[50]

To maintain their own profits, or simply to ensure their contract with buyers is honoured, producers attempt to grow as much produce as possible while ensuring that a high percentage attains the highest cosmetic appearance. Techniques used to achieve these goals may include extending the growing season, extending the shelf life, improving shipping qualities, improving produce appearance, reducing costs of production and enhancing yield. These techniques may involve the use of greater concentrations of pesticides than the production of less cosmetically perfect crops.

Although consumers' perception of fruit and vegetable quality has come to be based, in part, on cosmetic quality, whether consumers asked retailers for produce of such high cosmetic quality is debatable. Such produce may be easier to transport and store and has a longer shelf life, but it may also taste bland and use of pesticides to achieve this cosmetic quality raises uncertainties for environmental and public health. Addressing this issue will require a substantial change in marketing practices and consumer preferences. Some supermarkets have begun to stock misshapen fruit at a reduced price.

## Seasonality

Seasonality may be an aspiration in affluent society cuisine today but, historically, it has been associated with famine, at worst, and dearth or restriction, at best. It troubles low-income country households on a mass scale in modern times.[51] There are more contemporary academic studies of seasonality effects on wild animals than on human diet. Has seasonality's importance thus been consigned to the history books by technology, as some of its prophets wished? As with many other aspects of quality, seasonality is not as easy to define as might appear. Its interpretation may depend on who is using the term and the context in which it is being used. Many consumers, for example, associate seasonal with locally produced food but, by other definitions, local is not a necessary criterion for seasonal food. For many people seasonality is associated with fruit and vegetables but not linked to other crops or animal food production. Difficulties in definition also arise when considering food produced in the natural growing season in one country then imported and consumed in another country, or food grown locally in the natural growing season then stored and eaten several months later in the same country, as can happen with, say, English apples.

A study commissioned by the UK Department for Environment, Food and Rural Affairs (Defra) proposed two definitions of seasonal food, the first based on where the food is produced, and the second on where it is produced and consumed.[49] In the first definition, food is grown or produced outdoors during the natural growing/production period for the country or region where it is produced.

It need not necessarily be consumed locally to where it is produced. This is defined as global seasonality. Apples grown in season naturally outdoors in New Zealand and eaten in Europe in the spring and summer by this definition would be globally seasonal. In the second definition, food is produced and consumed in season and in the same climatic zone without high energy use or storage. This is described as locally seasonal food, but this leads to a further debate on what constitutes 'local'. For example, are raspberries grown in season in Scotland and consumed in Wales locally seasonal? The most important aspect of both these definitions of seasonality is that the food is grown or produced outdoors in its natural season without the use of additional energy, thereby not creating additional greenhouse gas emissions.

Although these definitions may appear straightforward, specific aspects of them have been questioned,[52] particularly those related to being produced 'outdoors' and the 'natural growing/production season'. So, do unheated plastic tunnels constitute outdoors or should seedlings started in heated greenhouses then grown outdoors in the natural growing season be excluded? Would crops bred to extend the natural growing seasons be included?

Given these complexities, it is difficult to reach conclusions on the relationship between seasonal food and sustainable diets. If one wants to eat strawberries throughout most of the year, it is best to eat them grown outdoors far away and trucked to you than more locally under heated (and therefore high GHG-emitting) conditions locally.[53] That said, if you ate strawberries grown in your own garden, their GHGs are likely to be even lower. There is no iron rule that favours seasonality above other considerations. A paper by Macdiarmid concluded that relying on local, seasonal food year-round could reduce fruit and vegetable consumption, but the environmental impacts on water stress, land-use change and biodiversity could be less than for a globally seasonal diet.[39] It could, however, limit international trade with implications for economic stability and resilience within the global food market. Global seasonality has the nutritional benefit of providing a more varied and consistent supply of fresh produce year round, but this increases demand for foods that in turn can have a high environmental cost in the country of production (for example, water stress, land-use change with loss of biodiversity). Greenhouse gas emissions of globally seasonal food are not necessarily higher than food produced locally as GHGEs depend more on the production system used than transportation. Locally seasonal food is often perceived to be more expensive and less convenient to source. However, it is likely to be fresher and have a better flavour than food transported long distances.[54] Overall, eating seasonal food is not without benefits in terms of sustainability but is not likely to be as important as other aspects of sustainable diet such as reducing meat consumption and reducing food waste. The Swedish government's National Food Administration and Environmental Protection Agency produced the first open published evidence-based sustainable dietary advice. It recommended that Swedes should eat seasonally and locally where possible (see Chapter 8).[55] Despite some conflict with the European Food Safety

Authority (EFSA) over this package, the Swedish government has reiterated that advice.[56]

## Provenance

Provenance refers to place of origin and is derived from the French verb *provenir*. In relation to food and cuisine, provenance refers to the geographical origins of a particular product, including ingredients and dishes or style of cooking or cuisine. It is closely related to authenticity, evoking a relationship between food and place and has similarities with ideas of heritage and tradition. In many cases, food producers have sought to gain the weight of legal authority for their claims of provenance. Within the European Union, for example, a variety of acronyms have been developed under the overall legal framework of Protected Geographical Status. These include the Protected Designation of Origin (PDO) and Protected Geographical Indication (PGI). A PDO must have a place link at all stages of production whereas a PGI has a link at only one stage. Similar labelling schemes exist in North America. Although these schemes are relatively recent, they are related to concepts of brands and branding that have a longer history, being originally applied to the ownership of cattle and horses and now applied to a variety of products, including cheese, wine, smoked fish and so on. Protecting particular products using legal sanctions such as *Appellation d'Origine Controlée* (AOC) are sufficiently widespread as to be taken for granted but many have distinctive histories. The AOC system, for example, was created in the early years of the twentieth century by French wine producers to protect themselves against cheaper imports from Algeria and Spain.

Provenance is also central to the French notion of terroir, where the value of a product is closely associated with the place it comes from. Provenance claims about terroir rest on the idea that the distinctive taste of particular products such as cheese and wine depends on local variations in climate, soil, the diet of the sheep, goat and cattle and the quality of milk they produce or the intimate connection between people and place. Provenance claims are advanced by producers as a way of adding value and can readily be exploited for commercial gain. This might involve the invocation of a loose connection between food and place. A retailer could market, for example, an 'Oakham' chicken, but not mean that the chicken had any real connection to the town of Oakham in the county of Rutland, England. Cheddar cheese now has little connection to the village of Cheddar. It has lost provenance. To convey authenticity, food companies sometimes invent 'mock' provenance. Governments have tried to introduce traceability and transparency in food chains to win consumer trust in what otherwise can become a provenance cat and mouse game.

It is for reasons like these that the issue of labelling is so sensitive. The matter becomes one of transparency. Market economic theory suggests that information flows to consumers enable market efficiencies to optimise. If provenance becomes part of a marketing or branding 'game', however, the flow is distorted and consumers are disempowered. This is why, for instance, the US FDA states that any processed product cannot be labelled as natural. [57]

## Authenticity

The concept of authenticity evokes a range of meanings, including that which is original, genuine, real, true or true to itself. Its meaning is applied across a range from purity to fraud. Here, again, the food chemist is present, with an important role of testing how authentic foods really are. They have a battery of modern techniques such as microbiological-based DNA testing to investigate whether that 'beef' is beef or horsemeat or something else.[58] Concerns about authenticity have contributed to the re-emergence of food scientists being overtly critical of food technology, or at least standing away from technology being used for its own sake.[59] Just because something can be processed or grown or reared does not make it right.

While authenticity is generally considered to be a positive trait, there is considerable scepticism about its use among some food scholars, in part because of the frequency with which restaurants and food products make claims about their authenticity in promotional materials.[60] Most international food brands insist they are the 'real thing'. Gastronomes, meanwhile, tussle over whether a cuisine can be 'authentic' if taken out of its original setting. Can an Indian restaurant serve authentic cuisine in New York? Does it matter if it tastes good?

American food writers Johnston and Baumann suggest that common criteria of authenticity include simplicity (hand-made, small-scale, lacking pretension), personal connection to specific people or places (including the work of named individuals), historicism and tradition (including 'age-old' or 'timeless' methods of production), as well as more general claims like closeness to nature (natural, organic), sincerity, honesty and integrity.[61] Some of the features of the production process are drawn into the value of the food, encouraging conversations between consumers, and consumers and producers, about the product's origins, how it is made and who made it. This can be contrasted with foods produced in the industrialised food system, where labels are used to provide consumers with information about the production process when direct contact with the producer is missing. Only the label can authenticate the foodstuff as organic, fair trade or a regional specialty. This is how alternative food organisations control their producers through marketing and licensing schemes, and it is why they are sensitive if questioned as to effectiveness. A study of fair trade produce conducted for the UK Department for International Development, for instance, found that, while the price premium did percolate to developing country primary producers, not all of the labour force benefited.[62] Some of the women and first-level workers were not as well remunerated as the image implied they should be. Embarrassing though this may have been, it meant the fair trade movement reviewed its practices. No consumer on his or her own could have checked the authenticity. It needed another process – inspection – in addition to buyer–producer relations. This was the rationale for Accum's exposés two centuries ago.

In a world where most people do not produce most of the foods they eat, there can be a sense of rupture or disconnection, since they may still associate authenticity with creation through production.[63] Consumers – particularly urban gardeners – may attempt to overcome this disconnection by growing some of their own food. Gardening can be a creative food act in a consumerist culture. It is in it, but at odds with it. The pursuit of the 'real' is an attempt to recapture the aura of authenticity through consuming foods that are valued precisely because their connection to the world of production is known. In that sense, the search for authentic foods may occur as a result of a shadow cast by an economy organised around monetary exchange value. One distinction has been offered to contrast consumption as the pursuit of 'value for money' rather than 'values-for-money'.[64] The former prioritises cheapness; the latter a variety of values in the exchange. Foods identified as authentic are also associated with a perceived dignity of labour, in contrast to mass foods produced in the industrial food system. Mass versus artisanal is the significant cognitive dimension here. This immediately raises more questions for the authenticity discourse. Why is simple, traditional or artisanal food more expensive and its consumption therefore restricted by price and what are the reasons for relative lack of availability in mainstream retail outlets? A persistent criticism of the pursuit of authenticity is that it is mainly available only to an elite. Authentic food items maintain social and cultural distinction yet are a brake on blandness.[61]

## The visibility of food quality: making the (un)sustainable obvious

A theme arising from the account of quality so far has been whether quality is or can be made visible. Branding is an attempt to claim it can be, but for commercial purposes, to associate previous happiness from a purchase and predispose the consumer to repeat – habituation again. The shape or colour or logo is a signifier, with the human eye, in evolutionary terms, acting as the gatekeeper of quality control. Does it look right? If a fruit is so rotten that it is inedible, the consumer can see it. If the meat is decaying, it smells bad. But, with the advance of biology and microbiology let alone atomic or gene-typing, the primacy of the human eye and learned cultural rules in policing food quality no longer apply so clearly. Branding may still use and appeal to the eye, but microbiological contamination is by definition unseeable without equipment. Is food quality therefore dependent on expert, arms-length expertise? Does this need the existence of an expert working for the consumer? Should sustainable diets come under the remit of contracts and specifications professionals?

Though certainly not new, microbiological contamination continues to be an issue in the modern food system with, for example, almost three quarters of fresh chickens in UK supermarkets found to be contaminated with Campylobacter in 2015. In the USA, there have been cases of green vegetables, including salad greens, being contaminated with Salmonella, and of frozen vegetables being contaminated with Listeria. Antibiotic resistance is also becoming a major concern worldwide, and antibiotic over-use on farm animals has increased risk of antimicrobial resistance (AMR).[65, 66] Methicillin-resistant staphylococcus aureus (MRSA) has emerged on, for example, pig farms and has been detected in retail meat products. Chemical contamination of food from pesticides, and substances such as acrylamide, formed by high-temperature cooking of mainly plant-based foods such as potatoes and grains, and bisphenol A, a component of some plastic beverage bottles and metal-can coatings, also raise questions for public health (discussed in Chapter 3). Chronic exposure of farm workers to pesticides is associated with increased risk of respiratory disease, blood disorders and neurological changes.[67] How can all this be made visible?

These questions take us towards the philosophy of science and to the issue of food governance (discussed in more detail in Chapter 8). The image of science is of the pursuit of objective, neutral knowledge and the accretion of an evidence base for policy and action. Dr John Snow is celebrated as a father of modern epidemiology and credited with ascertaining that water was somehow the cause of the cholera outbreak in London's Soho in 1854. He certainly did the right thing in halting use of the Broad Street water pump (reputedly taking off its handle), but he did this for entirely the wrong reasons.[68, 69] He subscribed, in fact, to miasma theory, which suggested the vector was in the air rather than what we now know were bacteria in the water. Although erroneous in his logic, his actions framed effective intervention.

The moral of the tale is that some kind of institutional capacity and role is needed to ensure quality and public health. The more evidence-based this can be the better, and it is inevitably political, as it requires funding and powers from the State. Equipment, professionals and monitoring powers are expensive, requiring finance such as by a levy or taxation. To detect dangerous levels of agrichemical residues, for example, requires special and expensive equipment. Instagram or Twitter might be good for fast communication, but they cannot provide what is needed for food quality control. This requires an infrastructure with longer time horizons and more depth of analytic skill. This is why, in the past, food inspectorates and public health agencies have been created and why sustainable diets need either to be placed with them or with new bodies.

Alongside such infrastructure, sustainable diets need to be supported by cultural 'rules' in everyday eating, if we are to take note of what anthropologists such as Claude Levi-Strauss and Mary Douglas unraveled.[70–72] They showed how humans learn within their culture what is 'good' and what makes up an acceptable meal.[73] The semi-cooked food that might be your delicacy might not be ours. The sheep's eyeball you think a delicacy might not be to someone from another culinary culture. Humans learn to distinguish between the raw and the cooked, the good and the bad.

## Ensuring quality in sustainable diets

How can the consumer gain (or reclaim, depending on one's perspective) control over quality? When applied to food and drink, quality means different things to different people. But what does it mean for sustainable diets? Quality is a term with almost universally positive connotations, unless it is prefixed with words like 'poor' or 'inferior'. How are taste, freshness, appearance, seasonality, provenance and authenticity linked with sustainable diets? It is becoming clear that they are not yet but they do need to be.

With regards to taste, there is no universal agreement on what tastes good to eat. However, energy-dense foods high in fat and sugar, including chocolate, cakes and biscuits, are generally widely enjoyed, even if people disagree over the types of energy-dense foods they like. However, the documentation of the global nutrition transition has shown how the supposedly innate taste for sugar and fat, which is tapped into by food industries, has serious consequences for public health. How can better tasting fruit and vegetables, beneficial for public health, be encouraged? It is known that the taste for sweet can be unlearned.[5]

Freshness is often linked to taste, particularly for fruit and vegetables, but fresh fruit and vegetables are not necessarily higher in micronutrients. Frozen vegetables such as peas, carrots and broccoli contain as much vitamin C as their freshly harvested equivalents and more vitamin C compared with fresh vegetables stored for more than 24 hours. In most cases, fresh vegetables eaten on the day of harvest, and harvested close to where they are consumed, which use no or limited energy for either freezing, transportation or refrigeration, are likely to offer the best micronutrient content and have the lowest environmental impact, but such fresh vegetables are not necessarily easily accessible to everyone.

The impact of choosing seasonal produce on sustainable diets is interesting. Local field-grown seasonal vegetables and fruit are likely to offer lower environmental impact than fruit and vegetables grown either locally or elsewhere in hot houses. However, storage of seasonal apples may have a higher requirement for energy use than freshly harvested apples shipped in from elsewhere. Field crops grown seasonally in another country may have a lower environmental impact than produce grown in hot houses in the region or country of consumption. However, limiting consumption of fruit and vegetables to those grown seasonally outdoors would reduce choice of these foods with potential impacts for public health.

One issue everyone agrees on is that grading food for its cosmetic appearance creates waste. Commercial rejection of food with blemishes has consequences for the livelihoods of producers, and this food may be perfectly fit to eat. At worst, such produce may be fed to livestock or, if unwanted at the retailer stage, it may be anaerobically digested or sent to landfill, the former having more benign environmental impact than the latter.

## Bridging personal and cultural preferences

Quality food for sustainable diets should have a low environmental impact, promote public health, be culturally acceptable, accessible and economical, fair and affordable. In this chapter we have highlighted the complexities of quality in relation to food and how the different aspects of quality pose questions for the pursuit of sustainable diets. In an ideal food world, everyone should have access to culturally acceptable quality food whatever their income, and it should be available not only in fine restaurants and households with comfortable food budgets but also in public sector dining facilities, street vendors and food retailers, both chains and independents.

We have noted, too, that food quality cannot simply be reduced to individual preferences. Quality characteristics are learned, culturally loaded and dependent upon hidden but shared norms. The pursuit of sustainable diets today comes on top of centuries in pursuit of better quality of food. Sustainable diet campaigners can take heart from this, and do not need to resort to the over-simplistic policy formulae such as of consumer sovereignty or market information efficiencies. The pursuit of optimum quality characteristics for sustainable diets requires championing by social movements as well as technical support from professionals. Over the last two centuries, the notion of food quality has exhibited some consistency, such as over contamination and fraud, but also some fluidity, such as over appearance. For decades, apparently, consumers did not want wobbly, knobbly vegetables until food waste campaigners pointed out the stupidity of rejecting raw foods on the grounds of shape.[74-76] The commercial view of quality can also be in tension with the public interest, so the challenge is how to align both. However, commercial views of 'quality' can easily slip into the world of brand protection and corporate risk assessment. The consumer, as ever, is prodded, inspected and controlled. But so is the food. This tension between technical and social approaches to food quality is deeply rooted and deserves attention in the transition to sustainable diets. The consuming public needs help to redefine what is acceptable and unacceptable, to recalibrate 'disgust', perhaps, as well as pleasure, and to set new norms and habits in everyday behaviour.

## References

1　Hassall AH. *Food and Its Adulterations: Comprising the Reports of the Analytical Sanitary Commission of 'The Lancet' for the Years 1851 to 1854*. London: Longman, 1855

2　Paulus ILE. *The Search for Pure Food: A Sociology of Legislation in Britain*. Oxford: Martin Robertson, 1974

3　Grunert KG. Food quality and safety: consumer perception and demand. *European Review of Agricultural Economics*, 2005; 32(3): 369–91

4　Brunsø K, Fjord TA, Grunert KG. *Consumers, Food Choice and Quality Perception*. Aarhus, Denmark: Aarhus School of Business, 2002

5　Wilson B. *First Bite: How We Learn to Eat*. London: Fourth Estate, 2015

6　Popkin BM, Hawkes C. Sweetening of the global diet, particularly beverages: patterns, trends, and policy responses. *The Lancet Diabetes & Endocrinology*, 2016; 4(2): 174–86

7　Hawkes C, Smith TG, Jewell J, et al. Smart food policies for obesity prevention. *The Lancet*, 2015; 385(9985): 2410–21

8　MacDougall W. *An Introduction to Social Psychology*. London: Methuen, 1908

9　James W. *Principles of Psychology*. London: Macmillan, 1891

10 Warde A. *The Practice of Eating*. Cambridge: Polity Press, 2016
11 Kahneman D, Tversky A. *Choices, Values, and Frames*. New York: Cambridge University Press, 2000
12 Thaler R, Sunstein C. *Nudge: Improving Decisions about Health, Wealth, and Happiness*. New Haven, CT: Yale University Press, 2008
13 Rozin P, Fallon AE. A perspective on disgust. *Psychological Review*, 1987; 94(1): 23–41
14 Rozin P, Haidt J, McCauley CR. Disgust, in: M Lewis, JM Haviland-Jones, LF Barrett (Eds) *Handbook of Emotions*, 3rd Ed. New York: Guilford Press, 2008: 757–76
15 Haidt J, McCauley C, Rozin P. Individual differences in sensitivity to disgust: a scale sampling seven domains of disgust elicitors. *Personality and Individual Differences*, 1994; 16(5): 701–13
16 Curtis V. *Don't Look, Don't Touch, Don't Eat: The Science Behind Revulsion*. Chicago: University of Chicago Press, 2013
17 Bourdieu P. *Distinction: A Social Critique of the Judgement of Taste*. London: Routledge, 1984
18 Accum F. *A Treatise on Adulterations of Food and Culinary Poisons*. London: Longman, 1820
19 Lang T. Food, the law and public health: three models of the relationship. *Public Health*, 2006; 120(October): 30–41
20 Sinclair U. *The Jungle*. Harmondsworth: Penguin, 1985 [1906]
21 Krebs AV. *The Corporate Reapers: The Book of Agribusiness*. Washington, DC: Essential Books, 1992
22 Wilson B. *Swindled: From Poison Sweets to Counterfeit Coffee – The Dark History of the Food Cheats*. London: John Murray, 2008
23 Giusti AM, Bignetti E, Cannella C. Exploring new frontiers in total food quality definition and assessment: from chemical to neurochemical properties. *Food and Bioprocess Technology*, 2008; 1(130)
24 Fischer Boel M. 'Just desserts': ethics, quality and traceability in EU agricultural and food policy, in: C Coff, D Barling, M Korthals, T Nielsen (Eds) *Ethical Traceability and Communicating Food*. Dordrecht: Springer: 260–3, 2008
25 Red Tractor Scheme. *Red Tractor Assured Food Standards*. Available at: www.redtractor.org.uk/choose-site (accessed July 5, 2016). London: Red Tractor Assurance, 2016
26 IPMINA. Integrated Pest Management Institute of North America. Available at: http://ipminstitute.org/faq/ (accessed July 7, 2016). Madison, WI: IPM Institute of North America, 2016
27 LEAF. *Linking Environment and Farming*. Available at: www.leafuk.org/leaf/farmers/LEAFmarquecertification/standard.eb (accessed July 30, 2016). Stoneleigh: LEAF, 2016
28 Elliott C. *Elliott Review into the Integrity and Assurance of Food Supply Networks: Interim Report*. Available at: www.gov.uk/government/policy-advisory-groups/review-into-the-integrity-and-assurance-of-food-supply-networks (accessed July 8, 2016 ). London: HM Government, 2013
29 Elliott C. *Elliott Review into the Integrity and Assurance of Food Supply Networks: Final Report – a Food Crime Prevention Framework*. Available at: www.gov.uk/government/policy-advisory-groups/review-into-the-integrity-and-assurance-of-food-supply-networks (accessed July 7, 2016). London: HM Government, 2014
30 Hawkes C. The worldwide battle against soft drinks in schools. *American Journal of Preventive Medicine*, 2010; 38(4): 457–61

31  Hawkes C, Blouin C, Henson S, *et al.* (Eds) *Trade, Food, Diet and Health: Perspectives and Policy Options*. Oxford: Wiley, 2009

32  Popkin B. *The World Is Fat: the Fads, Trends, Policies and Products That Are Fattening the Human Race*. New York: Avery/Penguin, 2009

33  Taylor AL, Jacobson MF. *Carbonating the World: The Marketing and Health Impact of Sugar Drinks in Low- and Middle-Income Countries*. Washington, DC: Center for Science in the Public Interest, 2016

34  Goodman D, Goodman M. Alternative food networks, in: Kitchin R, Thrift, N (Eds) *International Encyclopedia of Human Geography*. Oxford: Elsevier, 2008

35  Kneafsey M, Holloway L, Cox R, *et al. Reconnecting Consumers, Producers and Food: Exploring Alternatives*. Oxford: Berg, 2008

36  Dowler E, Kneafsey M, Cox R, *et al.* 'Doing food differently': reconnecting biological and social relationships through care for food. *Sociological Review*, 2010; 57(S2): 200–21

37  Burch D, Lawrence G (Eds). *Supermarkets and Agri-food Supply Chains*. Cheltenham, UK: Edward Elgar, 2007

38  Burch DR, Rickson RE, Lawrence G. *Globalization and Agri-food Restructuring: Perspectives from the Australasia Region*. Aldershot: Avebury, 1996

39  Macdiarmid JI. Seasonality and dietary requirements: will eating seasonal food contribute to health and environmental sustainability? *Proceedings of the Nutrition Society*, 2014; 73(03): 368–75

40  Blythman J. *Swallow This: Serving Up the Food Industry's Darkest Secrets*. London: Fourth Estate, 2015

41  Morgan K, Marsden T, Murdoch J. *Worlds of Food: Place, Power and Provenance in the Food Chain*. Oxford: University Press, 2006

42  Pyke M. *Industrial Nutrition*. London: MacDonald and Evans, 1950

43  Pyke M. *Technological Eating: Or Where Does the Fish Finger Point?* London: John Murray, 1972

44  Stuart T. *Waste: Uncovering the Global Food Scandal*. London: Penguin, 2009

45  Freidberg S. *Fresh: A Perishable History*. Cambridge, MA and London: Belknap, 2009

46  Jackson P. Fresh, in: Jackson P (Ed.) *Food Words*. London: Bloomsbury, 2013: 85–7

47  Food Standards Agency. *Criteria for the Use of the Terms Fresh, Pure, Natural etc. in Food Labelling*. Available at: www.food.gov.uk/sites/default/files/multimedia/pdfs/markcritguidance.pdf. (accessed September 16, 2014), 2008

48  Quested T, Ingle R, Parry A. *Household Food and Drink Waste in the United Kingdom*. Available at: www.wrap.org.uk/content/household-food-and-drink-waste-uk-2012 (accessed February 10, 2014), 2012

49  Defra. *Understanding the Environmental Impacts of Consuming Foods That Are Produced Locally in Season*. Project FO0412. Available at: http://randd.defra.gov.uk/Default.aspx? (accessed February 16, 2016), 2012

50  Fox T, Fimeche C. *Global Food: Waste Not, Want Not*. Institute of Mechanical Engineers, London, 2013

51  Longhurst R. Household food strategies in response to seasonality and famine. *IDS Bulletin*, 1987; 17(3): 27–35

52  Sumberg J, Sharp L. *Is It Possible to Find a Meaningful Definition of the Term Seasonal Food?* Available at: www.fcrn.org.uk/sites/default/files/NEF_What_is_seasonal_food_2009.pdf (accessed July 8, 2016), 2009

53  Smith A, Watkiss P, Tweddle G, et al. The Validity of Food Miles as an Indicator of Sustainable Development: Report to DEFRA by AEA Technology. London: Department for the Environment, Food and Rural Affairs, 2005

54  Dibb S, Collins J, Mayo E for the National Consumer Council. Seasons' Promise: An Enjoyable Way to Tackle Climate Change. Available at: www.consumerfutures.org. uk/wpfb-file/seasons-promise-an-enjoyable-way-to-tackle-climate-change-2006-pdf (accessed September 16, 2014), 2006

55  National Food Administration, Environment Agency. Environmentally Effective Food Choices: Proposal Notified to the EU. Stockholm: National Food Administration, 2008

56  Livsmedelsverket, National Food Administration. Find Your Way to Eat Greener, Not Too Much and Be Active. Stockholm: Livsmedelsverket/National Food Administration, 2015: 26

57  US FDA. What Is the Meaning of 'Natural' on the Label of Food? Available at: www. fda.gov/AboutFDA/Transparency/Basics/ucm214868.htm (accessed July 30, 2016). Washington, DC: US Food and Drug Administration, 2016

58  Woolfe M, Gurungb T, Walker MJ. Can analytical chemists do molecular biology? A survey of the up-skilling of the UK official food control system in DNA food authenticity techniques. Food Control, 2013; 33(2): 385–92

59  Arvanitoyannis IS. Authenticity of Foods of Animal Origin. Abingdon: CRC Press, 2016

60  Jackson P. Food Words: Essays in Culinary Culture. London: Bloomsbury Academic, 2013

61  Johnston J, Baumann S. Democracy versus distinction: a study of omnivorousness in gourmet food writing. American Journal of Sociology, 2007; 113(1): 165–204

62  Cramer C, Johnston D, Oya C, et al. Fairtrade, Employment and Poverty Reduction in Ethiopia and Uganda: Final Report to DfID. London: School of Oriental and African Studies, University of London, 2014: 143

63  Pratt J. Food values: the local and the authentic. Critique of Anthropology, 2007; 27(3): 285–300

64  Lang T. From 'value-for-money' to 'values-for-money'? Ethical food and policy in Europe. Environment and Planning A, 2010; 42: 1814–32

65  Review on Antimicrobial Resistance (Chair: Jim O'Neill). Securing New Drugs for Future Generations: The Pipeline of Antibiotics. London: Wellcome Trust and HM Government, 2015

66  Review on Antimicrobial Resistance (Chaired by Jim O'Neill). Tackling Drug-Resistant Infections Globally: Final Report and Recommendations. London: Review on Antimicrobial Resistance, 2016

67  Ye M, Beach J, Martin JW, et al. Occupational pesticide exposures and respiratory health. International Journal of Environmental Research and Public Health, 2013; 10 (12): 6442–71

68  Sandler DP. John Snow and modern-day environmental epidemiology. American Journal of Epidemiology, 2000; 152(1): 1–3

69  Johnson S. The Ghost Map: a Street, a City, an Epidemic and the Hidden Power of Urban Networks. London: Penguin Books, 2006

70  Douglas M. Food in the Social Order: Study of Food and Festivities in Three American Communities. New York: Russell Sage Foundation, 1984

71  Douglas M, Isherwood B. The World of Goods: Towards an Anthropology of Consumption. London: Allen Lane, 1978

72  Lévi-Strauss C. *The Raw and the Cooked: Introduction to a Science of Mythology: 1.* Harmondsworth: Penguin, 1966

73  Douglas M. Deciphering a meal. *Daedalus*, 1972; 101: 61–82

74  Oliver J. *Cutting Food Waste: Reclaiming Wonky Veg.* Available at: www.jamieoliver.com/news-and-features/features/reclaiming-wonky-veg/#SiOQ8PtZYCVUpU06.97 (accessed July 30, 2016). London: Jamie Oliver Organisation, 2016

75  Fearnley-Whittingstall H. *Hugh's War on Waste*, BBC TV. Available at: www.rivercottage.net/war-on-waste. London: BBC and The River Cottage, 2016

76  Stuart T. *The Global Food Waste Scandal: Food Waste Facts.* Available at: http://feedbackglobal.org/food-waste-scandal/ (accessed July 30, 2016). London: Feedback/Feeding the 5000, 2014

## Chapter 7

# Real food economics
## Runaway costs and concentration

### Contents

### Core arguments

There has been little mainstream economic analysis of sustainable diets, but the case for such analysis is growing. This chapter shows that sustainable diets require insights from food economics that go beyond the simple rhetoric that markets and prices will determine outcomes or allocate resources. There is strong evidence that food costs do not convey the true costs of production and consumption or of diet's impact on public health and the environment. The chapter reviews a number of key features of what is required from economics such as inequality of access, labour in the food supply chain, the persistence of low wages, the surprising and shocking state of slavery and poor working conditions in some communities, the hidden and often unpaid extra costs due to environmental and health externalities, and the burden of waste. It concludes that food economics has a useful role to play but cannot be the ultimate arbiter of the transition to sustainable diets and food systems if that economics is narrowly conceived. A broad-based food economics can help shift culture from a simplistic focus on 'value for money' to one based on 'values for money'.

## Why economics matters for the sustainable diets debate

As we wrote in Chapter 1, it would be impossible to do justice to the notion of a sustainable diet without facing the importance of economics. Food costs. It represents value-added. People make money from food. Consumer choices are shaped by its price, their incomes and by affordability. That much is both obvious but also central to the task of this book, which is to explore the role of diet and food in debates about sustainability in general and certainly about food sustainability. Discussion about food and health has had a patchy relationship with economics. The twentieth century's success was, in part, a result of how food production managed to increase output, industrialise food systems and lower costs so much that more people than ever in history were fed and fed more amply than before.[1,2] And yet, by the turn of the twenty-first century, the pursuit of cheapness as a prime motive had become problematic.[3] Food was so cheap that even relatively poor consumers in rich societies were wasting huge proportions of it, while poor consumers in low-income societies were still having to spend high proportions of their incomes on food, so did not waste food once they had purchased it.[4] Still the old truth remains that the poorer people are, whether in high- or low-income countries, the more of their income goes on food.[5] Moreover, as the nutrition transition swept across the world, ever more people were eating food so high in calories, because it had become more affordable and available, that overweight and obesity far exceeded the nightmare of previous generations – hunger – not that this was absent either. This indeed suggests a complex web of social and economic interactions. Yet, as we will discuss, some economists seem to claim that economics can be the ultimate arbiter of what a good diet is. We doubt that. We take a broader view of food economics as it affects the pursuit of more sustainable diets and food systems.

To some extent, the fact we describe the relationship of economics to food as troubled is because economists (rather than economics as an academic pursuit) have come to hold a powerful sway over what societies think of as good systems. This image has been dented considerably since the banking crash of 2007–8, the Great Recession that ensued and the exposé of the people and motives behind them.[6] The image of economics is now also tarnished by coverage of the lifestyles of flash 'money men' and financiers, the reality of speculative high-frequency trading and massive consumer debt while politicians discipline the public sector with homilies about 'balancing the books'. Meanwhile there is serious wage inequality within and between societies. This is the contrary world of economics into which the sustainable diet discourse has to fit.

The ancient Greek words *oikos* and *nomos*, which were combined to coin 'economics', suggest something more philosophical than modern economics might like to accept. As we have shown throughout this book, the debates about sustainable diets and food system sustainability do indeed raise highly philosophical issues – what is a good life or society? To analyse sustainable diet, one needs to retain a broad approach to economics, ranging from finance capitalism (because food is a commodity and is, historically and still today, much speculated on by investors)[7-9] to the domestic sphere of the home, people's lives and lifestyles.[10, 11]

The word 'economics' came to mean the 'rules of the house', the principles of domestic management, and only thence was it applied to the wider economy. This domestic focus was retained in the twentieth century in school education with the creation of a subject taught in many societies and known as home economics or, more grandly, as domestic science. This spawned a school curriculum and classes where young people (mainly women) were taught how to manage their (future) homes, and were taught the skills deemed appropriate to that end. Home economics grew dramatically from the mid-twentieth century, a time when industrial food was spreading in Western cultures.[12] Home economics, in this tradition, was about domestic skills; not just cooking but also management of clothes (and fashion), household goods (furniture, bedding, curtains), domestic finance and the choice of consumer goods.

This educational strand of food and domestic economics can be traced to the formal teaching of skills of household management in the Victorian era. *Household Management* was the title of a celebrated Victorian tome written by a young Mrs Isabella Beeton, first published by her husband in 1861 and then reproduced in instalments (a 'part-work') and, despite Mrs Beeton's death in 1865, in endlessly revised forms to the present day.[13] The Victorian age was when mass-processed foods and commodified goods gained a significant market presence. Some major food processing and retailing companies trace their origins to that period. By the mid-twentieth century, however, a new phase emerged in the industrialisation of food, with the mass uptake of many new technologies now taken for granted such as refrigeration and freezers, ready-made meals, new forms of packaging and storage. The rise of kitchen gadgets illustrates a theme to which we return later: the role of technology in replacing food labour. Indeed, a key battle in food economics that impinges on the sustainability debate is where that labour is based – in the factory or the home? – where it is most 'efficient', what is meant by that, and whether and how much it is paid. Is efficiency represented by the capacity of a person (male or female) to cook a meal from raw ingredients from scratch? Or is it measured by carbon emissions, in which case factory food may be more efficient due to the efficiencies of scale?

Domestic science and home economics can be tracked as reactions to and purveyors of how to address big change in food. Home economics in the 1860s targeted the middle-class women who ran households – and the messages were not just about thrift but also about managing servants and expressing the new opulence (multiple-course meals, etc.). The first colleges of domestic science began in the late nineteenth century. Home economics in the 1950s–70s, by contrast, was apparently more democratic. It was about managing one's own resources, appealing to modernity and running the simplified, smaller household with fewer children and no servants. The equipment – fridges, vacuum cleaners, cookers, gadgets, etc. – replaced the servants. But all these messages, trainings and advice were mostly oriented at women. Gone was the middle-class matriarch managing the large household and in came the self-servicing domestic goddess with multiple roles. This is sexist economics, accepting a conventional division of (domestic) labour, and it is why there is a strong strand of feminist critique of this version of home economics.[14, 15]

The US radical Charlotte Gilman Perkins had argued in 1898 that the sooner women abandoned the private kitchen and that food was produced in collective kitchens (almost on Scandinavian shared-kitchen lines), the better life would be for women.[16] Domestic work should be professionalised and paid. This would liberate women to be wage-earners themselves in the wider economy. Despite these views, Gilman Perkins rejected the feminist label, arguing that this was about progress in social evolution. She was not alone at that time in arguing the case that the industrialisation of food was an advance, laying out the parameters of a debate still running today: is domestic cooking a good thing,[10] and where and how do women spend their time? Gilman Perkins put great emphasis on the liberation potential of domestic technology and house design – notably kitchens.[17] Historically and to the present day, women have constituted a high proportion of workers in the food system. In some cultures, women do almost all domestic crop cultivation. One study estimated that women were 69% of the workers in South Africa growing food for the European market while, in the UK, women were only 31% of the waged labour force.[18] Almost everywhere women have lower wages and spend the most time on food preparation and shopping.

We have begun this chapter by locating economics in the domestic sphere for good reason. It reminds economists that their science has strong and honourable household and food roots. The language of economics is full of food references, especially from farming – 'ploughing back the profits'. Also, it is a reminder that some of the economic debates about sustainable diets – on affordability, costs, who pays, where the money goes – are not new. They are highly charged and also moral. Even those who see or saw home economics as the teaching of skills could not and cannot avoid the moral overtones. A good woman manages her house well. Eating thriftily is something that had to be taught, at odds with the 1960s consumerism and encouragement to spend, to waste, to consume.

Against this conceptual language, modern economists prefer to present themselves as quantitative arbiters of reality – 'the costs don't add up', 'face financial reality', 'don't spend what you haven't got'. Language and culture are replete with economic homilies. Yet, in reality, economists have rationalised (some might say created) bubbles in financial systems, contributed to awesome levels of monetary debt, and have redefined morality, not least in helping shape modern banking systems that determine national and international trade, debt and exchange. This is an approach to economics that has tried to sever overt ideological links, applying cool hard logic in the name of Adam Smith. Smith, however, did not see economics in this way. For him, as for the fellow architects, economics was a moral and political but rational pursuit.[19, 20] The 'rules' of living are malleable; they represent political choices. However, modern economics, as a social science, has become something different, trying to sever the politics and to claim value-neutrality. Apocryphally, Thomas Carlyle called Malthus a purveyor of 'dismal science', and not without reason since Malthus' prognosis about the nigh inevitability of famine and crisis if population growth outgrew food-growing capacity was indeed pretty 'dismal'; i.e., dismal in the sense of depressing and sobering. Sustainable diets, too, can be painted as moralist, saying 'no', 'eat less' and favouring restraint.[21] The optimistic message is that it provides the ultimate positive message of permanence, long horizons, quality, eating better, social solidarity and public health.[22]

There are many approaches within modern economics, from Right to Left in formal politics. Since the late 1970s and 1980s, neoliberal economic thinking has perhaps been the most powerful approach. This emphasises market discipline over state controls, and favours the price mechanism and financial mechanisms as arbiters of supply and demand. Competition is the normal route to efficiency and improvement. Bureaucracy, rules and regulations are the enemy of enterprise. Neoliberalism has gone through many phases and emphases; its home used to be Germany and Hungary but is today more associated with Chicago economics.[23, 24] Neoliberalism sought to replace the Keynesian approaches that had emerged in and after the Second World War, most famously articulated by John Maynard Keynes.[25, 26] Partly in reaction to the devastating effects of the 1920s and 1930s slumps and the 1929 Wall Street Crash, Keynes argued that the state had a key responsibility to even out capitalism's tendency to go from boom to slump – rising and then falling markets. His work echoed some of the experiments in state regeneration after the slump: a commitment to create employment, introduction of welfare (paid by taxes), marketing support (such as agricultural boards) and other interventions. These were anathema to neoliberals who saw them as drains on enterprise, intrinsically inefficient and a constraint on freedom.[27] They put civil servants in the way of consumer sovereignty, allowed the state to intervene in the dynamics of markets, putting burdens where there could be freedoms. The freedom of consumers to choose became a key theme for twentieth-century neoliberals; the individual is the key actor not the collective.[28] Given a political mandate, they saw their role as unwinding decades of institutional growth, the privatisation of public goods and the delivery of what has been termed the Washington Consensus.[29, 30] Neoliberals have pursued high economic growth, the opening up of markets, the removal of national barriers to trade and the creation of 'level playing fields'. Marketing boards created in the USA and Europe to support farming after the 1930s recession and the war were dismantled in the 1980s. Who needs a Mushroom or Milk or Potato Marketing Board? Let the retail supermarket buyers mediate between supply and consumer demand.

The reason why this divergence of opinion and this digression into political economic history matters to the sustainable diet issue is that the debate about sustainability raises fundamental criticisms of the impact of neoliberalism. By contrast, 'green' or environmental economics questions whether prices are true and whether cheap food is actually cheap. It may be cheap in the shop but the full costs are not being borne by the purchaser. The environment is being exploited and not recompensed. Pollution is dumped out there, with the ecosystem taking the negative impacts in the form of biodiversity destruction, polluted biosphere, water and air. This argument and the data generated in this vein have been major drivers of the sustainable diet approach, as we will show. Many studies show the cost of poor diets to healthcare systems and in lost quality of life.

Our argument here is that the economics of sustainable diets and sustainable food systems must discriminate between these two major positions, one the dominant norm of neoliberalism, the other the emerging powerful arguments about true cost accounting. In the rest of this chapter we explore this terrain.

## Economics of the food system: price or priceless?

The cost of food waste is enormous. In preparation for the Second International Conference on Nutrition in 2014, the FAO published a summary of what this is. It calculated that food produce that is not consumed has an annual 'bulk-trade value' of $964 bn annually. This is a huge sum but, just as significant in the FAO's view, is that these separate costs have knock-on or interactive effects. Lost food has also lost soil nutrients, which adds to soil depletion, which increases the likelihood of conflict from resource scarcity. Some FAO calculations are given in Table 7.1. Country case studies by the FAO show how significant this can be. One of milk wastage in Kenya, for example, calculated the actual loss of milk sales as 571,418 tonnes valued at US$151 m. But if the social and environmental costs due to GHGs, water, land, water pollution, soil erosion, water scarcity, biodiversity and human health were computed as well, this total loss rose to US$758 m.

The sums computed here are considerable but is this monetisation the best measure of efficiency? In our view, price remains a key indicator but does not capture everything. Money mediates between production and consumption. It encapsulates estimated value in a market. Price shapes what people can afford to eat. But there are other conventional measures too, such as productivity of labour and capital. How much food is produced per $ € £ invested? How much food is produced by each food worker? How good is company performance as measured on the stock exchanges? We also need different measures, not least land use, energy and resource use.

Both business and economists have nurtured the transfer of the language of capitalism into food thinking, but one notion has achieved particular resonance: the notion of capital. A distinction is often now made between finance

Table 7.1  Costs of societal impacts of food wastage ($bn per year, at 2012 value)

| Costs | Global | OECD countries | Non-OECD countries |
| --- | --- | --- | --- |
| GHG emissions | 394 | 85 | 309 |
| Deforestation | 2.9 | 0.3 | 2.6 |
| Water use | 7.7 | 2.2 | 5.5 |
| Water scarcity | 164 | 14 | 150 |
| Water pollution | 24 | 13 | 11 |
| Soil erosion | 34.6 | 16.4 | 18.2 |
| Biodiversity | 9.5 | 4.4 | 5.2 |
| Health (acute pesticide incidence cost) | 8 | 0.8 | 7.2 |
| Livelihood (adults) | 228.6 | 7.8 | 230.8 |
| Individual health (adults) | 102 | 2.8 | 99.2 |
| Conflict (adults) | 248.9 | n/a | n/a |
| Total | 1,224.2 | 146.7 | 838.7 |

Source: FAO 2014.[31]

capital (money), natural capital (eco-systems, nature), human capital (skills, education, etc.) and social capital (interactions, networks). In some respects this has been a demeaning transfer of language. Everything becomes 'capital' or it doesn't exist. However, it has had one good result in our view. It has meant that data and analyses from areas outside normal economic monetary discourse have been developed and the language of environmental capital has now become that of capital depletion, loss, asset squeeze, and so on. The UN, for example, has been able to engage with processes such as the System of Environmental and Economic Accounts, and the FAO and UNEP to work jointly on the ongoing Economics of Ecosystems and Biodiversity (TEEB) analysis.

If we take economics back to fundamentals, it is a lot about land. What is land for? Around 1.4 bn hectares of land is available for food growing on the planet. This varies dramatically in quality of soil, growing seasons, plant suitability and much more. But, taking that rough figure, one EU NGO in 2013 decided that this means each of the planet's current 7 bn people has about 2,000 square metres ($m^2$) to grow their food on or for the food they consume to come from.[32] This sobering figure led it to suggest a different, more intensive approach to food growing, with an emphasis on plants rather than animals; animals take a lot of food-growing space. Agronomists (agricultural economists) can help flesh out this kind of 'broad brush' approach, which is understandably designed to engage with public consciousness and to encourage behaviour change. A paper by Cassidy and colleagues tried to do this, also engaging with the land-use question; it proposed that the most useful metric in the future will be 'people fed per hectare', i.e., whether or how many people are actually fed, rather than the conventional agronomic measures of productivity or profit that indicate what the landowner gains.[33]

Cassidy and colleagues studied 41 crops produced globally, calculating that $9.46 \times 1{,}015$ calories are available in plant form, of which 55% feed humans directly, 36% are fed to animals, of which 89% is lost, and a further 9% goes into industrial use such as biofuels and is thus lost as human feed. In total, therefore, 41% of total crop calories are lost from the food system. If this crop production was fed directly to humans, they calculated that another approximately 4 bn people could be fed.[33] With its culinary culture historically based on using meat as flavouring (slivers of pork in a chow mein, for instance), China is estimated to feed 8.4 people per hectare, whereas Brazil, with far more land, feeds 5.2 people per hectare. The USA uses only 34% of the food it produces to feed humans directly, allocating nearly double (1.8) the amount of food to animals than does China. The conclusion of this study was clear: it would make sense to: (a) reduce the emphasis on producing ever more animals for meat or dairy; (b) use what feedstuff there was to feed the more efficient converters such as chicken and pigs; (c) shift consumer culture away from meat-centrism; and (d) make 'people fed per hectare' the most important metric.

They began with the important but old fact – forgotten by generations reared on thinking that food comes from supermarkets – that animals vary in their feed conversion efficiency. One kg of feed to an animal does not result in 1 kg of meat or produce for human consumption. The US Department of Agriculture estimates that 1 kg of beef has taken 12 kg of feed to be produced, while 1 kg of chicken used about 5 kg of feed, but even these figures can vary dramatically; much depends on the quality of the feed and how and the circumstances in which the animal is reared. There is agreement, however, that generally cows/beef take more feeding than sheep, and they more than pigs, and that poultry have the fastest feed-conversion ratio. All these animals can be used to convert food waste, of course, but the trend of recent decades has been for crops to be grown specifically for the animal feed market and for 'waste' to be unsafe. Fed on specially reared crops, meat production is a pretty inefficient way of producing food. But it is almost assumed to be, indeed it is being factored into, the case for neo-Malthusian urgency and prognostications of impending food crises. Rising meat consumption is assumed to be an unstoppable trend.[34] Table 7.2 gives some calorie and protein conversion efficiency percentages for dairy, eggs, chicken, pork and beef.

Table 7.2 Livestock conversion efficiencies

|  | Dairy | Eggs | Chicken | Pork | Beef |
|---|---|---|---|---|---|
| Calorie conversion efficiency % | 40 | 22 | 12 | 10 | 3 |
| Protein conversion efficiency % | 43 | 35 | 40 | 10 | 5 |

Source: Cassidy et al.,[33] based on Smil.[1]

Not all land is equivalent. Forage crops that a sheep or cow can graze cannot be eaten by humans, any more than humans can graze grass growing on a wild hillside. However, humans can eat grains that are so widely fed to animals but not the by-products of sugar cane production or industrial by-products. This is often given as the justification for animal production.[35] A commonly cited concern is that rising prosperity and rising populations require more meat and, in turn, more crops for animal feedstuffs.[36] Some analyse this as an ecological pressure; others as a rationale for new technologies. But when nearly half the grains grown on the planet are fed to animals,[37, 38] their usefulness as converters of what otherwise would be 'waste' or by-products is being somewhat distorted by using them as ends in themselves, and a rationale for industrialised factory farming.

One measure or term that has come into the sustainable food policy discourse is 'footprints'.[39] This was coined by researchers to capture how human activity left an impact on the earth.[40, 41] Originally it was used to convey how much land is used to support existence.[42] Thus London in 2002, then a city of approximately 7 m inhabitants, was estimated to need 6.63 global hectares (gha) to maintain each citizen, not just in food but in everything.[43] The study showed how a squeeze was underway. Londoners may have used 6.63 gha each, but their fair share globally would have been only 2.18 gha. Materials and waste accounted for 44% of the footprint, food for 41%, energy for 10%, transport for 5% and water for 1%. Later work in 2014 for London confirmed that food was an immense emitter and space user.

This kind of material analysis actually goes back to Malthus of course but also, in the 1960s and 1970s, to work by Georg Borgström who started analysing farm resource use for the amount of land it used in 'ghost acres' or hidden land use.[44] Your local chicken farm might only sit on a hectare or two but it uses tens of hectares elsewhere, hidden by trade, to feed the animals. The metaphor can be interpreted in different ways – a footprint in setting concrete (i.e., permanent) or a footprint in sand on the seashore (i.e., that will be erased by incoming tides) or something that can be swept over (i.e., restorative). In fact, the term has come to be used extensively to mean more permanent damage across sustainability topics from carbon to water.[45]

There is now a vast body of work measuring the carbon and water footprints of food products. UNESCO has published detailed work coordinated by a team of Dutch researchers on tens of thousands of food products.[46-48] It builds on the pioneering work of UK geographer Tony Allan who mapped how what he called 'virtual' water was traded across borders.[49, 50] He was concerned by the inevitability of water-scarce countries, for example in the Sahel, inevitably needing to import water in embedded form in foods. He proposed that this trade in hidden water should be made overt and rationally managed. The footprint approach has been enthusiastically adopted by cities and regions to audit their environmental impact and infrastructure, but also by food companies.[51] For instance, Tesco, the third largest food retailer in the world, publishes an audit of its energy footprint.[52, 53] The methodology can become sensitive over where the boundaries of responsibility are drawn. If a company sells refrigerators or dairy products, should its carbon or water footprint include the carbon and water that went into the making and transporting of the products? Is their responsibility only what happens within or proximate to the store?

Footprinting could become what critics decry as 'greenwash', used by corporate PR machinery, but it is useful in policy as a non-financial auditing tool. The Global Footprint Network, for example, runs a much-cited data set on each country and the planet monitoring whether countries are consuming within their biocapacity or exceeding it.[54] In 2014 it estimated that global consumption was at a level that implies there are 1.5 planets. There are not, of course, and that is the point being made; this cannot go on without catastrophic effects on biosystems. The 2007-8 banking crisis and subsequent recession was actually good news in resource use, because less was used but mainstream economists urged a return to 'growth'!

A key method within footprinting is life-cycle analysis (LCA) (discussed in Chapter 2); this audits the full 'career' of a product or food from inputs to waste. The European Union appears committed to some form of both LCA and the bigger goal of achieving a circular economy, in which waste is not wasted but recycled. The EU is in negotiation with big industrial sectors to agree methodology and data publication.[55] Its usefulness in the sustainable diet discourse can be illustrated by one Spanish study comparing its traditional Mediterranean diet with what the Spanish actually now eat (which it termed a 'Western dietary pattern', i.e., less desirable for health). The study suggested that if the Spanish population returned to the traditional diet, its dietary impact would reduce its greenhouse gas emissions (GHGEs) by 72%, land use by 58%, energy consumption by 52% and water consumption by 33%. The Western dietary pattern implied an increase in all those indicators of between 12% and 72%.[56] Footprinting, in other words, can be a useful measure alongside public health considerations. But where does it take discussion of prices?

## The big picture on food prices

Part of the threat of sustainable diets to conventional economics lies in the fact that it appears to confront what is meant by progress, and not without reason. In the USA or EU, food typically takes 10-15% of domestic expenditure, whereas in India, Russia or China it may be over 50%, and may be 75% in the poorest of low-income countries in Africa.[57] Progress can be measured by politicians and economists quantitatively. If, in the UK in 1885, the working classes spent 71% of their earnings on food and drink with bread being the main staple food and, by 1946, even after a punishing world war, food expenditure had dropped to 34% of average incomes, surely this was progress?[58] How much more progress if, by the turn of the millennium, food expenditure was under 10% of average incomes? But what lies behind this approach to food economic progress? Within the European Union, which operates a 'single market' in foods, there is considerable variation in how much consumers spend on food as a percentage of their

*Table 7.3* Percentage of total consumer expenditure on food and non-alcoholic beverages in the EU

| EU country | % share | Ranking | EU country | % share | Ranking |
|---|---|---|---|---|---|
| Luxembourg | 8.3 | 1 | Malta | 14.8 | 15 |
| UK | 9.3 | 2 | Slovenia | 14.9 | 16 |
| Austria | 10.0 | 3 | Czech Republic | 15.5 | 17 |
| Ireland | 10.2 | 4 | Greece | 16.2 | 18 |
| Denmark | 11.3 | 5 | Slovakia | 17.5 | 19 |
| Germany | 11.7 | 6 | Hungary | 17.6 | 20 |
| Netherlands | 12.0 | 7 | Portugal | 18.2 | 21 |
| Sweden | 12.1 | 8 | Poland | 18.5 | 22 |
| Finland | 12.5 | 9 | Estonia | 19.0 | 23 |
| Cyprus | 13.4 | 10 | Latvia | 19.2 | 24 |
| Belgium | 13.6 | 11 | Bulgaria | 19.7 | 25 |
| France | 13.7 | 12 | Lithuania | 25.4 | 26 |
| Spain | 14.2 | 13 | Romania | 27.5 | 27 |
| Italy | 14.4 | 14 | Croatia | n/a | |

Source: Eurostat 2012 figures, cited in Schoen and Lang, 2014.[58]

total expenditure. Table 7.3 gives Eurostat figures on the percentages and the ranking for the EU member states in 2012.[58] It shows that Luxembourg, a wealthy EU member state, spent 8.3%, compared with Romania, a new EU entrant, that spent 27% – a threefold difference.

Figure 7.1 is a graph produced by the USDA showing how food prices fell in real terms in the twentieth century, even as the population grew.[59, 60] The advantage of this food price drop, at the rate of 1% per year on average, is that it released spending for other goods and services and it transformed lives, enabling people living on restricted diets to eat more. So to argue that food prices are not accurate and do not reflect true costs undermines the view that this has been progress and a public good. This is a hard message to convey to consumers who have become used to 'cheap' food and who juggle domestic budgets, faced with competing demands and tensions between needs and wants.

Behind the steady drop in prices lies a picture in which the price of the main agricultural commodities, the primary foods before processing, have risen in nominal terms (the actual cash cost) but dropped in real terms and also relative to the cost of living. Figure 7.2 shows how, in real terms, food prices have actually been fairly constant over the last 50 years, or since the FAO monitored them. But there have been two 'blips'. The first coincides with the early 1970s oil crisis. The second with the banking crisis and the subsequent Great Recession. This latter period has weakened mainstream economic confidence in the long-term continuation of ever lower prices. Three analyses now vie for dominance. One sees the present as a temporary period of volatility but that long-term trends of price reduction will continue. The second sees this

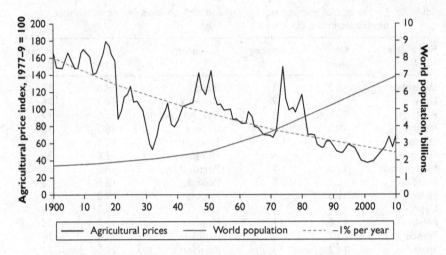

*Figure 7.1* Real agricultural prices and world population, 1900–2010

Source: USDA ERS/Fuglie and Wang 2012.[59]

Note: the agricultural price index used is the Grilli-Yang Price Index, which is a composite of 18 crop and livestock prices weighted by its share of global agricultural trade. World population estimates are taken from UN sources.

as the impact of 'new fundamentals' impinging on commodity markets, which now have to acknowledge finite resources, environmental uncertainties (notably climate change) and the effects of global economic restructuring.[61] After decades of being quiet cheer-leaders for conventional efficiency, the OECD, for example, began to support the latter interpretation, arguing that the new certainty was uncertainty and price volatility.[62] OECD and IMF data show how food prices closely follow the price of oil.[63] It also led to a third analysis that the rapid rise in prices and the volatility reflected speculation by financiers seeking a home for money after the collapse of value in the stockmarket.[7, 64, 65]

Figure 7.2 suggests that all these analyses might be right because the FAO's Food Price Index dropped seriously in 2014–15. This was due to a combination of factors: the oil price dropping as the USA's adoption of fracking kicked in, reducing its reliance on imported Middle East oil; Saudi Arabia allowing the base price of oil to drop to try to make fracking too expensive and thus undermine US self-reliance; and a slow-down in Chinese-led global economic expansion and search for resources. Be that as it may, this volatility after decades of relative passivity in food markets underlines new uncertainties about food prices,[66] and led the FAO's Director General to express concern about the impact on low-income countries.[67] This sober view was justified by a subsequent meta-analysis of 136 studies drawn from 164 countries that showed that price volatility hurt low-income countries the most and led to a drop in food consumption.[68] Table 7.4, just as Figure 7.2, takes the years 2002–4 as a benchmark of 100 and shows the fluctuations across the years 2000–15 in five crucial food commodities: meat, dairy, cereals, vegetable oils and sugar. The fluctuations are considerable and may be seen in the monthly breakdown July 2014–July 2015.

The price of raw commodities is only one part of the total cost of food, significant but, in fact, a shrinking proportion. Over the twentieth century, first in developed countries but now in developing countries, agriculture received a diminishing share of what consumers paid for food. Power and profits began to move off the land as populations urbanised, more processed food manufacturers emerged, retailers became larger chains and, latterly, with the explosion of eating out of the home. A useful account of who takes which share of the money US consumers spend is given in an annual summary by the USDA Economic Research Services.[70] In 2013, for example, of every dollar US consumers spent on US-produced food, farmers received 17.4 cents. Meanwhile their costs of production – what they had to pay for inputs – had risen from 8.3 cents in 2006 to 10.5 cents in 2013. The aggregated amount each sector in the food chain received in 2013 is given in Table 7.5.

In the UK the statistics are collected and presented differently but tell a not dissimilar story. The share received by primary growers, fisherfolk and farmers is small. In 2014 there were 64 m consumers in the UK who spent £198 bn on food, of which £86 bn was on catering services (i.e., food eaten out of the home) and £112 bn on food eaten in the home. Looking at the figures for gross value added by each sector – i.e., who added what value to that final figure of £198 bn spent by

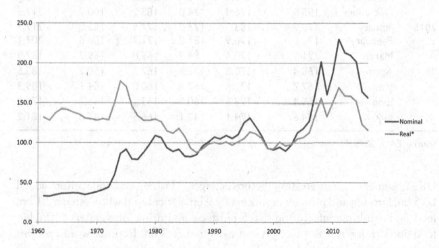

*Figure 7.2* FAO Food Price Index in nominal and real terms, 1961–2016

Source: FAO, 2016.

Note: * The real price index is the nominal price index deflated by the World Bank Manufacturers Unite Value Index (MUV).

Table 7.4 Food prices 2000–15 for five key commodities: meat, dairy, cereals,
vegetable oils, sugar

| Year | Month | FAO Food Price Index | Meat | Dairy | Cereals | Vegetable oils | Sugar |
|------|-------|----------------------|------|-------|---------|----------------|-------|
| 2000 | | 91.1 | 96.5 | 95.3 | 85.8 | 69.5 | 116.1 |
| 2001 | | 94.6 | 100.1 | 105.5 | 86.8 | 67.2 | 122.6 |
| 2002 | | 89.6 | 89.9 | 80.9 | 93.7 | 87.4 | 97.8 |
| 2003 | | 97.7 | 95.9 | 95.6 | 99.2 | 100.6 | 100.6 |
| 2004 | | 112.7 | 114.2 | 123.5 | 107.1 | 111.9 | 101.7 |
| 2005 | | 118.0 | 123.7 | 135.2 | 101.3 | 102.7 | 140.3 |
| 2006 | | 127.2 | 120.9 | 129.7 | 118.9 | 112.7 | 209.6 |
| 2007 | | 161.4 | 130.8 | 219.1 | 163.4 | 172.0 | 143.0 |
| 2008 | | 201.4 | 160.7 | 223.1 | 232.1 | 227.1 | 181.6 |
| 2009 | | 160.3 | 141.3 | 148.6 | 170.2 | 152.8 | 257.3 |
| 2010 | | 188.0 | 158.3 | 206.6 | 179.2 | 197.4 | 302.0 |
| 2011 | | 229.9 | 183.3 | 229.5 | 240.9 | 254.5 | 368.9 |
| 2012 | | 213.3 | 182.0 | 193.6 | 236.1 | 223.9 | 305.7 |
| 2013 | | 209.8 | 184.1 | 242.7 | 219.3 | 193.0 | 251.0 |
| 2014 | | 201.8 | 198.3 | 224.1 | 191.9 | 181.1 | 241.2 |
| 2014 | July | 204.3 | 205.9 | 226.1 | 185.2 | 181.1 | 259.1 |
| | August | 198.3 | 212.0 | 200.8 | 182.5 | 166.6 | 244.3 |
| | September | 192.7 | 211.0 | 187.8 | 178.2 | 162.0 | 228.1 |
| | October | 192.7 | 210.2 | 184.3 | 178.3 | 163.7 | 237.6 |
| | November | 191.3 | 206.4 | 178.1 | 183.2 | 164.9 | 229.7 |
| | December | 185.8 | 196.4 | 174.0 | 183.9 | 160.7 | 217.5 |
| 2015 | January | 178.9 | 183.5 | 173.8 | 177.4 | 156.0 | 217.7 |
| | February | 175.8 | 176.9 | 181.8 | 171.7 | 156.6 | 207.1 |
| | March | 171.5 | 170.4 | 184.9 | 169.8 | 159.7 | 187.9 |
| | April | 168.4 | 170.8 | 172.4 | 167.2 | 150.2 | 185.5 |
| | May | 167.2 | 172.6 | 167.5 | 160.8 | 154.1 | 189.3 |
| | June | 166.4 | 173.6 | 160.5 | 163.2 | 156.2 | 176.8 |
| | July | 164.6 | 174.1 | 149.1 | 166.5 | 147.6 | 181.2 |

Source: FAO, 2015.[69]

UK consumers – an interesting picture emerges.[71] Fishing and aquaculture added
£0.5 bn, farming and primary producers £9.9 bn, agricultural wholesalers £2.1 bn,
food and drink manufacturing £26.5 bn, food and drink wholesalers £10.7 bn,
food and drink retailers £29.1 bn and caterers £26.9 bn. In other words, returns
are sparse to primary producers. The big money as well as employment lies off
the land. The UK farm and fishing labour force in 2014 was about 0.5 m, slightly
more than food manufacturing at 0.4 m (yet this is now the UK's largest manufacturing sector), wholesalers 0.2 m, caterers 1.6 m and retailers 1.2 m. Food work in
developed and many upper-middle-income developing countries is urban.

*Table 7.5* Sector 'share' of the US Food Dollar, 2013

| Sector | Share of Food Dollar (%) |
| --- | --- |
| Farm production | 10.5 |
| Food processing | 15.5 |
| Packaging | 2.6 |
| Transportation | 3.3 |
| Wholesale trade | 9.2 |
| Retail trade | 13.1 |
| Food service | 31.5 |
| Energy | 5.2 |
| Finance and insurance | 3.2 |
| Advertising | 2.5 |
| Other | 3.4 |
| TOTAL | 100 |

Source: USDA ERS, 2015.[70]

Note: these figures are for domestically produced US foods.

## Subsidies

In the mid-twentieth century, as countries experienced deep recessions and post-war reconstruction, Keynesian economics argued that governments could and should support food production and help even out the 'boom and slump' production cycles that had been shown to blight farm incomes and security. Subsidy systems began to be put in place to incentivise production. Some of these subsidies were hidden in the form of market support and some were overt. By the mid-1970s the by then resurgent neoliberals saw subsidies as a barrier to competition and the operation of pure markets. The OECD has been a source of constant monitoring of producer and consumer subsidies, and has been a policy 'prod' for subsidy reduction. This has been a constant feature of international trade negotiations. The OECD calculated that, in 2012–14, the 49 countries, some developed and other developing, which it monitored gave subsidies that transferred $601 bn (€450 bn) to producers, and spent a further $35 bn (€103 bn) on support for the sector's general functioning; this amounted to 18% of all farm income in those countries.[72] This high level of support is actually down from the heyday of the 1990s, according to OECD data. Figure 7.3 gives the OECD findings on Total Support Estimate (TSE), comparing the mid-1990s with 2012–14. This dropped for all countries reported here except China, Brazil and Indonesia.

New Zealand famously completely removed all its farm subsidies in 1984. Neoliberals expressed delight and certainly the immediate collapse some farm jeremiahs predicted did not happened. Subsequently, however, evidence began to mount that this did not stop New Zealand farming from intensifying nor did it prevent environmental burdens.[73] Elsewhere, however, subsidies flourish, despite

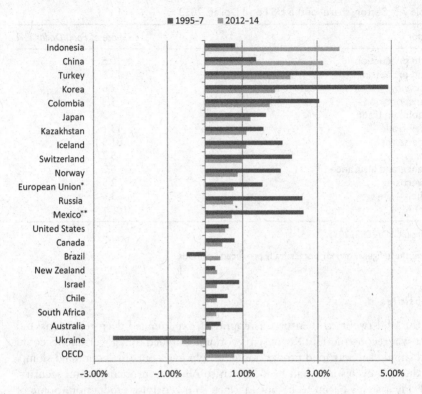

■ 1995–7   ■ 2012–14

*Figure 7.3* Total Support Estimate, by country, 1995–7 and 2012–14

Source: OECD, 2015.[72]

Notes:
 * The EU was 15 member states in the 1990s but 28 in 2014.
 ** Mexico figures are for 1991–3.

being neoliberal anathema. A Chatham House study, for example, suggested that China subsidised pig production by $22 bn in 2012 at the average rate of $47 per pig.[74] One of the iniquities of subsidies can be that those who need them least gain the most. In the USA it has been calculated that 10% of US farmers receive 75% of $15 bn subsidies, while 62% receive none at all.[75]

Another feature of real, as distinct from fantasy or theoretically 'pure', food markets is their tendency to concentrate. Big companies dwarf the others.[3] Four giants dominated the international grain trade: Cargill, Archer Daniels Midland (ADM), Louis Dreyfus and Bunge, whose revenues rose from $150 bn in 2005 to $318 bn in 2011.[76] The top food manufacturers globally by sales are Nestlé ($87,977 m), PepsiCo ($65,492 m), Coca-Cola ($48,017 m) and ADM ($46,289 m).[77] In 2012 the European food and drink manufacturing sector, for example, had 286,000 companies, employing over 4 m workers, at an average of

16 workers per firm, and had collective sales of just over €1 trillion. In this vast market 5% of these companies account for 77% of all turnover and 61% of all employment.[78] This high level of concentration is exceeded in other sectors. In seeds, for example, three companies have 53% of the market, in fertilisers and pesticides three have about the same, in grains and soya four companies have 75% of world trade.[79] Is this really a free or open market?

Food businesses whether giant or small are under great pressure to innovate. Huge numbers of food products are developed and marketed each year in consumer markets, which are already full by any definition of need. For instance, according to Nielsen data in 2011–13, in Western Europe alone, 65,725 new products were launched. Of these, only 55% lasted six months from launch and 73% were not on shelves after one year.[80] Think of all that wasted investment and effort.

## The real cost of food

The picture drawn so far is of a food system that bears little resemblance to that given in children's story books. Growers are a minority, catering and shop workers by far the majority. For sustainable diets, a key issue is how food is being processed, whether in a factory, the fast-food joint or the home. The resource use (carbon, water, land) varies but the trend is towards food and diets that are highly rather than lightly processed, re-made and designed rather than cooked fresh. The trend to ultra-processing gives the opportunity for nutritious ingredients to be accompanied by salt, sugar and fat to excess, and thus contribute to the health burden.

An international study by Wiggins and colleagues at the London-based Overseas Development Institute (ODI) explored the effects.[81] It reviewed the literature on how price affects the healthiness or unhealthiness of consumption, mostly drawn from UK and US studies, and summarised that, over the last 30 or 40 years, 'energy-dense, processed foods have become cheaper relative to less energy-dense fruit and vegetables'. Healthier diets cost more. They then looked at five countries: three of which are upper-middle-income countries – Brazil, China, Mexico – one of which is high-income, Korea, and the UK for comparison. They found that 'prices of fruit and vegetables have risen substantially since 1990, mainly by between 2% and 3% a year on average – or by 55–91% between 1990 and 2012. [. . .] Four of the six processed products for which estimates are significant show[ed] price falls since 1990. Most of the other foods have seen their prices rise by 1–2% a year, with the exception of the price falls for rice in Korea and chicken in Mexico.' The drop in price of ready-made processed foods accompanied by a rise in the cost of simple unprocessed 'raw' foods means that price signals favour the consumption of the former rather than the latter. Yet, the ODI researchers argued, the health consequences are not acceptable and are a burden on development. They concluded that 'a strong case emerges for using taxes and subsidies to offset these changes to encourage more consumption of healthy foods and less of unhealthy items.'

A separate systematic review of 24 studies found that fiscal interventions do have an impact on diet but noted that these were conducted only in affluent countries.[82] Despite the caveats, this is not a message neoliberal economists are likely to applaud. The pressure on their intellectual supremacy continues to build, however, not least over issues such as whether to tax 'unhealthy' foods,[83-86] and how to capture uncosted factors of production. We now turn to this latter point.

### Externalised and internalised costs

One measure for estimating the economic impact of human activity such as food on public health and the environment is what economists term 'externalities'. These are costs arising from the food system but not necessarily reflected in the price consumers pay. They include the impact of agricultural inputs, food production itself, transport, processing, packaging, waste, subsidies to health, and a whole range of environmental, health and social costs. In their pursuit of 'true' and pure markets, conventional economists have acknowledged that reality is distorted. Costs may even not be costed (who pays for air pollution?), and costs may be borne by one sector but caused by another, or created in one country but manifest in another. This last point has long been recognised within public health. Indeed, there was highly organised international cooperation on disease control in the late nineteenth century on zoonotics and contagious diseases. They knew food was a vector for costly cross-border spread of disease.

The calculation of externalised and internalised costs is the attempt to capture these tricky features. One incentive to do so has come from health economists concerned about the rising costs of healthcare, a considerable proportion of which is associated with diet and lack of physical activity due to changed lifestyles. In the USA, healthcare costs are stubbornly high; for decades, moreover, tens of millions of US citizens were not covered by healthcare insurance. For those that were the bill was considerable, $2.8 trillion in 2012, approaching a fifth of GDP, and generating highly charged partisan politics of healthcare reform from President Clinton to 'Obamacare' so hated by President Trump.[87, 88] Right across the developed world, even though the costs of ill-health vary by country, the full costs appear to be immense.[89]

One calculation is that, over the period 2010–30, non-communicable diseases (NCDs) will cost a cumulative total of US$30 tn, equivalent to 48% of global GDP in 2010.[90] The same study estimated that mental health problems will add an additional loss of US$16.1 tn in 2010–30. Within these costs, cardiovascular disease is set to rise by 22% to US$20,032 bn over the 20-year period. Diabetes is set to rise from $500 bn in 2010 to $745 bn by 2030. The greatest impact is expected to be in lower- and middle-income countries, such is the effect of the nutrition transition. Business optimists see this as a growth opportunity for expensive medical technology even in poor societies,[91] but can even affluent countries afford mounting healthcare costs, let alone low- and middle-income ones? In vastly expensive and wasteful private systems, such as the USA's, costs unaffordable to employers are being increasingly transferred to the public purse.[92] Such costs are brakes on the improvement in living standards and public goods that characterised the mid- to late twentieth century. In the twenty-first century the rise of wages and living standards appeared to stall, with US academics arguing that Americans had become over-worked and wages had frozen for the vast majority of the US workforce. Meanwhile political changes, shaped by neoliberal anti-state agenda, were reducing the 'social wage' – the welfare infrastructure put in place throughout the twentieth century to ease out booms and slumps and to provide support mechanisms and minimise personalised risk. Across the West, pensions, healthcare, housing, amenities, even cultural infrastructure (libraries, galleries) are being renegotiated, privatised, closed, monetised and often presented as unaffordable. This is a harsh economic context for the sustainable diet transition!

Making financial calculations of environmental or health costs requires clear analysis but is still partly a philosophical exercise. Costs can be physical and social, material and cultural. How can one calculate the loss of a view of the sky from a window or of prime agricultural land from being covered by a housing estate or factory or the destruction of a species?[93] Take the issue of fertiliser use, which has been the main driver of the twentieth-century rise in food production. The value of having a plentiful source of fertilisers had been shown by the nineteenth-century use of vast resources of guano (dried bird manure accrued over thousands of years). Mining guano made the traders rich and showed that spreading extra fertilisers on fields increased land outputs. Newly confident chemical scientists understood that nitrogen was plentiful in the air. The problem was how to 'fix' it. This was solved in Germany in 1909–10 where a technical process was developed, first in the laboratory in 1909 by Haber, and then in 1910 at industrial scale by Bosch working for the chemical giant BASF to create the cheap and plentiful Haber-Bosch process. The two Germans received the Nobel Prize for their efforts. But nitrogen-based 'artificial' fertilisers are oil-based, i.e., they use previously cheap, compressed energy from decayed plants trapped in the earth's geological strata. A century after Haber-Bosch, we now know this is a big factor in agriculture's impact on climate change. What initially was an advance is now an environmental threat.

Table 7.6 provides some current environmental costs and projections for 2050, drawn from the UN's TEEB project.[94] This suggests that total environmental costs are set to rise from $6,596 bn in 2008, equivalent to 10.97% of global GDP that year, to $28,615 bn by 2050, equivalent to 17.78% of global GDP in 2050. These are huge sums, stratospherically different from the humble world of the consumer juggling domestic budgets. The International Sustainability Unit of the Prince of Wales Charities conducted some case studies of very diverse food systems in 2010–11.[95] It reviewed these for a mix of impacts: subsidies, greenhouse gases, air pollution, water pollution, soil degradation, water depletion and biodiversity loss, and concluded that, for every $100's worth of food produced, the true costs were all significantly higher. Corn production in the USA had a true cost of \$135–150; all UK agriculture's real cost was \$144; beef production in Brazil was \$166–231; wheat in India was \$170–186; mixed agriculture in Ethiopia was \$154–240; Bluefin tuna production from the North East Atlantic was \$118; shrimp production was \$134; and coastal fish from Senegal was \$159.95. None was sold at the true cost.

True costing work is increasing, even within conventional business and economics, and has contributed to concerns about what are termed 'stranded assets', i.e., assets that carry such burdens that they might not be worth investing in. There is a strong case, for instance, for considering whether the supplies of oil remaining in the ground worldwide are not worth extracting simply because, if burned, they will tip the world into accelerating climate change and thus undermine their own 'value'.[96] In 2013 the Oxford University Smith School's Stranded Assets Programme conducted a high level systematic review of the effects across physical, material, human, social and financial assets of defined physical and economic risk (such as land degradation, biodiversity loss, overfishing, agricultural diseases, phosphate availability, water scarcity, regulations covering land use, biofuel, biotechnology, gas, etc).[97] It found a significant risk (0.5%) of annual losses of \$11.2 tn from stranded assets in agriculture alone. This did not cover the whole food chain. These are immense sums not included in the price of a cheap frozen pizza assembled and precooked from globally sourced ingredients and trucked across continents. And that is even before the consumer has got into his or her car to get to the supermarket and then return to 'cook' it.

Table 7.6 Annual environmental costs of the global economy in 2008 and projections for 2050

| Environmental impact | External costs in 2008 (US$bn) | External cost relative to global GDP in 2008 | Projected external costs in 2050 (US$bn) | Projected external cost relative to global GDP in 2050 |
|---|---|---|---|---|
| Greenhouse gas emissions | 4,530 | 7.54% | 20,809 | 12.93% |
| Water abstraction | 1,226 | 2.04% | 4,702 | 2.92% |
| Pollution (SOx, NOx, PM, VOCs, mercury) | 546 | 0.91% | 1,926 | 1.20% |
| General waste | 197 | 0.33% | 635 | 0.39% |
| Natural resources: | | | | |
| Fish | 54 | 0.09% | 287 | 0.18% |
| Timber | 42 | 0.07% | 256 | 0.16% |
| Other ecosystem services, pollutants and waste | n/a | n/a | n/a | n/a |
| TOTAL | 6,596 | 10.97% | 28,615 | 17.78% |

Source: Trucost plc/UNEP and PRI, 2010.[94]

## Food labour

This ought to be a central issue in the sustainable diet debate. The UN's International Labour Organization estimates that agriculture is the major employer on the planet, with 1.3 bn people working the land, of whom 500 million work on plantations. Tens of millions of these are unwaged.[98] Table 7.7 gives the regional figures from 1991–2013 and shows considerable variation. South East Asia has actually increased its farm labour. According to the World Bank and FAO, farming employs half the population in about 50 countries, although this proportion is slowly dropping with urbanisation and other trends. In 2000–2 agriculture employed 37% of the world labour force. By 2010–12 it was 30%.[99]

No food system is labour-free. Probably the hunter-gathering system is most labour-intense as it treats nature as the unpaid source,[100] but modern food systems vary in where and how they place and value labour. A characteristic of them all, however, is that the labour is cheap. Even expensive foods often have hidden labour that is low paid. Does it matter whether the workers are well paid? Just who is it who produces the food (whether sustainable or not)? These might seem naïve questions to some. Why, food comes from shops, and it is ultimately sourced from either the land or sea! All true. But this would not happen without labour and for centuries the status of that labour has troubled society. The history of sugar and slavery are inextricably entwined; unpaid slave labour made the brutal work and transport across the globe economically viable and highly profitable.[101] Less well acknowledged is how, when the British abolished slavery, it was replaced by punitive systems of indentured labour that, for example, took people from India to the sugar plantations of Guyana.[102] Supposed contracts signed labour to work for long periods. Even today, centuries after slavery had supposedly been outlawed, it still exists, as the US State Department's annual report shows.[103] Wage rates aside, the State Department report asserts

Table 7.7 Employment in agriculture, by region as % of total employment, 1991–2013

| Region | 1991 | 2013 | % change |
|---|---|---|---|
| World | 44.5 | 31.3 | −29.7 |
| Developed economies and EU | 6.9 | 3.6 | −47.8 |
| Central and SE Europe (non-EU) and CIS | 28.8 | 17.7 | −38.5 |
| East Asia | 56.8 | 30.3 | −46.7 |
| South East Asia and the Pacific | 58.9 | 39.3 | 33.3 |
| South Asia | 62.1 | 46.3 | −25.4 |
| Latin America and the Caribbean | 24.7 | 14.8 | −40.1 |
| Middle East | 24.5 | 14.3 | −41.6 |
| North Africa | 34.9 | 28.0 | −19.8 |
| Sub-Saharan Africa | 65.9 | 62.0 | −5.9 |

Source: ILO.[98]

the continued existence of what in Britain in the eighteenth century used to be called the 'truck' system, under which workers are made to buy food and other necessary objects from the company store 'at inflated prices'. Another problem is child labour, shocking anywhere but particularly, as the ILO notes, in one of the three most hazardous industries on earth – agriculture.[104] A study of the cocoa industry by academics at Tulane University, USA, estimated that 2.26 m young people aged between 5 and 17 years were working in Ghana and the Ivory Coast in 2013–14, a 21% increase since 2008–9.[105] Investigation by academics, NGOs and journalists keep unearthing poor to appalling labour conditions in places as diverse as English vegetable factories and Thai prawn farms.[106–110] The Joseph Rowntree Foundation, a highly respected charity, published a damning report in 2013 about forced labour in the UK food sector, based on interviews with migrant labour. Embarrassed about such exposés, the UK government passed a Modern Slavery Act in 2015.[111]

Sustainable diet advocates cannot ignore these issues. Consumers wanting local, seasonal and regional food in affluent countries are sometimes unaware that, with long supply chains and many 'actors' in the food system each taking their cut, there are pressures to use migrants as cheap but local labour, often picking in fields or working in packing houses. Some countries created formal structures for this – in the UK the Seasonal Agricultural Workers Scheme (SAWS, now disbanded) and in Canada the Canadian Seasonal Agricultural Workers Program (CSAWP). Studies of these schemes suggest the exploitation can be high and extensive. In 1978 Canada imported 5,000 seasonal workers. By 2009 it was 26,000.[112] Some of these 'temporary foreign workers' were made to pay for their own housing and paid fees to work (some equivalent to half the annual pay), according to the Canadian farm workers' union.

The conditions of labour are not just indicated by wages but by features such as dignity, right to unions, time off, work facilities (toilets, clean water, etc.) and noise levels. Everywhere these require constant monitoring and accountability. Even the 'purest' of foods in health and environmental terms can be sullied by poor labour conditions. On the positive side, there has been a rise in public policy (and also commercial policy) on how to make sure the food sector creates and maintains good jobs. Progressive elements in the UK industry and NGOs joined forces in 1998, for example, to create the Ethical Trade Initiative and this covered 9.8 m workers worldwide by 2015.[113] The fair trade movement has been particularly active in the food sector for the last two decades; its goal is to raise the incomes of primary producers. It has not been without critics, however. A large study funded by the UK Department for International Development (DfID) conducted by economists at London University's School of Oriental and African Studies (SOAS) found that the growth of earnings in two countries it studied – Ethiopia and Uganda – was not as significant as it could be for the waged labourers.[114] SOAS conducted detailed micro-studies of agricultural export commodities: coffee and flowers in Ethiopia and coffee and tea in Uganda. It concluded that the mainly female labour was not benefiting and still experienced deprivation 'in terms of educational attainment, restricted diets, and ownership of or access to many rudimentary assets'. It also concluded soberly that it was 'unable to find any evidence that fair trade has made a positive difference to the wages and working conditions of those employed in the production of the commodities produced for fair trade certified export in the areas where the research has been conducted'. This report led to a furious debate with the movement and anguished rebuttals.[115, 116] But it raised wider discussion about how to encourage the transition to a food system with 'better' economics, another old debate.[117] Was another route simply to sort out food employment back in the rich world rather than to try to do it through trade?

An example of this thinking is New York City's report on the potential of the food sector to increase good food jobs there. There had been a remarkable growth of food employment away from the farm already.[118] In 2001 NYC had 244,723 people employed in restaurants, retail, wholesale, manufacturing or agriculture. By 2011 this had risen to 326,059. This 33% increase was heavily due to the rise in restaurants, up 44% in the period 2001–11. The number of establishments, not just jobs, also rose, again with restaurants leading, but agriculture grew by 38% with the rise of trendy urban farms, albeit from a small number to start with. This 'good' news, however, was offset by a reduction in wages in the food system: down 5% in the restaurant trade, 6% in food retail and grocery wholesale, 19% in food manufacturing and 17% in agriculture. This pattern is visible in many developed countries and represents a shift in employment from the land to the urban context and considerable use of migrant labour.

### The social goal of a living wage

Most philosophical traditions make an important distinction between needs and wants. Needs are fundamental – they are what bodies need to survive let alone prosper; they are the basic requirements for life. Wants are what minds aspire to; these are cultural artefacts, sparked by opportunity and circumstance. A hunter-gatherer will not want a TV until s/he knows of it but few children can now avoid the power of advertisements; the systematic moulding of consciousness. 'I am hungry', a child might cry, but this is not starvation, it's more of a pang. In economics this distinction can easily be translated into a debate about wages. How much money does a worker need to live decently? Early nutritionists, such as the influential US scientist WO Atwater, tried to calculate basic nutritional needs in a series of papers for the US government.[119–121] This was before even vitamins had been discovered,[122] but enough was known about dietary intake to be able to estimate how much of particular foods a steelworker needed to be able to work regularly. The human body was conceived as an input–output organism: food in, work out.

Atwater's work was used by Seebohm Rowntree, a big UK chocolate manufacturer turned social researcher, to calculate how much money people living in his home city of York needed to exist. He used Atwater's calculations to create a stark but just sufficient diet, which he then costed and used to estimate how many people were poor in York.[123] Even using draconian standards he found far more poor people than he expected, and over the next half century he both studied them and softened his position, ending his life arguing that food was both a basic need and a cultural matter of dignity and decency; harshness of 'need' was not necessary.[124] Rowntree was trying to provide a scientific basis to an argument as old as the English Peasants' Revolt in 1381 or, in the nineteenth century, the rise of a mass industrial poorly paid working class that spawned the trades union movement to protect and improve its conditions. What does a household or person need? In a 1907 legal judgment, the Harvester Judgment, Australia took a social policy lead on this question by recognising that a 'basic and fair wage' for a husband, wife and three children should include 'enough wholesome food', decent shelter, provision for 'rainy days' and 'frugal comforts'.[125] This was an early statement of what is now termed the 'right to food' perspective. The 1948 UN Declaration of Human Rights stated that every person, irrespective of birth, gender, income or circumstance, had certain basic rights to existence, which implied a right to food. Over the next 60 years there was a gradual growth of specificity to that generalised right, summarised elsewhere,[126-128] culminating in the UN's 2004 Voluntary Guidelines for each country to enact the right to food.[129]

## Conclusions: fixing the economics for sustainable diets

The picture we have painted in this chapter is of economics as inevitably complex but with essential features for sustainable diets. Price is not the only useful indicator but, in a market economy where wages and incomes determine the food, the quality and the amount a person can buy, prices are clearly of great significance. But do they capture all that matters about sustainability? Not entirely. What, then, could or would the food system look like if it nurtured and delivered sustainable diets? This chapter has suggested that the economics of food would be more realistic if it broadened its criteria beyond a focus on price or, if price is a key criterion, for these to be true and fair. We have suggested that the fair distribution of earnings, for workers and across the sectors of (increasingly complex) supply chains, is a justified measure for judging whether a diet or food system is sustainable. If society wants a food system and consumption patterns that are better, then economics needs to reclaim its original late eighteenth-century roots in moral, domestic and political economy by giving more emphasis to issues such as justice, distribution of power, labour, conditions, security and time.

Some analysts think that technology will come to the rescue. Genetic engineering, nanotechnology, laboratory meat, robotics and other technical fixes are proffered as lowering food's environmental impact. We have here recognised the need to include long-term as well as short-term time horizons, as commentators such as the poet-farmer Wendell Berry and Herman Daly (when a World Bank economist) suggest.[130-132] The unintended consequences of hasty actions can come to haunt the policy maker. The dominant politics favour looking to companies and market mechanisms to resolve the unsustainability of food systems. The good news is that there are growing numbers of food companies who are genuinely troubled by food's impact on health and/or the environment. Corporate responsibility strategies grow in influence. Giant food companies that were hostile now grudgingly accept that they need to reduce their carbon or water footprint. Some of the world's largest food companies set up the Sustainable Agriculture Initiative in the early 2000s.[133] Companies now share good agricultural practice (GAP) through joint projects such as GLOBALG.A.P.[134] The World Economic Forum and McKinsey produced a roadmap for sustainable agriculture, arguing that companies needed to look after primary producers better or lose their resource flows.[135] Unilever, one of the world's food giants, now operates to a Sustainable Living Plan that commits it to improve the cash flow of its small farmers, lower its footprint and prioritise sustainability rather than short-term profitability.[136, 137] Tesco, the third largest food retailer in the world, has a commitment to lower the sugar content of its own-label soft drinks.[138] PepsiCo has experimented in the UK with reducing its carbon footprint by 50% in five years.[139] Environmental auditing is becoming more normal.

These are remarkable signs of corporate capitalism thinking aloud and acting, and are not to be dismissed lightly. And yet, and yet. The elephant in the sustainable diet room remains: how can over-consuming countries consume less while poor and developing countries are encouraged to consume more, better and more equitably? We discuss this in the next chapter but, meanwhile, we draw attention to an approach to food economics that is fast becoming central. This goes under the name of the circular economy.[140] Food epitomises waste, as we have shown. Some of this waste is sheer inefficiency – profligate use of energy, over-engineering – but much is failure to recycle, to re-use or to prevent. Plastic bottles and tin cans are thrown away, yet the embedded carbon is huge. The point of conducting water audits is to reduce water waste. The circular economy adherents argue that all resources should be viewed as 'borrowed' and to be returned. The EU has now adopted this as its general direction for economic and industrial policy.[141, 142] If this is truly followed through it could revolutionise the food system, but it would require the wholesale transformation of resource management. Would a throwaway plastic wrapper around a long-distance sandwich be conceivable under a circular economy? We doubt it. But the circular economy does not address the crisis or cost of diet-related ill-health or the social dislocation of poor land use. It sees food as a material entity. The challenge posed by our broad perspective on food economics remains.

One good example of such broad-based economic analysis is a 2014 report on the UK's food system by the New Economics Foundation (NEF), an environmental economics research body. Its report concluded that the UK food system was failing to meet good sustainability standards, by which it meant health, environmental and social measures.[143] It calculated the adverse environmental impacts as £5.7–7.2 bn per year, equivalent to 6.3–7.9% of the market price of food ('and probably higher'). Adding the cost of obesity and subsidies paid through the Common Agricultural Policy (CAP), the researchers estimated the total external cost of the UK food system to be between £11 bn and £26 bn. This means that the UK's food bill is actually at least 12–28% greater than the price consumers paid at the till. NEF's verdict was that the UK food system:

- used approximately eight calories of energy to produce every one calorie of energy from food;
- employed approximately 11% of the UK labour force, but most of them are in the least well-paid jobs, with salaries of less than half the UK average;
- gave a decreasing share of total value to farmers;
- had an opaque and complex structure;
- was unequal: all 17 million hectares of agricultural land is owned by about 0.25% of the UK population and the price of an acre of bare land has increased more than threefold from 2004;
- had volatile prices with particular pressures on low-income consumers.

Behaviour change is another solution or strategy being offered by and to policy makers.[144, 145] This recognises that current consumer eating and purchasing patterns must change. They are bankrupting healthcare and warping entire economies. But the usual approach is to adopt soft 'below the radar' nudge and advice techniques, when what is required is the reframing of the economy and setting tougher new norms for lifestyles. This cannot happen a bit here or there, and just at the individual level. It means changing norms, recalibrating what is acceptable behaviour, and altering cultural aspirations. Small changes are not enough, unless coordinated on a mass scale, which is not so far what is happening.

We have described this problem of food economics as one that is not just about money but also about people, roles, resources and time. Researchers are clear that food takes a lot of daily time. Hence technologists' appeal, alongside Charlotte Gilman Perkins cited early in this chapter, that equipment and engineering ingenuity can transform the quality of life and food. Arguably, there has not been enough contemporary discussion within the sustainability discourse about time. 'Time is money' is the old saying, but unwaged time is one area in lifespace that is not costed. Development, technology (home equipment), women's rights, smaller families, the rise of the oil-based and car-based food economy, all these have restructured where and how food time is spent. Less time is spent cooking but more travelling to the store, parking and returning. Shopping occurs more infrequently. Home delivery and online shopping is now changing time expenditure yet again. In developed economies more time is spent on eating out of the home than a century ago, but in many developing economies eating on the street is also common because it is cheap. US Government data show that, since 1960, Americans spend less money on food in the home but food out of the home has steadily risen. The time they spend on food is now considerable.

A USDA ERS study of time data found that, on an average day, Americans aged 15 and older spent 67 minutes eating and drinking as a 'primary' or main activity, and 23.5 minutes eating and 63 minutes drinking beverages (except plain water) while doing something such as watching television, driving or working.[146] Eleven per cent of the population – defined as 'constant eaters' – spent at least 4.5 hours on an average day engaged in eating and drinking activities. Lower-income Americans, those with household incomes less than 185% of the poverty threshold, spend less time engaged in eating and drinking activities than those with higher incomes.

Now, to end on a big question: what would the food economy look like if it met and delivered sustainable diets? Well, clearly it would be very different. Some foods and products would be more expensive. If US consumers want a tasty mango flown at peak season from Pakistan (arguably among the best!), they should probably pay prohibitively for it. If we want an ethical food economy then workers in the food system need to be paid more. Probably the only way this can be delivered is by shorter food chains and more culinary emphasis on cooking rather than eating pre-prepared foods. But that needs to be studied. Factories are more energy efficient than a domestic kitchen. But the cultural connotations are entirely different. So, if sustainability is about multiple factors, economics remains just one factor, and not the deciding one. Just one. Ultimately, what this chapter suggests is that the food economy needs to shift from a focus on delivering 'value for money' to one that incorporates multiple values. Helping the transition to this new 'values for money' food economy requires help from improved food governance, the topic of the following chapter. How food decisions are made, and by whom, is a crucial feature of better food system management. It is not acceptable to leave environmental or social or health issues in the antechamber of food governance while discussion and reality are shaped and maintained by existing narrow conceptions of markets and economics. Happily, increasing numbers of economists share this view and are contributing to the discourse, as this chapter has shown.

## References

1 Smil V. *Feeding the World: A Challenge for the Twenty-First Century*. Cambridge, MA; London: MIT, 2000

2 Foresight. *The Future of Food and Farming: Challenges and Choices for Global Sustainability*. Final Report. London: Government Office for Science, 2011: 211

3 Lang T, Heasman M. *Food Wars: The Global Battle for Mouths, Minds and Markets* (2nd Ed.). Abingdon: Routledge Earthscan, 2015

4 Gustavsson J, Cederberg C, Sonnesson U, *et al. Global Food Losses and Food Waste: Extent, Causes and Prevention*. Rome: Food and Agriculture Organization, 2011

5 Oxfam. *If Campaign*. Available at: www.oxfam.org.uk/get-involved/campaign-with-us/our-campaigns/if (accessed September 10, 2015). Oxford: Oxfam, 2013

6 Tett G. *Fool's Gold: How Unrestrained Greed Corrupted a Dream, Shattered Global Markets and Unleashed a Catastrophe*. London: Little, Brown, 2009

7 Oxfam International. *Not a Game: Speculation vs Food Security: Regulating Financial Markets to Grow a Better Future*. Oxford: Oxfam International, 2011

8  Murphy S, Burch D, Clapp J. *Cereal Secrets: The World's Largest Grain Traders and Global Agriculture*. Oxford: Oxfam Publications, 2012

9  Piesse J, Thirtle C. Three bubbles and a panic: an explanatory review of recent food commodity price events. *Food Policy*, 2009; 34(2): 119–29

10  Gussow JD. Does cooking pay? *Journal of Nutrition Education and Behavior*, 1988; 20(5): 221–6

11  Gussow JD. Dietary guidelines for sustainability: twelve years later. *Journal of Nutrition Education*, 1999; 31: 194–200

12  Tull AML. *Why Teach (Young) People How to Cook? A Critical Analysis of Education and Policy in Transition*. PhD thesis, July. London: Centre for Food Policy, City University London, 2015

13  Beeton IM. *The Book of Household Management*. London: SO Beeton Publishing, 1861

14  Attar D. *Wasting Girls' Time: The History and Politics of Home Economics*. London: Virago, 1990

15  Hunt F (Ed.). *Lessons for Life: The Schooling of Girls and Women 1850–1950*. Oxford: Basil Blackwell, 1987

16  Gilman Perkins C. *Women and Economics: A Study of the Economic Relation Between Men and Women as a Factor in Social Evolution*. New York: Harper and Row, 1966 [1898]

17  Hayden D. *The Grand Domestic Revolution: A History of Feminist Designs for American Homes, Neighborhoods, and Cities*. Cambridge, MA: MIT Press, 1981

18  Barrientos S. *Female Employment in Agriculture; Global Challenges and Global Responses. Small Change or Real Change? Commonwealth Perspectives on Financing Gender Equality*. London: Commonwealth Secretariat, 2008: 172–9

19  Smith A. *The Wealth of the Nations*. Harmondsworth: Penguin, 1776/1970

20  Smith A. *The Theory of Moral Sentiments*. Harmondsworth: Penguin, 2010 [1759]

21  Lang T. Sustainable Diets: hairshirts or a better food future? *Development*, 2014; 57(4): 240–56

22  Eating Better. *For a Fair Green Healthy Future*. Available at: www.eating-better.org/ (accessed October 12, 2015). Brighton: Eating Better, 2013

23  Friedman M. *Capitalism and Freedom*. Chicago, IL: University of Chicago Press, 1962

24  Friedman M, Friedman RD. *Free to Choose: A Personal Statement* (1st Ed.). New York: Harcourt Brace Jovanovich, 1980

25  Keynes JM. *The General Theory of Employment, Interest, and Money*. London: Macmillan, 1936

26  Keynes JM. *Economic Possibilities for Our Grandchildren. John Maynard Keynes: Essays in Persuasion*. New York: WW Norton & Co., 1963 (1930): 358–73

27  Hayek F. *The Constitution of Liberty*. London: Routledge, 1960

28  Cockett R. *Thinking the Unthinkable: Think-Tanks and the Economic Counter-Revolution, 1931–1983*. London: HarperCollins, 1994

29  Harvey D. *A Brief History of Neoliberalism*. Oxford: Oxford University Press, 2005

30  Williamson J. *A Short History of the Washington Consensus. From the Washington Consensus Towards a New Global Governance* (hosted by Fundación CIDOB). Barcelona: Institute for International Economics, 2004

31  FAO. *Mitigation of Food Wastage: Societal Costs and Benefits*. Rome: Food and Agriculture Organization of the United Nations, 2014

32  ARC2020. *2000m2*. Available at: www.2000m2.eu/ (accessed October 14, 2015). Berlin: Agriculture and Rural Convention, 2014

33  Cassidy ES, West PC, Gerber JS, *et al*. Redefining agricultural yields: from tonnes to people nourished per hectare. *Environmental Research Letters*, 2013; 8: 034015

34  Thornton PK. Livestock production: recent trends, future prospects. *Philosophical Transactions of the Royal Society B*, 2010; 365: 2853–67

35  Capper J, Berger L, Brashears MM, *et al*. *Animal Feed vs. Human Food: Challenges and Opportunities in Sustaining Animal Agriculture Toward 2050*. CAST Issue Paper 53. Ames, Iowa: Council for Agricultural Science and Technology 2013

36  Keyzer MA, Merbis MD, Pavel IFPW, *et al*. Diet shifts towards meat and the effects on cereal use: can we feed the animals in 2030? *Ecological Economics*, 2006; 55(2): 187–202

37  Gerber PJ, Steinfeld H, Henderson B, *et al. Tackling Climate Change Through Livestock: A Global Assessment of Emissions and Mitigation Opportunities*. Rome: Food and Agriculture Organization of the United Nations, 2013

38  Steinfeld H, Gerber P, Wassenaar T, *et al. Livestock's Long Shadow: Environmental Issues and Options*. Rome: Food and Agriculture Organization, 2006

39  Wiedmann T, Barrett J. A review of the ecological footprint indicator: perceptions and methods. *Sustainability*, 2010; 2(6): 1645–93

40  Wackernagel M, Rees WE, Testemale P. *Our Ecological Footprint: Reducing Human Impact on the Earth*. Gabriola Island, BC: New Society Publishers, 1996

41  Rees WE. Ecological footprints and appropriated carrying capacity: what urban economics leaves out. *Environment and Urbanization*, 1992; 4(2): 121–30

42  Frey S, Barrett J. *The Footprint of Scotland's Diet: The Environmental Burden of What We Eat*. A report for Scotland's Global Footprint Project. York: Stockholm Environment Institute, 2006: 13

43  GLA Economics. *London's Ecological Footprint: a Review*. London: Greater London Assembly Economics, 2003

44  Borgström G. *The Hungry Planet: Modern World at the Edge of Famine*. New York: Macmillan, 1965

45  Plassmann K, Edwards-Jones G. *Where Does the Carbon Footprint Fall? Developing a Carbon Map of Food Production*. London: International Institute for Environment and Development, 2010

46  Chapagain AK, Hoekstra AY. *Water Footprints of Nations, vols. 1 and 2. UNESCO-IHE Value of Water Research Report Series No. 16*. Paris: UNESCO, 2004

47  Chapagain AK, Hoekstra AY. *Water Footprints of Nations, vols. 1 and 2. UNESCO-IHE Value of Water Research Report Series No 16*. Paris: UNESCO, 2006

48  Hoekstra AY, Chapagain AK, Aldaya MM, *et al. The Water Footprint Assessment Manual: Setting the Global Standard*. London: Earthscan, 2011

49  Allan JA. Virtual water: the water, food and trade nexus: useful concept or misleading metaphor? *Water International*, 2003; 28: 4–11

50  Allan JAT. *Virtual Water: Tackling the Threat to Our Planet's Most Precious Resource* (1st Ed.). London: I.B. Tauris, 2011

51  Birch R, Ravetz J, Wiedmann T. *Footprint North West: A Preliminary Ecological Footprint of the North West Region*. Manchester and York: Stockholm Environment Institute (York), Centre for Urban and Regional Ecology, Action for Sustainability (North West Regional Assembly), 2005

52  Finch J. Tesco labels will show products' carbon footprints. Available at: www.guardian.co.uk/environment/2008/apr/16/carbonfootprints.tesco?gusrc=rss&feed=networkfront (accessed July 6, 2008). *The Guardian*, Wednesday April 16, 2008

53 Tesco plc. *Measuring Our Carbon Footprint*. Available at: www.tesco.com/climatechange/carbonFootprint.asp (accessed June 12, 2008). Welwyn Garden City: Tesco plc, 2007

54 Global Footprint Network. *Living Planet Report 2010: Biodiversity, Biocapacity and Development*. Gland, London and Oakland: WWF, Institute of Zoology, Global Footprint Network, 2010

55 DG Environment. *Environmental Footprint of Products*. Available at: http://ec.europa.eu/environment/eussd/product_footprint.htm (accessed July 10, 2016). Brussels: Commission of the European Communities DG Environment, 2015.

56 Sáez-Almendros S, Obrador B, Bach-Faig A, *et al*. Environmental footprints of Mediterranean versus Western dietary patterns: beyond the health benefits of the Mediterranean diet. *Environmental Health*, 2013; 12(118)

57 UBS. *CMCI Food Index: Drivers Behind Food Prices*. London: UBS, 2011

58 Schoen V, Lang T. *UK Food Prices: Cooling or Bubbling?* London: Food Research Collaboration, 2014

59 Fuglie K, Sun LW. New evidence points to robust but uneven productivity growth in global agriculture. *Amber Waves* (USDA), 2012, September. Available at: www.ers.usda.gov/amber-waves/2012-september/global-agriculture.aspx#.Vd76l5dZhLE (accessed August 27, 2015)

60 Fuglie KO, Sun LW, Ball VE, editors. *Productivity Growth in Agriculture: an International Perspective*. Wallingford: CAB International, 2012

61 Lang T. Crisis? What crisis? The normality of the current food crisis. *Journal of Agrarian Change*, 2010; 10(1): 92–102

62 OECD, FAO. *Agricultural Outlook 2013–22*. Paris: Organization for Economic Cooperation and Development and Food and Agriculture Organisation, 2013

63 Abbott P. *Development Dimensions of High Food Prices*. Paris: Organization for Economic Cooperation and Development, 2009: 97

64 World Development Movement. *Food Speculation: Stop Bankers Betting on Food – Our Campaign to Curb Commodity Speculation*. London: World Development Movement, 2012. Available at: www.wdm.org.uk/food-speculation (accessed October 12, 2015).

65 De Schutter O. *Food Commodities Speculation and Food Price Crises: Regulation to Reduce the Risks of Price Volatility*, briefing note by the Special Rapporteur on the right to food. Geneva: Office of the UN Rapporteur on the Right to Food, 2010

66 FAO. *Price Volatility in Agricultural Markets*. Rome: Food and Agricultural Organization, 2015. Available at: www.fao.org/economic/est/issues/volatility/en/#.Vd9EmpdZhLE (accessed August 27, 2015)

67 FAO. UN food and agriculture agency warns about negative impact of food speculation, 6 July. Available at: www.un.org/apps/news/story.asp?NewsID=42412#.Vd9FjpdZhLE (accessed October 12, 2015). Rome: UN News Centre, 2012

68 Green R, Cornelsen L, Dangour AD, *et al*. The effect of rising food prices on food consumption: systematic review with meta-regression. *BMJ*, 2013; 346(f3703)

69 FAO. *Food Price Index*. Available at: www.fao.org/worldfoodsituation/wfs-home/foodpricesindex/en/ (accessed August 27, 2015). Rome: Food and Agriculture Organization, 2015

70 USDA ERS. *Food Dollar Series*. Available at: www.ers.usda.gov/data-products/food-dollar-series/documentation.aspx (accessed June 11, 2016). Washington, DC: United States Department of Agriculture Economic Research Services, 2015

71 Defra. *Agriculture in the UK 2014*. London: Department for Environment, Food and Rural Affairs, 2015

72  OECD. *Agricultural Monitoring and Evaluation 2015*. Paris: Organisation for Economic Cooperation and Development, 2015: 35

73  MacLeod CJ, Moller H. Intensification and diversification of New Zealand agriculture since 1960: an evaluation of current indicators of land use change. *Agriculture, Ecosystems & Environment*, 2006; 115(1–4): 201–18

74  Bailey R, Froggatt A, Wellesley L. *Livestock – Climate Change's Forgotten Sector: Global Public Opinion on Meat and Dairy Consumption*. London: Royal Institution of International Affairs, 2014

75  Environmental Working Group. *US Farm Subsidies Database*. Washington, DC: EWG, 2015

76  McMahon P. *Feeding Frenzy: The New Politics of Food*. London: Profile Books Ltd, 2014

77  Rowan C. The world's top 100 food and beverage companies. *Food Engineering*, 2013: 68. Available at: www.foodengineeringmag.com (accessed July 19, 2014).

78  FoodDrinkEurope. *Data and Trends of the European Food and Drink Industry*. Brussels: FoodDrinkEurope, 2013

79  Exonexus, Berne Declaration. *Agropoly: A Handful of Corporations Control World Food Production*. Zurich: Berne Declaration, 2013

80  Nielsen. *Looking to Achieve New Product Success. Listen to Your Consumers*. Available at: www.nielsen.com/content/dam/nielsenglobal/dk/docs/Nielsen%20Global%20New%20Product%20Innovation%20Report%20June%202015.pdf (accessed December 2, 2016). Denmark: The Nielsen Company, 2015

81  Wiggins S, Keats S, Han E, *et al*. *The Rising Cost of a Healthy Diet*. London: ODI, 2015: 64

82  Thow AM, Jan S, Leedeer S, *et al*. The effect of fiscal policy on diet, obesity and chronic disease: a systematic review. *Bulletin of the World Health Organisation*, 2010; 88(8): 609–14

83  Strnad JFJ. *Conceptualizing the 'Fat Tax': The Role of Food Taxes in Developed Economies*. Stanford Law and Economics Olin Working Paper No 286. Palo Alto, CA: Stanford Law School, 2004

84  Caraher M, Cowburn G. Taxing food: implications for public health nutrition. *Public Health Nutrition*, 2005; 8(8): 1242–9

85  Cornelsen L, Carreido A. *Health-Related Taxes on Foods and Beverages*. London: Food Research Collaboration, 2015

86  Jacobson MH, Brownell KD. Small taxes on soft drinks and snack foods to promote health. *American Journal of Public Health*, 2000; 90: 854–7

87  Starr P. Professionalization and public health: historical legacies, continuing dilemmas. *Journal of Public Health Management and Practice*, 2009; 15(6): S26–S30

88  Cuckler GA, Sisko AM, Keehan SP, *et al*. National health expenditure projections, 2012–22: slow growth until coverage expands and economy improves. *Health Affairs*, 2013; 32(10): 1820–31

89  UNEP Finance Initiative, PRI. *Universal Ownership: Why Environmental Externalities Matter to Institutional Investors*. Geneva: United Nations Environment Programme (UNEP) Finance Initiative and The Principles for Responsible Investment (PRI), 2010

90  Bloom DE, Cafiero ET, Jané-Llopis E, *et al*. *The Global Economic Burden of Noncommunicable Diseases*. Geneva: World Economic Forum and Harvard School of Public Health, 2011

91  Manson K. Ethiopia's middle class rises, with western diseases in tow. *Financial Times*, February 27, 2014

92　Wilson R. Health care spending still rising for states and cities. *The Washington Post*, January 31, 2014

93　Hirsch F. *Social Limits to Growth*. Cambridge, MA: Harvard University Press, 1976

94　UNEPFI & PRI. *Universal Ownership: Why Environmental Externalities Matter to Institutional Investors*. Nairobi: United Nations Environment Programme Finance Initiative & Principles for Responsible Investment, 2011

95　International Sustainability Unit. *What Price Resilience? Towards Sustainable and Secure Food Systems*. http://pcfisu.org/wp-content/uploads/pdfs/TPC0632_Resilience_report_WEB11_07_SMALLER.pdf (accessed October 11, 2015). London: Prince of Wales' Charities International Sustainability Unit, 2011

96　Carbon Tracker, LSE Grantham Institute. *Unburnable Carbon 2013: Wasted Capital and Stranded Assets*. London: Carbon Tracker and Grantham Research Institute on Climate Change and the Environment, London School of Economics, 2013

97　Caldecott B, Howarth N, McSharry P. *Stranded Assets in Agriculture: Protecting Value from Environment-Related Risk*. Oxford: Smith School of Enterprise and the Environment, Stranded Assets Programme, 2013

98　International Labour Organization. *Agriculture; Plantations; Other Rural Sectors*. Available at: www.ilo.org/global/industries-and-sectors/agriculture-plantations-other-rural-sectors/lang--en/index.htm (accessed August 27, 2015). Geneva: ILO, 2015

99　World Bank. *World Development Indicators: Agricultural Inputs, Table 3.2*. Washington, DC: World Bank, 2015. Available at: http://wdi.worldbank.org/table/3.2 (accessed 16 May 2016).

100　Tudge C. *Neanderthals, Bandits and Farmers: How Agriculture Really Began*. London: Weidenfeld and Nicolson, 1998

101　Mintz SW. *Sweetness and Power: The Place of Sugar in Modern History*. Harmondsworth: Penguin Books, 1985

102　Bahadur G. *Coolie Woman: The Odyssey of Indenture*. London: Hurst & Co, 2013

103　US Department of State. *Trafficking in Persons Report 2015*. Washington, DC: State Department, 2015: 384

104　Hurst P, Termine P, Karl M. *Agricultural Workers and Their Contribution to Sustainable Agriculture and Rural Development*. Rome and Geneva: Food and Agriculture Organization, International Union of Foodworkers, International Labour Organization, 2005

105　Bertrand W, de Buhr E, Dudis S. *Final Report 2013/14: Survey Research on Child Labor in West African Cocoa Growing Areas*. New Orleans: School of Public Health and Tropical Medicine, Tulane University, 2015

106　Lawrence F. *Hard Labour*. Harmondsworth: Penguin, 2004

107　Lawrence F. The exploitation of migrants has become our way of life. *The Guardian*, August 17, 2015: 23

108　Hodal K, Kelly C, Lawrence F. Revealed: Asian slave labour producing prawns for supermarkets in US. *The Guardian*, 10 June. Available at: www.theguardian.com/global-development/2014/jun/10/supermarket-prawns-thailand-produced-slave-labour (accessed July 23, 2015), 2014

109　Simpson DC. *Salads, Sweat and Status: Migrant Workers in UK Horticulture*. Brighton: University of Sussex, 2011

110　Geddes A, Scott S. UK food businesses' reliance on low-wage migrant labour: a case of choice or constraint?, in: M Ruhs and B Anderston (Eds) *Who Needs Migrant*

*Workers? Labour Shortages, Immigration, and Public Policy.* Oxford: Oxford University Press, 2010: 193–221

111 Foster A. How modern slavery act affects food and drink firms. Available at: www.foodmanufacture.co.uk/Regulation/Modern-Slavery-Act-what-it-means-for-food-firms (accessed July 10, 2016). *Food Manufacture,* 2015

112 UFCW Canada, Agriculture Workers Alliance. *The Status of Migrant Farm Workers in Canada, 2010–2011.* Rexdale, Ontario: United Food and Commercial Workers Canada, 2011: 25

113 ETI. *Ethical Trade Initiative: About Us.* Available at: www.ethicaltrade.org/ (accessed August 30, 2015). London: Ethical Trade Initiative, 2015

114 Cramer C, Johnston D, Oya C, *et al. Fairtrade, Employment and Poverty Reduction in Ethiopia and Uganda: Final Report to DfID.* London: School of Oriental and African Studies, University of London, 2014: 143

115 Fairtrade International. *Statement on SOAS Report: Fairtrade, Employment and Poverty Reduction in Ethiopia and Uganda,* 16 May. Available at: www.fairtrade.net/single-view+M5a2383b864f.html (accessed October 12, 2015). Bonn: Fairtrade International, 2014

116 Sylla NS. *The Fair Trade Scandal: Marketing Poverty to Benefit the Rich.* London: Pluto, 2014

117 Barratt Brown M. *Fair Trade: Reform and Realities in the International Trading System.* London: Zed Press, 1993

118 New York City Food Policy Center. *Jobs for a Healthier Diet and Stronger Economy: Opportunities for Creating New Good Food Jobs in New York City.* New York: Hunter College and City University of New York School of Public Health, 2013

119 Atwater WO. Investigations on the chemistry and economy of food. *US Department of Agriculture Bulletin 21.* Washington, DC: Department of Agriculture, 1891

120 Atwater WO. Foods, nutritive value and cost. *US Department of Agriculture, Farmers Bulletin 23.* Washington, DC: US Department of Agriculture, 1894

121 Atwater WO. Methods and results of investigations on the chemistry and economy of food. *US Department of Agriculture Bulletin 21.* Washington, DC: Department of Agriculture, 1895

122 Hopkins SFG. *Nobel Prize in Medicine 1929: Nobel Biography.* Available at: www.nobelprize.org/nobel_prizes/medicine/laureates/1929/hopkins-bio.html (accessed October 15, 2015). Oslo: Nobel Prize Committee, 1929

123 Rowntree BS. *Poverty: A Study of Town Life.* London: Macmillan, 1902

124 Rowntree BS. *Poverty and Progress.* London: Longmans, 1941

125 Dixon J, Isaacs B. Why sustainable and 'nutritionally correct' food is not on the agenda: Western Sydney, the moral arts of everyday life and public policy. *Food Policy,* 2013; 43(December): 67–76

126 Lang T, Barling D, Caraher M. *Food Policy: Integrating Health, Environment and Society.* Oxford: Oxford University Press, 2009

127 De Schutter O. *The Right to Food and the Political Economy of Hunger.* Twenty-Sixth McDougall Memorial Lecture. Opening of the thirty-sixth Session of the FAO Conference. Available at: www.srfood.org/images/stories/pdf/other documents/20091118_srrtf-statement-wsfs_en.pdf (accessed October 15, 2015). Rome: Food and Agriculture Organization/UN Special Rapporteur on the Right to Food, 2009

128 De Schutter O. *End of Mandate: Looking Back – and Onward.* Available at: www.srfood. org/en/end-of-mandate-looking-back-and-onward (accessed October 15, 2015). Geneva: UN, 2014

129 FAO. *Voluntary Guidelines to Support the Progressive Realization of the Right to Adequate Food in the Context of National Food Security.* Adopted by the 127th Session of the FAO Council, November. Rome: Food and Agriculture Organization, 2004

130 Berry W. Discipline and hope, in: W Berry (Ed.) *A Continuous Harmony: Essays Cultural & Agricultural.* New York: Harcourt Brace, 1972

131 Daly HE, Cobb JB, Cobb CW. *For the Common Good: Redirecting the Economy Toward Community, The Environment, and a Sustainable Future.* London: Green Print, 1990

132 Daly HE, Farley JC. *Ecological Economics: Principles and Applications* (2nd Ed.). Washington, DC; London: Island Press, 2011

133 SAI. *Sustainable Agriculture Initiative Platform.* Available at: www.saiplatform.org/ (accessed August 10, 2016). Brussels: Sustainable Agriculture Initiative, 2016

134 GLOBALG.A.P. *What Is GLOBALG.A.P.?* Available at: www.globalgap.org/ (accessed July 7, 2014). Cologne, Germany: GLOBALG.A.P., 2014

135 World Economic Forum, McKinsey & Co. *Realizing a New Vision for Agriculture: a Roadmap for Stakeholders.* Davos: World Economic Forum, 2010

136 Unilever. *Sustainable Living Plan 2010.* Available at: www.sustainable-living.unilever. com/the-plan/ (accessed December 12, 2010). London: Unilever plc, 2010

137 Unilever. *Sustainable Living: Greenhouse Gases.* Available at: www.unilever.co.uk/ sustainable-living-2014/greenhouse-gases/index.aspx (accessed October 13, 2015). London: Unilever plc, 2014

138 Tesco. *Tesco and Society Report 2014.* Available at: www.tescoplc.com/index. asp?pageid=81#ref_society (accessed July 27, 2014). Welwyn Garden City: Tesco plc, 2014

139 PepsiCo UK. *50 in 5 Commitment: We Plan to Reduce Our Water Use and Carbon Emissions by 50% in 5 Years.* Available at: www.pepsico.co.uk/purpose/environment/ reports-and-updates/2010-environment-report/passionate-about-growing/50-in-5 (accessed October 13, 2015). Richmond, Surrey: PepsiCo UK, 2010

140 Ellen Macarthur Foundation, McKinsey & Co. *Towards the Circular Economy.* Cowes, Isle of Wight: Ellen Macarthur Foundation, 2013

141 European Commission. *Communication from the Commission: Closing the Loop: An EU Action Plan for the Circular Economy, COM/2015/0614 final.* Brussels: Commission of the European Communities, 2014

142 European Commission. *The Circular Economy: Communication 'Towards a Circular Economy: A Zero Waste Programme for Europe'.* Available at: http://ec.europa.eu/ environment/circular-economy/index_en.htm (accessed November 14, 2015). Brussels: European Commission, 2014

143 Devlin S, Dosch T, Esteban A, *et al. Urgent Recall: Our Food System Under Review.* London: New Economics Foundation, 2014

144 Rayner G, Lang T. Is nudge an effective public health strategy to tackle obesity? No. *British Medical Journal,* 2011; 342: d2168-d68

145 Thaler R, Sunstein C. *Nudge: Improving Decisions about Health, Wealth, and Happiness.* New Haven, CT: Yale University Press, 2008

146 Hamrick KS, Andrews M, Guthrie J, *et al. How Much Time Do Americans Spend on Food?* Washington, DC: USDA Economic Research Service, 2011

# Chapter 8

# Policy and governance
## Will anyone unlock the consumption lock-in?

## Contents

## Core arguments

This chapter considers how the issue of sustainable diets might be addressed. Governance, instead of being about resolving problems, has itself become part of the problem. The chapter outlines what is meant by the word 'governance'. By this we mean not just government or the state, which has historically been seen as the source of policy change. Governance is now the actions, decisions and process roles of many actors, all of whom have a stake in the food system. This chapter considers the decline of state influence over society and the rise of neoliberal consumerist thinking. This has seen a shift from 'old', top-down forms of governance to 'new' more complex and multi-level ones, based on markets. Modern policy actors therefore now include companies, civil society organisations, consumers and professions, as well as the weakened state. Governance levels include the local, national, regional and global. This modern governance affects the pursuit of sustainable diets and more beneficial food systems. 'Multi-criteria' and 'single' criteria approaches see the issues differently. The former sees sustainability as complex and therefore subject to endless juggling. The latter suggests concentrating on one important element of the overall problem – often nutrition. It's better to achieve change on one front and have knock-on beneficial environmental effects. Food waste is widely agreed to be a top priority. Waste lends itself to technological or economic efficiency arguments for addressing sustainable diet but the cost is the marginalisation of issues such as culture and social values. Another big theme is the delicacy of translating sustainable diets into everyday behaviour for ordinary consumers. Many points of engagement are emerging on sustainable diets. A period of democratic experimentation is already underway. Some nation states have tried to give overt sustainable dietary advice but often this has met resistance. Pressure for change continues, not least from civil society, scientists, city-regions and some sections of the food industry. There is some support at the international level. The chapter concludes that a key to good governance is a whole food-system approach. The transition requires long commitments and time horizons, plus transition processes that are inclusive and democratic. Food culture is a key tension point. The chapter considers an SDG² strategy – Sustainable Dietary Guidelines to deliver on the food elements of the UN's 2015 Sustainable Development Goals. This is a strategy to operationalise tasks, set clear goals and engage with not just some but all aspects of food supply and cultural change. This chapter suggests that the outcome of contemporary governance will be shaped by the degree of coordination and organisation of social forces who want dietary change in line with ecosystems health.

## What is meant by policy and governance?

As we noted at the end of Chapter 1, the term 'food governance' means more than simply what government does. It refers to the entire process of decision-making: how decisions are made, by whom and with what effect. Governance includes the style and mode of decision not just the decision itself, and draws attention to the role of values not just facts. Whether decisions are about sustainable diets or genetic modification, governance analysis requires us to consider whether the discourse and process are completely open and transparent, and to be clear about their moral as well as material context. Governance is particularly sensitive over food matters and, as a result, is much analysed by food academics.[1,2]

To approach any food problem through the lens of governance means that we ask a number of broad as well as specific questions. Whose interests are at the table where decisions are being made and futures mapped out? Is the process subject to audit and accountability? Is this transparent? What is shaping the discussion and outcomes? Who leads on the transition to more sustainable diets, how and why? Much of the food governance challenge raised by questions such as these dissolves down to whether policy makers think the issue is just too complex or whether it actually can be translated into practical change. If so, how is this to come about? Led by whom, where and with what legitimacy? Can this be left to consumer choice or market power? These are intriguing, important and sometimes ideologically influenced questions, but they make a difference in what and how people grow, process and eat food. This requires interdisciplinary analysis and thought.[3] No one food culture is 'correct'. Societal development over at least 10,000 years has left humanity with many thousands of cuisines and tastes, all derived from different economies, lifestyles, social structures and eco-system locations. Their governance varies as a result.

This chapter lays out some of the themes that have emerged as decision-makers face the complexity of sustainable diets, and it outlines the terrain and levels where the action is. There is no one 'answer' to governance. Indeed, governance can itself become the battleground, as the various battles that have already occurred show. There is strong resistance to sustainable diets. Neoliberals argue that the transition to more sustainable diets is not necessary in the first place. Others argue over means and modes. But, as these arguments are being fought over, we can note that, while there might not be agreement on what a sustainable diet is, there is some degree of consensus about the criteria by which it may be judged. This chapter summarises various attempts to capture the middle ground – what some authors have referred to as the 'principles' to guide the transition to food sustainability.[4, 5] But the challenge remains as to how to achieve this change, and how to negotiate through the messiness of the transition? In democratic societies these are no light issues. Just because there is evidence does not mean decision-makers will push through change to address it. Governance frameworks shape the options, alliances and dynamics, all of which are affected by events. (We write as UK researchers whose decades of experience was changed by the 2016 UK referendum vote to leave the European Union.)

One of the reasons academic studies of public policy introduced the term 'governance' was to capture a shift from an 'old' politics to a 'new' politics, from top-down governance to more fluid and contested processes. With spreading democracy from the nineteenth century to today, and with twenty-first century rapid access to multi-channel media, the web and information flows across borders, ordinary people can see political processes and rights differently to how their forebears did. Power relations have changed, say some, but the world remains highly unequal; the realities have come closer and become more visible. Television and films can convey yet confuse these realities. The medium can become the message. Complex processes are hard to capture in a 140-character tweet. Big Data concentrates power yet drowns the citizen with knowledge.[6, 7] What sociologists describe as 'choice world' for affluent consumers can be remote and debilitating to low-paid slum workers in developing countries despite – or even because – it is available on screens where they live.[8, 9] This is a paradoxical state of existence. No wonder so many political scientists agree political processes have become more diffuse, more complex and more multi-level.[10] National governments today sit in a web of international, cross-border and bi-lateral agreements on everything from trade to civil liberties and information flows.[11] These shape the world of food and it is this which the word 'governance' tries to capture. Food illustrates this diffusion of power while exposing fissures in where and how power operates.

### Why the term 'governance'?

The term 'governance' came into policy language in the late twentieth century because the role of the State came under concerted and deliberate political attack.[12] From the 1940s an emerging neoliberal (politically right-wing) analysis argued that the then dominant (now 'old') policy and politics were too top-down, the actions mostly of the State. These were a drag on economic efficiency and human liberty. Whether the State was benign, authoritarian or democratic was almost beside the point, the neoliberals argued. They saw the State as intrinsically too powerful, too patronising and as undermining the purity and benefits of market relations.[13, 14] Bureaucracies should be dismantled. Consumers should be sovereign, allowed to make their choices.[15, 16] There is no need for a paternalistic or patronising State to defend people's interests. Let consumers decide in the marketplace. This position rejected the counter view (first articulated by the UK Cooperative Movement in the nineteenth century and by the fledgling consumer movement in the USA in the twentieth century) that consumers were not really in control,[17] and that they are manipulated, bombarded with messages and desires, torn between conflicting motives and realities.

These are competing views with different demands of society and the political economy. This debate has been particularly resonant in the world of food, over issues such as food quality, value-for-money, standards, consumer rights, information, costs and power.[3, 18] What seems a simple matter can easily become ideological. To the neoliberal, for example, food's carbon footprint might be less important – perhaps even a myth that must be questioned. Indeed, some see it as a conspiracy pedalled by statist tendencies in science, seeking big grants and influence. To the social democrat, however, the refusal to contain food's carbon emissions or its impact on the biosphere (extraction of water, destruction of biodiversity, etc.) exemplifies the inflexibility of unregulated markets. They would work better if 'framed' by better regulations.

Keynesian thinking, forged prior to the Second World War, gave the State the key role in easing out the booms and slumps that had accentuated the 1930s recession. States since the Second World War should lead the reconstruction of the West, shaping markets.[19] In China and the USSR, different and more authoritarian states took even stronger roles. For all the differences between East and West, the State took a leading role in re-energising food and farming, to prevent failures in supply and to champion new efficient farming systems.[20] By the 1970s, the neoliberal critique was questioning Keynesian orthodoxy in the West, while communist inefficiencies were troubling the East. Government spending was high. Regulations were presented as blocking innovation and investment. The New Right emerged.[12, 21] Actually, like Keynesianism, it too had roots in the 1930s, with economic liberals who wanted a mid-course between authoritarian state-led socialism (associated with a ruthless state power in the Soviet Union) and the harshness of classical liberalism (associated with nineteenth-century Europe, a world prior to welfare safety nets).[22]

These roots are relevant to our concern for governance of sustainable diets because these arguments have had profound effects on food governance. If there is a real problem in addressing diet's impact on health, environment, justice, quality, affordability and so on, who is responsible for change? What kind of change is desirable? Can anyone or anything exert sufficient leverage to make a difference? Does anyone have the power? Indeed, some argue that modern governance is so complex that there is a problem of 'ungovernability'.[23] Others, neoliberal purists, always ask whether government has a place in a discourse in the first place.

From the 1970s these new politics of more reluctant, pared-down government emerged. Blaming government for ills gave legitimacy to those who preferred the primacy of market relations and the value of commerce. Companies, markets and consumers are more nimble than cumbersome government processes. Even within government, these views took hold, and there was a rise of consultation politics in which stakeholders and round tables were created, trying to gain consensus without too many shocks, but in which government ceded its primacy.

Government adopted a facilitator rather than a dirigiste role.[24] But this could be superficial. Political analysts detected, by the mid-1980s, the emergence of what is known as the Washington Consensus.[25, 26] This term was coined by a US policy analyst, John Williamson, commenting on the US approach to Latin American politics, at a time when there was hostility between North and South America, an era of liberation politics on that continent (as in Africa). Williamson argued that a new set of principles had emerged in Washington/US politics. This included: an emphasis on fiscal discipline; cutting of subsidies; tax reforms; trade liberalisation; privatisation of state enterprises; removing controls on externally derived investment; deregulation; and support of property and intellectual property rights.

These policies had considerable traction in the food system, shaping how, for example, the World Bank or International Monetary Fund (IMF) promoted liberalisation of trade and demanded more open markets in debtor developing nations.[27, 28, 29] The Uruguay Round of General Agreement on Tariffs and Trade (GATT), the set of world trade rules, concluded by bringing food and farming under its new rules, committed to tariff cuts. It created binding global structures under the World Trade Organization, replacing the GATT Secretariat in 1994.[30, 31] While globalisation was the mantra, in fact there was a strong trend to create inter-regional trade blocs. The European Union expanded from 9 to 28 countries by 2010. The North American Free Trade Agreement (NAFTA) and Asia-Pacific agreements were concluded. Such agreements altered the post-Second World War food regime which had given the State key leverage in the form of subsidies. The 1990s saw these cut, with the OECD advising their reduction. The OECD was and remains a strong champion of low subsidies, producing annual reviews of how farmers are subsidised by consumers.[32, 33]

While this anti-statism became so influential, and as its language of markets became the governance centre of gravity, evidence began to rise on the problems summarised in previous chapters. Cheaper food prices may make energy-dense foods and drinks more accessible and affordable but this cheapness does not take account of food's full or hidden costs – the 'externalities' discussed earlier (see Chapter 7). The widening of food choice – a dream of progress to previous generations – made highly processed foods ubiquitous and restructured cultural norms (see Chapters 5 and 7), but didn't pay for the health or environmental consequences. Intensification of food production raised yields but also eco-systems damage (see Chapter 4). The globalisation of brands, tastes and life-styles, together with lower food prices, helped generate rapid rises in overweight and obesity across the world. Heavy burdens of disease emerged (see Chapter 3). Instead of being expensive and partial on the plate, meat and dairy production rose and consumption grew. Culinary cultures altered (see Chapter 5). While hypermarkets gave consumers previously unimaginable choice, consumers were unable to fathom their collective impact. The nature of food itself changed (see Chapter 6). The world-wide web has produced astonishing information about food, yet food sales are still dominated by massive advertising budgets, which far outweigh information from teachers or nutritionists, let alone health education departments. Food labels cannot convey the complexity supposedly sovereign consumers might want to know.

If governments have become more hesitant and less prepared to lead let alone confront consumers into shifting to sustainable diets, how can consumers be encouraged to make the changes indicated by the evidence?[34] Consumers are the voters both in the ballot box and at the supermarket checkout. Politicians and businesses are reluctant to question them. The few studies that have looked at what consumers are prepared to do when they learn of diet's impact on health, the environment, culture, suggest some level of shock and 'willingness to change'.[35-38] But these are studies or consultations rather than mass-scale reality.

### Parallel systems of governance: public/private/civil

Trying to understand these realities and tensions, social scientists began to argue that in food, as in other sectors, new parallel systems of governance – public and private – had emerged.[39] The public framework of global trade rules now managed by the World Trade Organization (WTO) was being stretched to suit large private interests. In the early 1990s, the Codex Alimentarius Commission, the world body setting food standards in the name of the UN, was given responsibility to be arbiter in any trade disputes, in effect taking the role of providing benchmark standards for food. But big food businesses actually had a sizeable presence in what were supposedly national delegations making these decisions.[40] This embarrassed the UN and led to some tightening of the rules, but the tone was set.

More importantly, corporations began to bypass public accountability completely. Private consortia and alliances emerged to set food standards. Sometimes these actually exceed governmental standards. Some companies, for example, are tougher on pesticide residues than are governments. But the point is that the parallel systems of governance are being enshrined. An example is GLOBALG.A.P. (where 'GAP' stands for Good Agricultural Practice).[41] This is now a consortium of hundreds of companies working in over 100 countries agreeing standards that are 'voluntary' but can be specified in contract-tendering processes. Its existence partly reflects frustration with the slowness of public government, and partly with a desire to get into the 'nuts and bolts' of details that matter. Civil society organisations have also entered this world of private governance, cutting agreements on issues as diverse as fish capture standards, water extraction, forest management, biodiversity protection and food product reformulation.[42] Also, some big food companies worked with NGOs and some parts of government, coordinated by an industry research body (the IGD), to develop and promote Guideline Daily Amounts (GDAs) as a framework for nutrition labels.[43] In deciding matters such as labels, one sees the altered power relations between state, companies and public. The definition of the public good shifts.

Many academics have become critical of the blurring of lines between sectors as public–private partnerships (PPPs) emerge.[44-46] A major concern is about lost public accountability – not least with regard to accusations of 'air-brushing' cartels and anti-competitive behaviour (a big sin in the neoliberal canon). As states retreat from providing social safety nets, civil society organisations are also sometimes used to provide cheap and arms-length functions previously performed by the State. Some big NGOs, for instance, have developed their own food standards in the sustainable diet terrain on issues as diverse as sustainable fish (for example, the Marine Stewardship Council)[47], biodiversity protection (for example, forest-friendly coffee)[48], fair trade (to improve rural livelihoods)[49] and employment (for example, the Ethical Trade Initiative).[50]

The criticism is that, while these private and civil standards may be fine in themselves, they collectively reinforce the weakening of elected government.[51] The situation can reverse, however, if there is a crisis of public confidence over food. Then companies usually quickly want government to 'sort it out'. In the 1980s there were many such crises over food safety, public health, environmental damage and inappropriate corporate power.[18, 52–54] Some of these crises remained national, while others spilled over borders. In Europe, mad cow disease in the 1980s and horsemeat masquerading as beef in 2012 shook European consumer confidence and led to the downfall of the Commission itself.[55] In China, adulteration of milk with melamine not only shook consumer confidence but led to the head of food safety being executed.[56, 57]

## Different positions emerge on what to do

A fairly stark situation has emerged. On the one hand there is considerable evidence pointing to the need for serious change in diet. On the other hand, there is some reluctance to address the transition to sustainable diets. Do we need strong intervention or more 'leave it to markets'? Proponents of more sustainable diets are learning old lessons, that progress does not happen easily.[58] Public health and environment groups are beginning to work together and learn they are powerful together. As we will see below, there is also a growth of policy formulation, awareness and experimentation that we see as a positive democratic process. These suggest coordination of multiple actions is what is needed to shift unsustainable diets, not a single policy 'silver bullet'.

Table 8.1 gives an overview of positions on sustainable diets. This is schematic. In practice, these positions may overlap or fuse, or jostle for policy attention.

The first has been to question whether the issue can or should be tackled at all. Some say it is too complex; others are ideologically opposed in the first place.

The second is to accept that there is a problem but sees technology as the source of solutions. It does not question current eating patterns. Attempts range from improving farm productivity, to developing alternative animal-feeding sources,[59] to seeking new food products with lower impacts. The key word inside companies is 'reformulation', altering products to change their ingredients and reduce perceived threats.[60] Engineering takes a central place in this vision of sustainable food systems, for instance in resolving food waste.[61]

The third sees sustainable diets as a deviation from what should be the priority for food policy makers, namely preventing and resolving hunger. Some are wary on the grounds that, if sustainable diets are mainly championed by the affluent West, it might be a fig-leaf for rich society protectionism.

A fourth position puts responsibility on to consumers, by promising (if not fully providing) tools for change within the market model such as food labelling. There is no need for regulation; soft policy measures such as information and labelling would be sufficient to make consumers responsible.

The fifth response is to apply 'choice editing', below the consumer radar. Choice editing constrains the range of choices on the shelves or the manufacturer reformulates the ingredients before the consumer gets to see or buy the food.[62] It gives the consumer no option to reverse how the choice is structured other than to purchase elsewhere.[63]

The sixth response is to focus on high-risk and impact aspects of sustainable diets such as waste or meat. Research can inform policy makers as to what matters. It is better to focus on high-impact issues and to get some progress incrementally than to drown in trying to resolve everything.

The seventh policy response comes from within the public health sector. It is an appeal not to dilute the health message about diet by injecting complicating environmental concerns. It suggests that if consumers in the developed world were to follow current official health advice their dietary environmental impact would improve.[64, 65] A study of English school meals, for instance, found that if the meals met nutrition guidelines, their GHGEs declined.[66]

The eighth approach is to create new integrated dietary guidelines. These have the advantage of helping consumers in a holistic way and in sending clear signals throughout the food system as to best land use, production and consumption, and what is required from technology.[67, 68, 69, 70]

What determines how a particular position 'wins'? They might be championed by people with influence on a scientific committee but be curtailed by politicians higher up or rejected by industry. It matters whence they emerge and whether this is on the 'inside' or 'outside' track of policy-making. At the same time, experience suggests that one can never be certain where change will stem from. Animal welfare campaigners, for example, might have expected that giant fast-food companies would not take a progressive line on battery hens. Yet, in 2015, McDonald's made a commitment to go 'cage-free' in all its US and Canadian restaurants by 2025.[72] By 2016 105 US food companies had followed suit.[73] A market giant had led. It matters who sets standards, using which methods, because the implications for food management can be immense and costly.

In 2002 shockwaves went through the food-processing industries when acrylamide, a carcinogen, was found to be widely present in commercially fried and baked fatty foods following a surprising detection by Swedish researchers of worrying levels in people with no known exposure to the chemical. It turned out it was in widely consumed foods.[74] A massive industry effort then went into reducing

Table 8.1 Eight broad policy responses to dietary (un)sustainability

| Policy position | How manifest | Example(s) | Rationale | Comment |
| --- | --- | --- | --- | --- |
| There is no problem (or, if there is, it's 'not your business'). | Marginalisation of the agenda associated with sustainable diets. | Downplay food and climate change, or stress the costs of action. | This is progress; broadly neoliberal trust in market dynamics. | Business-as-usual. This is tantamount to 'this is none of your business'. |
| There is a problem but it can be addressed by technical solutions. | Search for new foods, ingredients and technical infrastructure. | Developing insects as a source of animal feed or nanotechnology in food processing. | This opens up new business opportunities while keeping the general business model in place. | Technology can be helpful in addressing sustainability but it downplays the social aspects. |
| This is a rich society problem. | A persistent focus on under-consumption/hunger. | The focus is on hunger; down-playing complex health and environmental implications. | Retain Western model of eating as the ideal; choice, if one has little, would be progress. | Ignores growing evidence of nutrition transition and food-related environmental problems in global South. |
| It is a consumer responsibility. | If consumers are to make informed choices they need help. | UK carbon labelling of selected food products. | Consumer choice depends on education; self-interest. | This assumes food markets work with maximum flow of full information. |
| Choice-editing. | Product reformulation; new supply-chain efficiency goals. | Smaller product size to cut carbon, packaging or calories. | Corporate responsibility. | Brand protection; prevention of future litigation; 'below the radar' actions. |
| Focus on high-risk issues/hotspots. | Particular issues are championed as 'the key'. | Cut waste, or reduce/contain meat and dairy consumption. | Data on impact is strong whether measured by science or finance. | This is critical-control-point thinking borrowed from HACCP in food safety. It misses the systemic nature of the challenge. |
| Stick to the health message. | Follow health advice and the environmental impact will fall. | Reduce meat and dairy. | There is no need to confuse signals to consumers with environmental or cultural norms. | It ignores the cultural dimension of food. It also assumes consumers are driven by health. |
| Provide clear advice on sustainable diets. | National guidelines. | National – for example, Sweden (2011), Germany (2013); intergovernmental – for example, Nordic Council (2012). | Food citizenship should replace consumerism. | Has cost implications and also requires changed policy frameworks beyond diet. |

Source: Lang, 2016.[71]

acrylamide but firmly out of the public eye. Meanwhile, mass withdrawal of mainstream brands was considered unacceptable and no label warnings were considered necessary despite US NGOs and a few independent academics pushing hard. The issue surfaced again when the UK Food Standards Agency issued advice to consumers in 2017 to beware acrylamide.

## Themes that have emerged in sustainable diet governance

Some themes, stances and cross-cutting questions have emerged from across academic and other literature on sustainable diets. This section gives more detail and direction to the broad positions outlined in Table 8.1 above. It summarises some key terms and arguments that have featured in discussions about what to do about sustainable diets, and which are therefore elements in the governance discourse.

### Reconnection with tradition and culinary history

It can be argued that sustainability requires food culture to reconnect a runaway consumerism with the realities of land use, food production and seasonality. If so, one interpretation is for rich societies almost to go back in food time, to eat simpler or less. Michael Pollen's much-cited summaries are apposite: 'Eat food. Not too much. Mostly plants', and 'Don't eat anything your great-grandmother wouldn't recognise as food', and other cultural 'rules' or norms.[75, 76] These suggest that twentieth-century food systems took a false route. Planetary limits have been ignored. Food choice needs to be recalibrated. Other versions of progress need to be charted to help consumers eat and live within resource boundaries. While recent years have seen the modern food system's reliance on material resources (goods, minerals, energy) taken more seriously, more thought needs to be given to culture. Hence the appeal to 'old ways'. Brazil and Sweden, in fact, have both published dietary guidelines appealing to tradition.[77, 78] Social scientists and the food industries, however, both agree that 'traditions' can and do change.[79] Culture is malleable. 'Traditions' can be invented and hard-wired quite quickly. The issue for governance is why and how should traditions change for sustainability.

### Modernisation: technical fixes and the role of science, technology and engineering

As the agricultural commodity and banking crises unfolded in 2007–8, the argument was made that this exposed a failure to maintain investment in food and farming output. There were calls for another bout of investment in agricultural productivity gains and for technical solutions to food waste.[80–82] Productivity gains had indeed been allowed to slow.[83] But was a new era of 'modernisation' required? If so, should this be hi-tech or low-tech, agro-ecological or focused on winning efficiency gains for conventional farming?[84] More organic farming or a rush into wide-scale biotechnology? Off-farm efficiency-oriented or land-use-focused? The FAO accepts that livestock emissions urgently need to be reduced, and could be by between 18% and 30% if best practice was adopted.[85] But, as a goal, modernisation became a battle about what is meant by 'sustainable intensification'. It could be interpreted in many ways, as pro-biotechnology or agro-ecology.[86, 87]

There is a strong strand of analysis that seeks 'technical fixes' for sustainable diets, the pursuit of single factors or intervention that could resolve wider socio-economic problems. The sustainable diets discourse is not immune from this and some wariness is in order. One US 2015 start-up saw the future in ending the meal itself – arguing it is a relic of industrialisation and affluence. Far better to eat soylent, a powdered combination of soy, lentils and other ingredients, it argued. This product raised over \$100 m in venture capital investment.[88] Others look to technical solutions not in single products but categories. Genetics can often be a policy 'white knight on a charger'. Despite strong evidence that obesity, for example, cannot be reduced to one factor but is the result of a complex of factors – the obesogenic environment[89] – a cohort of scientists still get funds to search for the obesity gene.[90] Food manufacturers have an obvious interest here, which is presumably why Nestlé searches for an enzyme 'which "tricks" the body into burning more fat',[91] or why the crisp/chips manufacturer researches a low-fat product with the same 'mouthfeel'. At the global scale there are engineers researching how they could 'cloud seed' or conduct some other intervention to mitigate climate change.[92] These technical fixes deviate attention from the quicker 'solution' of consuming less.

### Consumer behaviour change

How can consumers be helped to shift to sustainable diets? An international study by Chatham House suggested that consumers are prepared to move towards meat-reduction, but it and other studies have asked whether the public is actually receiving sufficient information to help people do so.[93] One country in Chatham House's study did subsequently give firm advice to reduce meat consumption. China set a remarkable target of 50% meat reduction in June 2016.[94, 95] As a controlled economy it may be able to deliver, but in looser political cultures there is likely to be a gap between any formal advice and subsequent behaviour. India also recognises its self-interest in containing food-related $CO_2$e emissions.[96]

Politicians generally do not want to be seen dictating what to eat to consumers. Even though meat reduction is a key finding from science,[69, 97, 98] this often meets resistance.[99, 100] Consumption change is politically delicate. That is why there has been a growth of interest in behavioural economics, the conflation of consumer psychology and economics. This has been popularised by 'nudge' thinking.[101]

## Protecting the poor

Much of the discourse about sustainable consumption emerged from the developed rather than developing world. Some champions of low-income country development are wary of ideas such as sustainable diets being yet more imposition on already stretched food systems. But there is also strong evidence that the nutrition transition now blights middle-income and many countries moving from low-income to middle-income status.[102, 103] They are in the front line of climate change and often least well-resourced to adapt to it. A concern that the sustainable diet issue might deviate attention from economic disadvantage was one factor behind reluctance at the UN's International Conference on Nutrition (ICN2) to face sustainable diets squarely.[104] The case for getting nutrients to the poor is, of course, unanswerable.[105] But the transition to sustainable diets and food supply is surely part of that process. The governance question is: what is the best way to do this? Is it through targeted welfare such as Scaling Up Nutrition which targets low-income countries,[106] or grand political declarations such as global conferences are wont to end with, or can it be left to big companies?[91] Most independent people think not.

## Dietary guidelines

Sweden was the first country to give clear, detailed, evidence-based advice in 2009.[107] This was subsequently retracted under pressure from within the European Commission on the grounds that the Swedish advice to eat locally and seasonally infringed the EU single-market rule. However, Sweden did not give up. Five years later it came back with deliberately looser but cultural rather than nutritional advice.[78] The loss of its national guidelines' specificity and detail was a great shame, although not its fault. Germany, meanwhile, had taken a different, softer route. Its Council of Sustainable Development first gave sketchy advice in 2003, based around alerting consumers to sympathetic 'sustainable' logos. Over time, with each new edition, this has strengthened and become more detailed.[108–110]

Advice on diet and how food can help health is almost as old as written records. The term 'dietary guidelines', however, refers to formal, scientifically based guidance at the population level. Dietary guidelines are meant to set food goals for a society. Most US nutrition history refers to the (still much cited) formal advice by Wilbur Olin Atwater, a pioneering professor of nutrition who advised the US government's Department of Agriculture at the end of the nineteenth century.[111] Atwater laid out nutrition goals for US farming. This policy approach spread to Europe in two ways, first as a way of calibrating nutritional needs for workers and the poor, best illustrated in the work of Seebohm Rowntree in the 1900s in York, UK.[112, 113] Second, it was used to set ration levels in times of war.[114–116] The USA began to offer dietary guidelines in publicly accessible form in 1916, always through the USDA (production to the fore) but latterly jointly with Health and Human Services. Dietary guidelines have been produced in the current format since 1980, revised by law once every five years.[117] Since the early 1900s, guidance has subtly changed through distinct phases, from an initial focus on children (1916–30s), to 'protective foods' and 'good eating' (1940s), to 'fitness' and 'hassle-free food' (1950s–70s), and then to 'choice' (1980s), 'adequacy and moderation' (1990s) and 'healthy eating' (2000s).[118] This evolution is itself fascinating, not least for how the messages were represented visually.

Dietary guidelines have been a key mode for public health nutrition influence globally. Many countries now issue nutrient and food based guidelines, encouraged by the WHO (see Chapter 3). So far, with the exception of Qatar (discussed later), these have downplayed any environmental dimension, but do appeal to national culinary culture. China, for example, has a Food Guide Pagoda. And Sweden which tried to produce real sustainable diet guidelines retreated to the cultural.

There is some debate about how effective dietary guidelines are. Some argue that they are too abstract and go over people's heads, while others think they do provide a basis for evaluating how good or distorted food supply is. US studies by a Harvard team have shown that other indices are rather better predictors of ill-health outcomes.[119] These apply more detailed nutrition data to nutrition advice. Nonetheless, our view (like the Harvard team's) is that it is sensible for societies to set national dietary guidelines, but these should be continuously tested and fine-tuned. They serve little purpose if ignored or are unrealised.

### Balancing universal and bioregional culinary rules

There is some discussion about whether sustainable diets can be universal or are inevitably context specific. What is the point in advising 'eat less meat' if a society is vegetarian but eating more dairy, or if it is a low-income society where meat is more rare? Surely advice must be context-related? Yet nutrition scientists tend to argue that human physiology is broadly the same everywhere and that advice need only be specific with regard to the very young or for women, pre-conception to post-parturition. Some traits may be ethnic-group specific, such as lactose intolerance, but, generally, the same messages are appropriate almost everywhere. The only difference is how to translate the science into the culinary culture. This is a sensitive issue.

People don't tend to think that they are eating nutrients, even though they are. They eat food. They enjoy tastes they know. They follow norms, and these norms and tastes vary remarkably worldwide. Any pursuit of sustainable diets, therefore, must take account of cultural differences. If the evidence is so clear that food supply will alter, then cultural rules are likely to alter too. Here is where the sustainability issue comes to the fore. Population and land-use pressures mean that food supplies will inevitably alter. Advice therefore must take account of ecosystems and demographic realities. Policy makers seem wary of entering this territory.

## Economic cost and feasibility

The 'bottom-line' test in much governance is cost. Ministers and CEOs alike will ask: how much will action X cost compared with action Y? A change may be feasible but is not fundable, or both feasible and fundable but not politically realisable. The 'dismal science' of economics is often invoked as the arbiter of policy options. It is generally supportive of the status quo, arguing that in richer societies the decline in cost of food has been a consumer benefit. Whereas consumers in Kenya, Egypt or Cameroon spend about 40% or over of their income on food, in the USA, Sweden or the UK it is nearer 10%.[120, 121] Health and environmental economists have worked with scientific colleagues for decades to create methodologies for estimating the externalised costs of food systems, and particularly its impact on ecosystems and population health (see Chapter 7). They counterargue that the drop in food expenditure is not the whole story. Within the UN, UNEP has championed this approach through its The Economics of Ecosystems and Biology (TEEB) study,[122] and its follow-up TEEB Agriculture and Food (TEEBAF) study.[123]

Indicators are produced by such economic analyses that are not simply monetary. An example is the World Bank and WHO Global Burden of Disease calculus, begun in the 1990s but now widened.[124, 125] Such studies have consolidated the critique of current dietary patterns, but they have not necessarily altered the status quo, let alone persuaded policy makers radically to change course. In the early 2000s, the UK government did two major studies, chaired by a banker, of the future costs of UK healthcare. The studies concluded that non-communicable diseases would have a rising cost to the National Health Service.[126, 127] Yet no shift in national diet strategy ensued. Only when the oil-market price rocketed in the banking crisis of 2007–8 was a strategic review of the food system made by the Cabinet Office. This concluded that a new direction was needed, around the goals of decarbonisation and health.[128] For two years the beginnings of a new strategy was worked on,[129, 130] only for this to be halted by the new Coalition Government elected in 2010. That incoming government reverted to a narrower policy, focused on agricultural technology and trying to expand UK exports, downplaying the environmental or health considerations.[131] That strategy in turn was thrown into abeyance by the UK's 2016 vote to leave the European Union.[132] Events and politics like these can and do trump even the economic argument about costs. While cost studies may provide sound evidence, they do not necessarily lead to evidence-based change. The economics are often not the clinching factor in governance. Other problems arise such as trade-offs, lock-ins and tipping points (see the next sections).

## Trade-offs

The issue of 'trade-offs' is much debated: if we get improvements in one aspect of eating, will it lead to the worsening of other aspects? Must we therefore trade-off some gains for those losses?[133] If we encourage people to eat less meat, for example, will that lead to a nutritional problem of iron deficiency? Does that matter? The answer is yes for some sectors of populations. So how can that be dealt with? The classic illustration of trade-offs as an issue for sustainable diets is fish. Nutrition science recommends consumption of fish, yet stocks are in some crisis.[134] Over a decade ago, the UK's Royal Commission on Environmental Pollution urged the Food Standards Agency to revise its fish consumption advice.[135] Today the FSA does recommend consumers choose sustainable fish. But changing the advice does not lever actual behaviour or prepare for a world of 9 bn consumers.[136] Another problem is palm oil, a plant with one of the highest yields in the world. Its use has been highly profitable to planters but its arrival in massive plantations has been associated with losses in biodiversity and hard times for labour and small farmers. Could nutritional critics of palm oil as a fat in cooking or food processing be mollified by genetically modified palms? And would this offset concerns about the high level of market concentration? These trade-off problems can be addressed by sophisticated modelling but such exercises are often only done by the powerful; what small farmer organisation can get modelling done to a level of robustness that powerful commercial bodies could not counter?

### Lock-ins, tipping points and the Anthropocene: is it possible to get adequate change?

As data on food's impact on health, environment and society have grown, so attempts to achieve preventive change have followed. Some analysts argue that small changes are all that is needed, which over time give incremental benefits. Others argue that big rather than small changes are needed, that the environmental clock is ticking, and that there needs to be rapid systemic change. This divergence of analysis has been a theme throughout this book. Among the supporters of systems change, a corollary debate has arisen. If the evidence for considerable change is so strong, yet comparable action is so limited, what stops the change? Does this mean that the impacts of failing to get sufficient change soon mean more dramatic and uncontrollable change becomes more likely later?

The notion of 'tipping points' has been prominent in the discourse.[137, 138] This came from physics – where addition of extra mass literally tips the scales – into both ecological and systems thinking. In these, the notion of tipping point is used to indicate the moment when the capacity of a system to bounce back or correct itself after change is impaired by the scale of change and, instead, it moves into a new equilibrium or balance of forces and relationships. Wars can be tipping points for food – they are events that reconfigure normality and force new rules and patterns to appear.[139] The language of tipping points can be apocalyptic – Professor Sir Martin Rees, former British Astronomer Royal, suggests that the twenty-first century is humanity's last century[140] – but it can also simply point out that equilibrium may change to a different plane. The concept of the Anthropocene contributes here, proposing that human activity has now shifted Planet Earth into a new era, the human-made era or Anthropocene. Industrialisation and burning of carbon on a massive scale began climate change, but other activities such as plastics in the environment and mass destruction of biodiversity mean there has been a quantitative and qualitative shift.

The notion of 'lock-in' has also been introduced to explain the resistance to change. A 2015 global study of consumers' willingness to change meat consumption concluded that they were prepared to, but there was a cycle of inertia at the policy level: (a) inaction by government, industry, media and civil society feeding (b) low public awareness feeding (c) low policy priority feeding (a), and so on.[93] A lock-in happens when forces supporting the status-quo are stronger than those pushing for change. Lock-ins can take many forms: technological (for example, consumers lack equipment for home cooking) or political (for example, they are relatively powerless) or cultural (for example, consumer understanding is shaped by marketing) or economic (for example, cheap prices entice them) or ideological (for example, they cannot conceive of eating a simpler diet, let alone of why they should). The International Panel of Experts on Sustainable Food Systems (IPES-Food) has outlined at least eight lock-ins that reinforce the industrialised model of agriculture.[84] These include: path-dependency (reliance on investment and equipment to maintain a chosen mode of farming), concentration of power and short-term thinking.

## The role of standards

Should there be standards for sustainable diets? Almost certainly yes. So far, science and the policy debate has done no more than map the criteria for sustainable diets and explore their general principles. But could this all be clarified by a bout of operationalisation? If something is measured, then performance can be monitored. Vice versa, as US President Dwight Eisenhower is reputed to have said, 'the uninspected quickly deteriorates'. Surely it would help if indicators for sustainable diets could be set. At present, most attention is on GHGs or nutrient profiles but, if other broader measures are included, national sustainable dietary change could be more accurately monitored. Two studies of the UK's diet found that when measures were included for land use and imports, its food system's footprint grew considerably.[141, 142] In other words, its unsustainability was higher than might have been expected by taking only face-value indicators.

Food standards can be a delicate matter politically. Developing countries complain that they can be a barrier to entry.[143] A review by FAO of the literature on small farmers' access to international markets and whether production standards act as barriers to entry found that most formal studies tended to have researched a surprisingly narrow set of standards mostly for organics, fair trade and GLOBALG.A.P. and, even then, disproportionately in the coffee and horticulture sectors.[144] The FAO review concluded that, intrinsically, standards need not be barriers to market access. Indeed, the FAO suggests that the key issue might be not so much standards or criteria but the democratic processes. Small farmers need to be included in, rather than at the edges of, sustainability govern-ance. Participatory governance is what is needed in the setting of standards.

## Measurement for measures

One issue raised throughout this book is measurement. What is meant by sus-tainable diets shapes what one wants to measure and vice versa. Whether it is possible to measure something is a different matter. Values are ideas and moral rules. They can be measured – by polls, by attitude surveys, by specialised value studies – but they don't tend to be what governments judge food systems by. Within the sustainable diet discourse there is an agreed need to put some 'edge' into vague goals. Commitments in other areas show the value of creating indica-tors. There are many. Since 2013 the Hunger and Nutrition Commitment Index (HANCI), for example, has been produced by an academic institute, funded by governments. It is used to rank and measure the political commitment by 45 developing countries at risk of hunger, to compare performance. The index is the outcome of 22 other indicators. Countries are ranked as high, moderate, low and very low. Could there be a Sustainable Diet Index that focuses on the affluent world and not just the poor world? Yes.

A systematic review of measurement used in empirical studies of sustainable diets found most studies were conducted in affluent countries and, although there were about 30 indicators used, the most used were headline indicators, notably GHGs. The researchers concluded – in line with the position taken in this book – that this unduly narrows the conception of sustainability.[145] They suggest that there are three broad approaches to measurement: modelling, integrated indi-cator and participatory. The FAO and Bioversity International hosted a large conference in 2010 that recognised the problem of sustainable diet, outlined some thinking and generated the much-cited definition. This needed specific follow-up across the UN system and ought to have been addressed in the WHO/FAO International Conference on Nutrition in 2014. Alas, it wasn't, although there was a later push in that direction with the proposal to address issues through a Decade of Action on Nutrition 2016–25, agreed in April 2016. Just before that, in September 2015, the UN did however give a strong lead with the 17 Sustainable Development Goals agreed in New York.

These 17 SDGs were translated into 169 Targets. Food was one cross-cutting element. UNEP's World Conservation Monitoring Centre, for example, pro-posed the Ecological Footprint as an SDG metric for Goal 12.2: 'by 2030 [to] achieve sustainable management and efficient use of natural resources'. It saw this as within the longer-term aspiration, articulated back in 1991, as 'improving the quality of human life while living within the carrying capacity of supporting eco-systems'.[146] This is living within environmental limits. The most common measurements are now well-known, notably $CO_2$ or $CO_2e$, often using life-cycle analysis. Policy analysts like figures that can be benchmarked and used as targets to measure performance. The UK's Public Health England, for instance, used the

Carbon Trust to calculate the carbon footprint of different diets when making its 2016 nutrition advice which for the first time added an environmental element to the national advice on eating meat.[147, 148]

## Resource use and limits to growth: food in the 'circular economy'

Engineers look at sustainability as a matter of resource management.[61] Food is always about resources – inputs and outputs. Food is biological but is a material entity. It has mass. It is wasted. It has presence with impacts – putrefaction, garbage, pollution, health contagion. When modern food systems, often held up as paragons of efficiency, began to be audited for their use of resources, their energy inefficiency and their wastefulness in the 1970s,[149, 150] the results failed to get much interest except from the already sceptical – supporters of alternative technology or small-scale food systems.[151] It was seen as too critical. Spurred on by the concerns voiced by the 1972 *Limits to Growth* report,[152] a thorny but brilliant question was posed by environmental economists about whether economic growth can be de-coupled from resource use.[153–155] Could there be capitalism without destruction of eco-systems? This question continues today.[156, 157]

At the 1992 'Rio' UN Conference on Environment and Development, the EU offered to take a lead on resource efficiency, with Sweden leading for the EU. By the 2000s the EU charted resource efficiency as a key factor in what political scientists call ecological modernisation. The European Commission published a Roadmap to a resource-efficient Europe in 2011.[158] This applied life-cycle analysis and thinking to energy, buildings, transport, fish, land use, food and beverage, agriculture and soil. It argued the advantage for price security, risk reduction and resource availability by creating foods whose materials could be fully recycled.[158] In the 2010s the circular economy became a new language in boardrooms and capitals.[159, 160] Food should be recycled, turned back into energy or fertiliser. Entire food systems should be designed to circulate materials (but not capital). This is a step forward, without doubt, but is in fact an old idea, arguably just a fancy version of domestic economy, thrifty Victorian household management, an appeal to 'sensible' pragmatism, but is an advance for recognising that waste cannot be dumped. It cements the 'cradle-to-grave' approach to product development, the obligation on producers to manage how the inputs to finished products can be re-used. It has particular resonance in packaging. To give an example, in 2002 Innocent, a successful UK firm making fruit-based 'smoothies', bought out and globalised by Coca-Cola in 2013, first introduced 25% recycled plastics into its bottles. By 2007 all its bottles were made from 100% recycled plastics. In 2012–13 it cut the weight of packaging for its 900 ml fruit juice carafes by 10%, saving an estimated 1,000 $CO_2$e per year. This approach made the company highly critical of the lack of uniformity in the UK's 433 local authority recycling schemes.[161]

### The case for 'contract and converge'

What can be done about sustainable diets at the macro-level? One clear position was given by the UK's Royal Society, one of the oldest scientific bodies in the world, which, in 2012, proposed that the unequal distribution of resources, access and wealth means that the only fair route ahead is to apply the 'contract and converge' approach in food and consumer goods.[162] In this proposed transition, borrowed from energy analysts,[163] the goal is to get affluent economies to reduce their consumption and resource-use (not least since they over-use and waste them), while allowing lower-income societies to raise their standards of living (not least since deficiencies lead to ill-health, economic under-performance and lost potential). While this 'contraction' phase runs, all types of society 'converge' to a steady state level of consumption within environmental limits. The implications of contract and converge are immense, not least for politics. It requires strong buy-in from political leaders and their citizens, and it is a serious medium-term framework for how to tackle the unsustainability of diet.

### What works? Interventions and 'natural' experiments

The goal of evidence-based policy and behaviour is tantalising but, as we show in the section 'Governance in practice' below, it is frustratingly slow and meeting resistance in the case of sustainable diets. So far.

Interventions can range from soft to hard, from top-down to bottom-up, from consumer-oriented to industry-oriented. Generally, interventions in the broad area of sustainability of food consumption have remained at the soft end of intervention, i.e., appeals, information and a very few labels, but there has been little tough intervention such as taxes, laws, regulations or mixed measures to deliver systems-wide food change. A 2015 review by the Food Climate Research Network and Chatham House concluded that there was insufficient data to show if anything worked, but it was possible to review different interventions such as for healthy eating or recycling.[164] The study concluded that awareness raising does not work or work enough to make a difference. A sugar tax on soft drinks (sodas) can work as Mexico shows[165] but, while lowering consumption of these drinks is valuable for health, it doesn't address the totality of dietary change. The key is to achieve framework change, to ensure that multiple interventions recalibrate social norms. This requires governments to govern, and that requires pressure on governments.

## Governance in practice: who has tried to do what?

This section outlines the basic architecture of who is doing what to address the sustainable diet agenda, and at which institutional level.

## Intergovernmental/global

The UN missed an opportunity to engage with food and sustainability at its big International Conference on Nutrition (ICN2) in 2014.[104] Surely, this huge intergovernmental conference on public health nutrition was the occasion to merge nutrition and environmental strategy – not least since the UN was itself actively creating the Sustainable Development Goals (SDGs) that were agreed the following year and which saw the importance of food? Nevertheless, it didn't. The following year, however, the Paris Climate Change Accord did respond to pressure by producing a new framework for sustainable or decarbonising consumption and production. Pressure from big business was an undoubtedly important factor in committing 195 signatory governments to keep climate change within two degrees.[166] This will be nigh impossible without the food system reducing its emissions.[167, 168] Twelve of the 17 Goals in the SDGs agreed a few months later require action on food.[169]

The SDGs and Paris Accord are welcome but late. In the years before, frustration at the weak level of governmental response spawned many other initiatives. A number of 'high level' panels emerged, some with the blessing of the UN and others at arms-length. The International Panel of Experts on Sustainable Food (IPES-Food), launched in 2014 and chaired by former UN Rapporteur on the Right to Food Professor Olivier De Schutter and Professor Olivia Yambi, is in fact aiming to develop an alternative, more people-oriented approach. That panel is composed of many respected people and part-funded by the Franco-Spanish Carasso Foundation.[170] The panel's first major report argued they are key to paradigmatic change.[84]

Other panels are both 'blessed' by and familiar with official channels and see their function as to inject thinking at the top level. The Global Panel on Sustainable Agriculture and Nutrition started in 2013, was chaired by former Kenyan President Kufor and former UK Chief Scientist Sir John Beddington, and funded by the Gates Foundation and UK Government to be 'an independent group of influential experts advising decision-makers, particularly governments, on generating nutrition-enhancing agricultural and food policy and investment in low and middle income countries'.[171] Earlier, in 2010, the High Level Panel of Experts on Nutrition and Food Security had been created by the FAO itself to be the science–policy interface for the reformed Committee on World Food Security.[172, 173]

The EAT Forum takes a different tack again. This is an annual global conference on food and sustainability based in Stockholm and is a partnership between and co-chaired by a Norwegian Foundation and the Stockholm Resilience Institute at the University of Stockholm. The EAT Forum aims to foster collaboration between science, progressive business and public interest organisations. It encourages brainstorms and ideas exchange on sustainable transition in the food system. It partly focuses on the high-level (prime ministers and CEOs) but also on encouraging and representing social movements. In 2016, with The Lancet, it co-created the EAT-Lancet Commission to propose new advice on how healthy diets could be generated by sustainable food systems.[174] This was pitched at collating best evidence on sustainability and healthy diets to garner support within the public health world. IPES-Food, by contrast, was more interested in civil society, and an early paper argued they are key to paradigmatic change.[84]

This mushrooming of initiatives can be seen both as a sign of interest and as non-governmental actors filling policy space not being filled by governments internationally. Governments sometimes actually encourage such arms-length processes as they can be ignored if the messages are unacceptable and claimed if approved. Their ideas and analyses can be cherry-picked and incorporated in part if not as a whole. Much depends on how and where such panels or commissions are positioned. Are they 'inside track' close to the power brokers? Or are they focused on a different policy community? Whom do they want to influence and how? Wherever they are located, these short-term rather than standing commissions are interesting actors in the modern complex governance terrain.

Within formal state governance, the 'highest'-level actors are at the WTO level. Here headline agreements frame issues such as finance and trade. The incorporation of food and agriculture under the GATT/WTO in 1994 was intended to create a new level playing field for food trade. But in the decades since, the complexity of sustainability has intervened and the realities of globalisation have been less rosy than proponents promised. World Trade Organization processes became ground down in global politics, and a new wave of regional agreements ensued, such as the North American Free Trade Agreement (NAFTA) and the extension of the EU, and a new focus was given to existing international forums such as ASEAN and APEC. In the 2010s the USA undertook particularly expansionist regional agreements such as the Trans Pacific Pact (TPP)[175] and a Transatlantic Trade and Investment Partnership (TTIP) with the EU.[176] These were to be a new phase in globalisation – rejected by President Trump anyway – in which sustainability was side-lined, generating considerable opposition as a result.[177, 178, 179]

## National government

For historical reasons dietary guidelines have tended to be the preserve of governments. Most set these as nutrition guidelines. From the 2000s there has been a useful if limited experience of some governments trying to add an environmental and/or cultural dimension into their formal nutritional advice. The approaches vary. Some are in the form of general advice. For example, Germany's Council for Sustainable Development began giving advice very simply, but has expanded that advice over time.[108–110] It requests German consumers to do the right thing by eating well for the environment. Sweden, however, raised the bar with its 2008 science-based formal guidelines.[180] This was the result of years of working through the data by its National Food Administration and Environmental Protection Agency. It was diplomatically made to withdraw them at EFSA, with the argument that the advice to eat locally and seasonally infringed EU non-discrimination rules within the market. In Australia, the committee of experts charged to update Australia's dietary guidelines set out to inject environmental considerations and began that process, but was reined back by the powerful meat industry and farm interests who involved their political contacts to put a halt to the process. The dietary advice report that was eventually published put environmental considerations into an appendix rather than at the core of public advice.

A not dissimilar fate was inflicted on the committee producing the US 2015 Dietary Guidelines for Americans. The Scientific Advisory Committee for the revisions produced a comprehensive overview of (some but not all) environmental factors in diet and proposed that US DGAs should now be environment-proofed.[181] Its advice was rejected by the US Secretary of State for Agriculture. The powerful US meat lobby used its influence effectively.

The tiny oil kingdom of Qatar surprised many when, in 2014, it produced one of the first national dietary guidelines to integrate principles of food sustainability.[182, 183] What lay behind this statement was an interesting policy mix of motives: national interest in environmental sustainability and food security, population concern over food waste (reinforced by Islamic religious law), the strong authority of the Supreme Council of Health (supported by an Emirate government), a small domestic food industry and therefore a lack of any countervailing food industry influence on the guidelines. These all contributed to the inclusion of sustainability principles within the document.* It set out some principles that echoed the Swedish advice (bar the last one):[184]

- emphasise a plant-based diet, including vegetables, fruit, whole-grain cereal, legumes, nuts and seeds;
- reduce leftovers and waste;
- when available, consume locally and regionally produced foods;
- choose fresh, home-made foods over highly processed foods and fast foods;
- conserve water in food preparation;
- follow the recommendations of the Qatar Dietary Guidelines.

Table 8.2 provides an overview of some government-level initiatives: Germany's Council for Sustainable Development in 2014, Sweden's National Food Administration and Environmental Protection Agency in 2008 (withdrawn), the Netherlands Health Council in 2011, the UK's Defra Green Food Project in 2014, the Brazilian Ministry of Health in 2014 and Qatar's Supreme Council of Health in 2014. These vary but all combined either nutrition and environment or cultural reasons. We see important differences between how governments engage with environmental and cultural aspects of sustainable diets. Some are fully engaged, while others keep these issues low key, and others (the majority)

---

* Our thanks to Dr Barb Seed who advised the Qatari Government.

Table 8.2 Six examples of government sustainable dietary advice

| Source/ country | Environmentally effective food choices (Sweden)[180] | Sustainable Shopping Basket (Germany)[110] | Guidelines for a healthy diet: the ecological perspective (Netherlands)[185] | UK Green Food Project, 8 principles[34] | Brazilian Food-Based Dietary Guidelines[77, 186] | Qatar National Dietary Guidelines[182, 183] |
|---|---|---|---|---|---|---|
| Date | 2009 | 1990s→2013 (4th Ed.) | 2011 | 2013 | 2014 | 2014 |
| Lead body | National Food Administration & Environmental Protection Agency. | German Council for Sustainable Development. | Health Council of the Netherlands. | UK Government working party. | Ministry of Health, Brazil. | Supreme Council of Health, Health Promotion and Non-communicable Diseases. |
| Prime concerns | Pro health and environment to reduce climate change and promote non-toxic environment. | To integrate advice from many sources for daily food shopping. | Linking gains in public health nutrition to lower ecological impact. | To combine health and environmental advice. | To promote public health and to realign health and food culture. | To integrate principles of sustainability into the Qatar Dietary Guidelines. |
| Actual advice | Eat less meat. Replace it with vegetarian meals; choose local meats or organic if available. Eat fish 2–3 times a week from sustainable sources. | Follow the food pyramid. Eat less meat and fish but savour them. | Move to a less animal-based, more plant-based diet – this is the key advice. Lower energy intake and eat fewer snacks. | Eat a varied balanced diet to maintain a healthy body weight. Eat more plant-based foods, including at least five portions of fruit and vegetables per day. | 1 Prepare meals from staple and fresh foods. 2 Use oils, fats, sugar and salt in moderation. | 1 Emphasise a plant-based diet, including vegetables, fruit, whole-grain cereal, legumes. 2 Reduce leftovers and waste. |

| | | | | | |
|---|---|---|---|---|---|
| Eat fruit, vegetables, berries: a good rule of thumb is to choose seasonal, local and preferably organic products. | Follow 5-a-day on fruit and vegetables. | Eat two portions of fish a week but from sustainable sources. | Value your food. Ask about where it comes from and how it is produced. Don't waste it. | 3 Limit consumption of ready-to-consume food and drink products. | 3 When available, consume locally and regionally produced foods. |
| Choose locally grown potatoes and cereals rather than rice. | Eat seasonally and regionally as your first choice. | Reduce food waste. | Moderate your meat consumption, and enjoy more peas, beans, nuts and other sources of protein. | 4 Eat regular meals, paying attention, and in appropriate environments. | 4 Choose fresh, home-made foods over highly processed foods and fast foods. |
| Choose pesticide-free or organic when possible. | Eat organic products. | | Choose fish sourced from sustainable stocks. Seasonality and capture methods are important here too. | 5 Eat in company whenever possible. | 5 Conserve water in food preparation. |
| Choose rapeseed oil rather than palm oil fats. | Choose fair trade products. | | Include milk and dairy products in your diet or seek out plant-based alternatives, including those that are fortified with additional vitamins and minerals. | 6 Buy food at places that offer varieties of fresh foods. Avoid those that mainly sell products ready for consumption. | 6 Follow the recommendations of the Qatar Dietary Guidelines. |

(continued)

Table 8.2 (continued)

| Source/country | Environmentally effective food choices (Sweden)[180] | Sustainable Shopping Basket (Germany)[110] | Guidelines for a healthy diet: the ecological perspective (Netherlands)[185] | UK Green Food Project, 8 principles[34] | Brazilian Food-Based Dietary Guidelines[77, 186] | Qatar National Dietary Guidelines[182, 183] |
|---|---|---|---|---|---|---|
| | Eat fish 2–3 times a week from sustainable sources. | Choose drinks in recyclable packaging. | | Drink tap water. | 7 Develop, practise, share and enjoy your skills in food preparation and cooking. | |
| | | Use designated certification schemes (many are cited in the document). | | Eat fewer foods high in fat, sugar and salt. | 8 Plan your time to give meals and eating proper time and space. | |
| | | | | | 9 When you eat out, choose restaurants that serve freshly made dishes and meals. Avoid fast-food chains. | |
| | | | | | 10 Be critical of the commercial advertisement of food products. | |

Source: the authors.

are not engaged at all. We note, too, a difference in how formal or informal the embryonic guidelines are. There are considerable political sensitivities to this. The Nordic countries are currently taking a lead on progressive engagement, with the Nordic Council playing an interesting international role with its 2012 guidelines, after which Finland's 2014 'Eat Good' guidelines, for example, took steps in this direction.

## City regions

The role of cities as champions of health has long been established. They either sought or were given public health powers from the nineteenth century to address the ill health and environmental impacts of rampant industrialisation. There is a Healthy Cities network, approved by the WHO since the 1990s. While so far, as we have shown above, few governments have taken a lead on sustainable diet advice, there has been a recent rise of interest at the city region level. Milan City Council, led by Mayor Giuliano Pisapia, over the two years leading up to the World Expo 2015 in Milan, brought together what became 100 world cities to sign a Milan Urban Food Policy Pact on October 15, 2015.[187] By 2016 120 cities had signed. Signatory cities made a commitment to sustainable diets. Subsequently, for administrative reasons, this pact was subsumed into the C40 network of world cities concerned about climate change, numbering 80 city members. The C40 had an existing secretariat and, in 2016, it set up a subsidiary C40 Food Systems Network to champion this and other food sustainability commitments in the pact.

Table 8.3 gives more detailed examples of different city- or city-regional initiatives that consider food within their remit. For some, food is more central than for others. A declaration was signed at the 2015 ICLEI Local Government network conference in Seoul, Korea, with the aim for their cities to be '[. . .] low-carbon, resilient, productive and resource-efficient, biodiverse, ecomobile, economically sustainable, smart, happy, healthy, and inclusive'.[188] These are grand-scale aspirations. More specific case studies of cities of some developed countries such as Bristol, Ghent, London, Melbourne, Milan, New York, San Francisco, Toronto and Vancouver have been produced.[189] These tend to set up food policy councils (or something equivalent) to champion changes in supply and consumption. They champion food as an opportunity to deliver something practical for sustainability. In the UK, a network of 50 Sustainable Food Cities shares experience of structures, projects and reach.[190] An international study of three affluent cities showed that there can be considerable variation between cities of comparable wealth in how sustainable their food supplies are. Comparing Canberra, Copenhagen and Tokyo, researchers found that, while Canberra produces the majority of its most common foods in its regional hinterland, Tokyo primarily ensures its food security through import and Copenhagen's hinterland produces less than half of the consumption of its most common foods. The study also found that self-provision had declined in Canberra and Tokyo over the last 40 years as their populations expanded, while Copenhagen's self-sufficiency had risen with its population staying more constant.[191]

In the 2000s, the City of Surakarta in Indonesia used food for urban revitalisation and development. Following his election in 2005, Mayor Joko Widodo decided to support street vendors and the informal food economy – previously seen as troublesome actors and blocks on 'progress'. He said that they needed investment and infrastructural support to achieve higher standards, and for their food to be a centrepiece in the city's cultural liberalisation. [192, 96] He was elected President of Indonesia in 2014.

Table 8.3 also provides an overview of both specific new commitments to sustainable diets or food, and where existing governance systems are engaging with food as an opportunity to deliver more sustainable urban performance. International and historical lessons are already being learned from this unfolding collective experience. One lesson is that interest needs to be woven into the formal municipal structures if there is to be lasting effect. Unless there is funding and accountability, food easily suffers from 'projectitis' – short-term funded projects that may be imaginative and gain grassroots interest but have little lasting effect. Having leverage inside municipal structures is essential. It also means that food sustainability and performance are subject to political review and accountability.

We should not be surprised by the growth of activity at this city and urban level of governance. Big problems are always manifest at the local level. Demands to tackle poor public health, environmental degradation and social problems are hard to contain. History suggests that the value of investing in prevention ultimately wins, but only if there is pressure. Better transport infrastructure, housing and food all make sense. They make localities better. That is how and why the big municipal investments were made in the nineteenth century. They were reactions to the degradation, squalor and pollution of unfettered industrialisation. Berlin, London and Paris learned from each other. Amsterdam shared with New York. Boston pioneered public health intervention. Today, a not dissimilar exchange is developing about cities' modern food role. It can also happen out of the limelight, for instance in what one researcher has called a 'quiet food sustainability' being delivered by city-approved schemes such as the food self-provisioning in Hungary.[193] The case for more sustainable food systems and sustainable diets brings together good people in the name of the locality.

## NGOs

Malthus first outlined the population case for sustainable eating and food production in 1798. Of course, his case was based on a fixed view of social structures and ecological capacity. There have also been many periods of major dietary change in times of war and rationing.[194–197] In the modern food discourse, however, it was a small and then fledgling US NGO, now known as Food First, that captured the consumer-facing agenda in 1971. *Diet for a Small Planet* sold three million copies. It was written by Frances Moore Lappé and Joe Collins for the small but still active Californian NGO/think-tank they founded, and it set the tone for

Table 8.3 Multi-level institutional engagement with sustainable food: some examples

| Level | Name | Policy actor | Year started | Focus/function/comment | Weblink |
|---|---|---|---|---|---|
| Global | ICLEI | Cities | 1990 | Founded by 43 local governments, this became 1,500 by 2016. These are local governments for sustainability. | www.iclei.org/ |
| | RUAF | NGO | 1999 | Global partnership for urban agriculture and food systems as key to urban sustainability. | www.ruaf.org/ |
| | FAO Food for the Cities Initiative | UN FAO | 2001 | City-region as focus for urban-rural connection. | www.fao.org/fcit/fcit-home/en/ |
| | Food for Cities Dgroup | FAO | 2009 | Online platform set up by FAO. | https://dgroups.org/fao/food-for-cities |
| | International Urban Food Network | Research for local government | 2012 | City regions as drivers of alternative food systems. | www.iufn.org/en/ |
| | Milan Urban Food Policy Pact | Cities | 2015 | Agreement by 120 world cities to act on food. | www.foodpolicymilano.org/en/urban-food-policy-pact-2/ |
| | C40 Food Systems Network | Cities | 2016 | New 'channel' within C40 Network founded 2005 to address climate change. Food agreed to be key within that following Milan Pact. | www.c40.org/networks/food_systems |
| | United Cities and Local Governments | Urban | 2004 | Global network of cities and towns (re)created from nineteenth-century International Municipal Movement. | www.uclg.org/ or https://issuu.com/uclgcglu/docs/uclg_who_we_are |

(continued)

Table 8.3 (continued)

| Level | Name | Policy actor | Year started | Focus/function/comment | Weblink |
|---|---|---|---|---|---|
| Regional | EUROCITIES | EU cities | 1986 | Founded by six cities (130 in 2016) to focus on common issues in six themes (food as cross-cutting). In May 2016 a new EUROCITIES working group, FOOD, was formed, bringing together the 41 Euro cities members that signed the Milan Pact, and committed to follow up on European commitments and cross-collaboration. | www.eurocities.eu/ |
| | Nordic Cities EAT Initiative | Nordic | 2015 | Food as key action point for Nordic cities to build health and happiness. | http://eatforum.org/article/cities-are-where-the-future-happens-first/ |
| | African Centre for Cities | Mainly African cities, also Global South | 2007 | Interdisciplinary research and training programme. Home of the Hungry Cities programme, which looks at urban food security in cities across the Global South, including Mexico City and Bangalore. | www.africancentreforcities.net/ |
| | URBACT | EU | | Aims to foster sustainable and integrated urban development. One theme is on urban–rural connections. | http://urbact.eu/ |
| National | Michigan Center for Regional Food Systems | University academic support | n/a | Michigan and US research and advice. | http://foodsystems.msu.edu/ |

| Name | Country | Year | Description | URL |
| --- | --- | --- | --- | --- |
| UK Sustainable Food Cities Network | UK | 2013 | Fifty UK towns and cities working on six themes: health, poverty, waste, skills, procurement/catering, economy. | http://sustainablefoodcities.org/ |
| Windhoek Declaration on Food and Nutrition Security | Namibia | 2014 | Signed by 51 local authority representatives. It recommends the establishment of food banks, the promotion of urban and peri-urban agriculture and the reduction of food loss and food waste. | www.worldfuturecouncil.org/windhoek-declaration/ |
| Citydeal | The Netherlands | 2016 | Currently (June 2016) 12 Dutch cities having joined forces to further develop and exchange on urban/city regional food agendas. | |
| Network for sustainable cities | Argentina | 2015 | A network of Argentinian cities working on sustainability issues. Food has been integrated as one of the working topics. | |

Source: authors, with thanks to Florence Egal, Kazie Flanagan and Marielle Dubbeling.

sustainable diet thinking. That book with multi-million sales proposed a simple policy recipe: a good society is one whose food system grows and supports plant-based diets, with low/no meat, and combining health, environment and social values.[198] It cut across the American mythologies of cattle-ranging cowboys and urban burgers, and argued that there was no shortage of food or Malthusian threat if people ate plant-based foods. It articulated a policy position that bridged hippie-dom and 'back to the land' and new urban lifestyles.

Other NGOs have followed in the same vein more recently, offering specific culinary 'rules' or guidance. The Vancouver 100 Mile Diet from British Columbia in 2005 recommended eating food from within a geographically bounded food-shed.[199] The Fife Diet was developed by a group of households in Scotland who, from 2007, committed to eat 80% of their diet from food grown within their county of Fife, not known for its benign climate or 'Mediterranean' growing condi-tions.[200, 201] These exemplify the localist or bio-regional perspective on sustainable diets. They are locavores who put a premium on locally sourced food. This has been a particularly rich source of engagement, often favouring the small-scale and direct link of grower to consumer. In London, a group of consumers placed their own contracts with growers and became Hackney Growing Communities, now an established food delivery scheme. France was the inspiration for the Food Assembly, a cross between farmers' markets and buying groups.[202, 203] These NGOs are democratic experimentation.

The NGOs within conventional or mainstream governance tend to be already well-established such as Greenpeace[204] or Friends of the Earth,[205, 206] and con-servation organisations such as the US Sierra Club or UK's National Trust, or ornithological organisations such as Birdlife International.[207, 208] These have engaged with food as a vector for sustainability by using food within their exist-ing lobbying or ownership to redefine policy and direction. The UK's National Trust, for example, is a huge landowner with 4.5 million members. In the 2000s it reviewed its food provision and took a stronger line in its own purchasing to support local food systems. This informed its lobbying, both for lowering its own farm-ing's environmental impact and for reform of fisheries policy (it owns vast tracts of coastline).[209–211] The Center for Science in the Public Interest in Washington, DC, which already focused on food and health, engaged with sustainability issues through the lens of food, urging its one million-plus supporters to eat well for health and environment.[212] Others have been created solely to focus on food and sustainability or food and health. Meatless Mondays, founded in 2003, spawned Meat-Free Mondays in 2009, funded by former Beatle Paul McCartney and family. They aim for meat reduction, particularly in public meals.[213] Eating Better, a coali-tion of 38 food-related UK NGOs, was created in 2013 to promote a reduction of meat and focuses on policy change.[214] In Boston, USA, City Growers and City Fresh Foods of Boston produces and delivers fresh, locally sourced, nutritious and culturally appropriate food for a range of community institutions, while demon-strating the possibilities for inter-cultural approaches.[215, 216] In Wales, the Centre for Alternative Technology, a medium-sized NGO set up in the 1970s to focus on low-tech technology, developed the pioneering Zero Carbon Britain project in the 2000s, a modelling exercise to see how diets could be zero carbon.[70] It concluded that the UK could eat at zero carbon, but only with a radically different diet.

The World Wide Fund for Nature (WWF), the world's largest conservation NGO, has championed sustainable diets consistently since the 2000s. Its motive for this work is and was that agriculture and food pressures are major threats to biodiversity.[217–220] The WWF has worked with academics to model 'realistic' sustainable diets and trialled them in different national contexts. Based upon work in four EU countries, WWF produced a set of six Livewell Principles for consumers:

1   Eat more plants – enjoy vegetables and whole grains!
2   Eat a variety of foods – have a colourful plate!
3   Waste less food – a third of food produced for human consumption is lost or wasted.
4   Moderate your meat consumption, both red and white – enjoy other sources of proteins such as peas, beans and nuts.
5   Buy food that meets a credible certified standard – consider Marine Stewardship Council (MSC labelled), free-range and fair trade.
6   Eat fewer foods high in fat, salt and sugar – keep foods such as cakes, sweets and chocolate as well as cured meat, fries and crisps to an occasional treat. Choose water, avoid sugary drinks and remember that juices only count as one of your 5-a-day however much you drink.

## Companies

The corporate and commercial food sectors have responded to and contributed to the governance map of sustainable food and diets. Their think-tanks, PR companies and lobbies have had to engage, partly defensively (for example, resisting labelling or regulations) but often now pro-actively. There is no one corporate view; they vary widely. Business has created alliances. The B20, for example, is a grouping of giant companies (not all food) that shadows the intergovernmental G20 meetings and sets out to ensure a business input to such talks, working with others such as the International Business Leaders Forum, whose interests lie in corporate ethics, preventing corruption and good governance.[221] Such groupings are flexible.[222] Some, like the Business and Industry Advisory Committee (BIAC), affiliated to the OECD, have been 'the officially recognized representative of the OECD business community' since 1962.[223] Such influence can be considerable and these formations have taken a close interest in the development of evidence on food and sustainability – particularly resource-reliance and climate change – for decades.

Perhaps the oldest corporate position on food sustainability is that on oil-dependency. The 1972 *Limits to Growth* report coincided with the Middle East oil crisis.[152, 156] It highlighted the dependence of modern agriculture and transportation on oil. This productionist focus has continued within business generally and particularly within the food sector. In 2002, Unilever, Nestlé and Danone, in the top ten largest global food companies, frustrated at inaction and lack of coherent leadership from governments and international bodies, set up their own Sustainable Agriculture Initiative.[224] By 2016 it had 80 members, all big food and drink corporations across the world. Investors have encouraged such initiatives and investment houses have created measures such as the Dow Jones Sustainability Indices.[225]

The World Business Council for Sustainable Development (WBCSD), which first became an active player on food and sustainability in the 1987–94 GATT talks, which brought food into the World Trade Organization remit, and at the Rio UNCED talks in 1992, has brokered long-term commitments from its 200 global members for lower carbon and product reformulation.[226, 227] It played a 'crack the whip' function at the 2015 Paris Climate Change talks, frustrated at the prospect of inaction on the scale of what happened in Copenhagen when the 2009 talks achieved little but frustration.[228] The WBCSD promised stronger ·actions for the food sector ahead and stated a goal 'to build a future in which 9 billion people can live well within the planetary boundaries by 2050'. This requires food and dietary change.

The role of corporate think-tanks cannot be underestimated. They attract high quality staff and are almost always well-funded. They have 'hot lines' into corporate decision-making, often helped by inside-track consultants. For instance, one of the most influential, McKinsey, charted a direction for sustainable agriculture in 2010 for the World Economic Forum.[229] There is also a vast web of less high-profile work conducted for individual firms, advising firms on corporate strategy. From seeing sustainable diets as threats in the 1970s, they now also see market opportunities. One such is in meat-free products. A study by UK market researchers explored which kind of consumer is most amenable to cutting back meat and concluded that 'stridently lecturing the consumer citizen is not effective; only soft and targeted encouragement is likely to work'.[230] The transition to sustainable diets presages new routes to profitability.

In the 2000s, the 1992 UNCED legacy began to flower, not least in the EU which championed sustainable consumption and production. The initial corporate focus on agriculture and production began to move downstream to address consumption. Unilever, for example, launched its Sustainable Living Plan in 2010, committing to support its small business suppliers and to reduce its footprint.[231] PepsiCo set up 50-in-5, a plan to use the UK sales to reduce its carbon footprint by 50% in five years. Nestlé (a founder of SAI) reviewed risks from water to its operations worldwide and found threats in 100 countries.

Strategies on food and sustainability proliferated, to the approval of mainstream thinking and ethical investors but to some scepticism from those wary of 'green-wash' or 'health-wash'. Questions arose: how is corporate progress on sustainability measured and is it monitored independently? Are these actions mainly driven by self-protection (and does that matter)? Is this really to reduce liability, and what does it mean in practice? What are the companies actually doing? Is the promise to reformulate products no more than an opportunity to reduce size, maintain prices and rationalise ingredients, or even to increase sales? Internal company dynamics shape the answers to these questions. If the company board 'gets it', the performance is likely to be tougher and less cosmetic.

A company that made a clear commitment was Marks & Spencer, the iconic UK retailer. In 2007 it launched Plan A – 100 commitments to lower its environmental footprint.[232] By the mid-2000s it had met most of those and was on to a third phase, now convinced that sustainability made financial savings as well as good corporate citizenship.[233] Barilla, the large Italian pasta company, has a smaller product range. It funded academics at Bocconi University, Milan, to produce the much-cited Barilla Double Pyramid, which suggests nutrition and environmental impacts can be inverted (see Figure 8.1). Although pasta is relatively low carbon, the company does make biscuits and other higher carbon goods. Despite that, it has taken a lead within business in pushing a broader approach to sustainability than simply decarbonisation, by stressing the cultural and biodiversity elements of sustainable diets.[234] It has also taken a strong public lead, providing books and also a yearly forum on food and sustainability at Bocconi, helping to push for the Milan Urban Food Policy Pact signed by 100 Mayors in October 2015 (see above) by launching a Milan Protocol with support of Milan's Mayor and the Italian Prime Minister in 2014.[235]

The catering industry was perhaps slower to wake up to the sustainability challenge than either food manufacturers or retailers. But it is a huge employer and has a growing share of consumer spending worldwide. In the USA, the Culinary Institute of America (the other CIA) worked with Harvard University's School of Public Health to create the innovative Menus for Change programme.[237, 238] This focuses on improving the taste appeal of food while both improving its nutrition and environmental profiles. This is choice-editing, and its attraction to caterers is that academics help them deliver evidence-based change.[237]

Like all sectors, catering is fragmented. Street food alongside *haute cuisine*. *Relais et Chateau*, the alliance of 540 top culinary establishments, restaurants and hotels, worked with UNESCO and in 2014 published a set of cultural commitments to commit members' food 'offer' to environmental protection.[239] Originating in France but now global and, given its market and clientele, targeting the high-quality end of food provision, it recognised that issues such as cultural diversity and waste reduction could be tackled by chef leadership as 'practice leaders'. The manifesto urged chefs to protect and enhance environmentally and territory-appropriate cuisines.

An interesting cross-sector alliance on sustainable diets emerged when Sodexho, one of the two global giant foodservice companies, worked with WWF and the UK's Food Ethics Council to review what catering could do to engender sustainable diets. They saw three business arguments.[240] Sustainable diets are a channel for: (a) delivering turnover growth by differentiating the product offer, enhancing brand reputation and building customer loyalty, stimulating customer

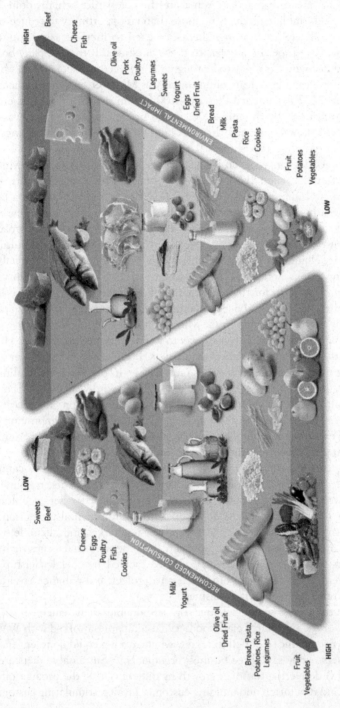

## ENVIRONMENTAL PYRAMID

HIGH

Beef

Cheese
Fish

Olive oil
Pork
Poultry
Legumes
Sweets
Yogurt
Eggs
Dried Fruit
Bread
Milk
Pasta
Rice
Cookies

Fruit
Potatoes
Vegetables

ENVIRONMENTAL IMPACT

LOW

## FOOD PYRAMID

LOW

Sweets
Beef

Cheese
Eggs
Poultry
Fish
Cookies

Milk
Yogurt

Olive oil
Dried Fruit

Bread, Pasta,
Potatoes, Rice
Legumes

Fruit
Vegetables

RECOMMENDED CONSUMPTION

HIGH

*Figure 8.1* The Barilla Double Pyramid

Source: Barilla Center for Food & Nutrition Foundation, 2014.[236]

demand and securing investment; (b) mitigating risks and increasing resilience by ensuring quality and security of supply, increasing the integrity of supply chains, reducing regulatory risks, reducing the risks to reputation and maintaining the licence to operate; and (c) maintaining and improving profit margins by improving staff motivation and retention, making efficiency savings, using lower- or same-cost ingredients and reframing costs. The alliance was concerned, however, about poor understanding within the industry and staff, and a perception that sustainable diets cost more.

Horticulture is probably the commercial sector with most to gain from more sustainable diets. This has not been lost on champions of sustainable diets. Older horticulturalists were slow to see this, but newer enterprises were not. One is Riverford, a £50 m turnover (in 2015–16) UK farm-to-consumer business, which sells vegetable and fruit boxes in its weekly deliveries to 55,000 UK consumers. It began to offer meat too. In a consultation with its consumers it mooted selling only grass-fed meat, to raise prices while reducing land use (on the argument that nearly half of grain grown is fed to animals). Riverford's founder, farmer Guy Watson, twice winner of the BBC's Farmer of the Year award, favours a multi-criteria approach to sustainable diets. Greenhouse gas emissions are not the sole indicator of sustainability, he has argued. Citing a talk by one of the present authors, he thinks the goal might be 'to return animals to their ecological niche',[241] and '[. . .] feeding grain and soya to ruminants, like beef and dairy cows, is insane'.[242] Businesses like his are not just thought-leaders but practice-leaders. Aarstiderne is a larger and similar operation in Denmark. This is a network of local organic supply delivering to 65,000 households weekly.[243] It provides 160 recipes a week to accompany its deliveries and makes videos to illustrate the recipes, all based on different preferences. These range from vegan or vegetarian to people wanting 'fast food' or even 'super-fast food'. It hosts an open weekend annually to engage its consumers with primary producers and to educate them, for example, on the case for eating less meat. It has helped 15,000 school children have gardens in 20 Danish cities, encouraging them to learn the new skills for a more sustainable eating culture. Enterprises like Aarstiderne and Riverford offer different links of consumption to production, and alternatives to mainstream food system messages. They are engaged in governance, providing not just food but messages (books, recipes, videos), and opportunities for debate and education.

### Science, technology and academia

Evidence-based policy is a mantra in policy circles – who wants to deny basing their actions on evidence? Yet experience suggests the link of evidence to policy is messier than the theory implies.[18] Evidence can be ignored, distorted, taken only in bits, and more. Sadly, wars and military conditions can offer bizarre opportunities to narrow the evidence–policy gap. In the Second World War, rationing in the UK actually narrowed inequalities in health and was a time when nutrition had enormous influence over food supply.[244] Also, in the early twentieth century, the British state was so shaken by defeats by healthy South African Boers that it was forced to recognise the need to improve the nutrition of its population if it wanted good healthy recruits for the armed forces.[245] In such historic moments the impact of scientific and expert advice can be considerable.[195]

But is the evidence on unsustainability of diets at such a juncture? Perhaps not yet, although strong pressure across the sciences on sustainable diets has been building up for 30 years. There are surprisingly few statements from academics, however, as to what sustainable diet advice ought to be. Mostly, the role of academics has been either to produce discipline-based analyses (to contribute to the collective 'body of knowledge'), or to contribute evidence for government and other official advisory functions. These may or may not be listened to. This has been the fate of attempting to 'green' national dietary guidelines, if we note the experience of scientific committees advising Sweden (2008–9), the UK (2008–10), Australia (2011–13) and the USA (2013–15). These met either fierce sectoral lobbying opposition or ultimate government refusal, or both.

Standing back, over the last half century, there have been distinct phases of scientific involvement in the emerging discourse on sustainable diets:

- Phase 1 in the 1970s saw the rebirth of interest in food's impact on the environment and health. The environment was the noisiest, shaped by the world oil/energy crisis and scientific environmentalism.[152] Neo-Malthusian demographic questions about population excess re-emerged.[246, 247] The first modern formulations of sustainable diets appeared in the West at this time from civil society rather than science, although influenced by the data. These broadly favoured vegetarianism, simplicity and wholefoods.[198]

- Phase 2 in the 1980s saw the emergence of fully fledged scientific public health nutrition interest, articulated by pioneering academics Joan Gussow and Kate Clancy. This was framed by the notion of responsible science, citizenship and food rights.[248–250] It built on emerging public health data about diet's effect on non-communicable diseases in the West and the need to tackle the food system in developing countries.[251–253]

- Phase 3 was in the 1990s when the discourse was dominated by regionalism and whether the Mediterranean Diet in particular was the diet to which to aspire.[254] Meanwhile a global nutrition transition was underway, hitting developing countries, itself a manifestation of globalisation.[255, 256]

- Phase 4 was in the 2000–10s and was initially dominated by data on food and farming's role in climate change.[85, 257] But data on the growth of mass obesity and overweight, not just in developed high-income countries, pushed public health concerns into the policy frame,[258] and generated serious institutional engagement. Could even rich societies afford to continue eating in excess? This was the moment when health, environmental, economic and international concerns began to come together. In the SDGs, for instance, the UN recognised food systems had to change. Tentatively, the first sustainable dietary guidelines emerged (see Table 8.2). As this official kind of engagement grew, a counter narrative also emerged, focusing more on individual behaviour change.

Academics have played a role in this policy evolution. Over time, they have demonstrated to policy makers the complexity of the sustainable diet challenge and collectively pushed policy makers towards multi-criteria thinking. Climatologists wanted action on greenhouse gas emissions. Health specialists wanted dietary transformation.[259] Biodiversity specialists pointed to the fact the planet is now in its sixth phase of mass extinction.[260] Social scientists highlighted the gross inequalities and maldistribution of consumer culture.[120] There might have been tensions between those with a farm or land focus compared to those with a food focus, and between those who look to technical rather than societal solutions. Gradually they realised the common interest expressed as sustainable diets. The reality is that a food system or sustainable diet perspective joins these discrete issues up.

Interdisciplinary rivalries weaken their messages and, in Phase 4, from the 2000s, there was emerging unanimity of diagnosis, if not of solutions. The good news is that some consistent messages have come out. A 2015 literature review by Hallström, Carlsson-Kanyama (a long-term analyst in this field) and Börjesson found that the more meat was consumed in a diet, the higher the $CO_2e$ emissions are; and the closer to a vegan diet it became, the lower they fall.[261] On land use a not dissimilar position emerged: the 'healthier' and/or low meat + high plant-based a diet becomes, the lower that diet's impact on land use. But will these cross-over messages gain policy traction? So far they have not. But some common frameworks are now in the scientific literature such as, for example, One Health,[262-264] which integrates human and animal health,[265] and Ecological Public Health,[266, 267] a social science perspective linking the material, cultural and bio-physiological levels of existence. These provide theoretical integration.

Technical and engineering approaches have developed a strong presence in the discourse, particularly over food waste.[61] Engineers sense the need for technical solutions and have promoted small-scale and large-scale solutions to recycling and GHG emissions: bio-gas plants, recycling, product reformulation in the factory and zero-carbon closed-engineering hydroponic systems. They have been particularly active in supporting the notion of the circular economy. One interesting focus has been on phone 'apps'. Might these help consumers change? They take different forms. Some assume the consumer is already interested and help them gain access to the foods and diets they want. Thus there are vegan or vegetarian food apps. The Guardian published a list of top 10 sustainable food apps which varied from calorie counters to the location of sustainable restaurants.[268] The Centre for Alternative Technology (CAT) in Wales has developed an app, Laura's Larder, to help people find out how good their diets are for their health and the planet.[269] Researchers, however, are more interested in the potential of Big Data to analyse and promote behaviour change at the population level.[7, 270, 271]

Table 8.4 Some cultural 'principles'/'rules'/guidance from academics on sustainable eating compared

| Source/ country | New Nordic Diet's 10 principles[284] | Barsac Declaration: Principles[285, 286] | Harvard T.H. Chan School of Public Health[287, 288] | Centre for Food Policy Tips for Eco-Nutrition[289] | Food Climate Research Network[133, 290] |
|---|---|---|---|---|---|
| Date | 2010 | 2009 | 2016 | 2007 | 2014 |
| Lead body | University of Copenhagen project | Nine international research groups of scientists | Harvard nutrition and other scientists | Centre for Food Policy, City University, London | Food Climate Research Network, University of Oxford |
| Prime concerns | To combine health and environmental advice. | To reduce nitrogen emissions and to encourage better food provision. | To (1) provide tips (T) for sustainable eating, and (2) promote sustainable consumption (PSC). | To formulate new twenty-first century cultural 'rules' (norms). | To identify the characteristics of diets that are both healthier and have lower GHG and land-use impacts. |
| Actual advice | More fruit and vegetables every day (berries, cabbages, root veg, legumes, potatoes and herbs). | Encourage the availability of reduced portion sizes of meat and animal products, compared to local norms. | Tip 1. Prioritise plants: fill half your plate with vegetables and fruit. | Eat a plant-based diet, eat flesh sparingly, if at all. | Diversity – a wide variety of foods eaten. |
| | More whole grain, especially oats, rye and barley. | Eat 'demitarian' meals containing half the amount of meat or fish compared with the normal local amount. | Tip 2. Minimise meat. This is good for health. Treat it more as a condiment than a main dish. | Eat simply as a norm and eat feasts as celebrations, i.e., exceptionally. | Balance achieved between energy intake and energy needs. |

| | | | | |
|---|---|---|---|---|
| More food from the seas and lakes. | Tip 3. Select new seafood. Avoid endangered fish. | Eat a correspondingly larger amount of other food products. | Drink water not soft drinks; if you drink alcohol, use it moderately. | Diet based around: minimally processed tubers and whole grains; legumes; fruits and vegetables – particularly those that are field-grown, 'robust' (less prone to spoilage) and less requiring of rapid and more energy-intensive transport modes. |
| Higher-quality meat, but less of it. | Tip 4. Think local. Eating from local farmers is an opportunity to meet and learn from and about them. | In social situations (for example, public eating or conferences) always offer 'demitarian', vegetarian and vegan alternatives. | Celebrate and eat biodiversity (from inside the field to your plate). | Meat eaten sparingly if at all – and all animal parts consumed. |
| More food from wild landscapes. | Tip 5. Eat mindfully: savour your food. | Ensure clear labelling of menu options, especially in buffet meals. | Eat locally where possible to support local suppliers and resilience. | Dairy products or alternatives eaten in moderation, for example, fortified milk substitutes and other foods rich in calcium and micronutrients. |
| Organic produce whenever possible. | PSC 1: Examine your personal food choices. | | Eat seasonally if possible to keep embedded energy in the food low. | Unsalted seeds and nuts. |

(continued)

Table 8.4 (continued)

| Source/country | New Nordic Diet's 10 principles[284] | Barsac Declaration: Principles[285, 286] | Harvard T.H. Chan School of Public Health[287, 288] | Centre for Food Policy Tips for Eco-Nutrition[289] | Food Climate Research Network[133, 290] |
|---|---|---|---|---|---|
| | Avoid food additives. | | PSC 2: Eat less red meat. | Choose your diet carefully and beware of hidden ingredients in food, especially salt and sugars. | Small quantities of fish and aquatic products sourced from certified fisheries and certified aquaculture systems. |
| | More meals based on seasonal produce. | | PSC 3: Practise mindful eating. | Eat equitably: (a) Eat no more than you expend in energy; (b) build exercise into your daily life. | Very limited consumption of processed foods high in fat, sugar or salt and low in micronutrients, for example, crisps, confectionery, sugary drinks. |
| | More home-cooked food. | | PSC 4: Choose a food guide that enhances both personal and planetary health. | Eat less but better: go for quality, not quantity; be prepared to pay the full (sometimes hidden) costs of producing and transporting the food. | |
| | Less waste. | | | Enjoy food in the short-term but think about its impact long-term. | |

To their credit, climate change scientists have been very active dietary change advocates in recent years, as their data showed agriculture and food to be key sources of GHGs. Professor Kevin Anderson of the Tyndall Centre, an authority on climate change, is one. He has put it clearly: '[. . .]even a slim chance of "keeping below" a 2°C rise, now demands a revolution in how we both consume and produce energy. Such a rapid and deep transition will have profound implications for the framing of contemporary society and is far removed from the rhetoric of green growth that increasingly dominates the climate change agenda.'[272] Bajželj and colleagues have also argued that big gains in tackling climate change can be made by improving diets and reducing food waste.[167, 273] The advantage of the West changing its diets from heavy reliance on meat and dairy products is that this would bring a double gain for both health and climate change, and therefore the wider environment. They modelled these gains as following from a pretty reasonable diet of two 85 g portions of red meat and five eggs per week, as well as a portion of poultry per day. They showed that if current food consumption trends continue food production alone would match if not exceed the global targets for total GHGEs by 2050.

Social science presence has been sparser, with notable long-term exceptions such as Annika Carlsson-Kanyama in Sweden[64, 68, 274] and Tara Garnett in the UK.[34, 86, 275–278] Yet the cultural and behavioural aspects of dietary change are without doubt the key to progress. That's why projects like Harvard and the Culinary Institute of America's Menus for Change are so important. They shift behaviour. Policy makers, however, are reluctant to be seen to shift consumers despite adopting the language of behaviour change in the 2010s. They don't mind others being seen to 'nudge' as long as they are not seen to do so.[101, 279] Actually, what the evidence suggests is needed is not 'nudge' but 'shove' – big change, pretty quickly.[280, 281] Reisch and colleagues, for example, have suggested many ideas about what to do on sustainability and food, distinguishing between information-based approaches, market-based approaches, regulatory measures and self-committing measures.[282, 283] Most people favour combinations of all, in which case this is hardly 'lite' policy. It is big change time.

To illustrate how academics can offer public advice on sustainable diet, Table 8.4 gives four sets of academic-derived advice or guidance. These are among the few contributions in cultural and everyday terms offering guidance or 'rules' or 'principles' to the public in the name of the transition to sustainable diets.

## Governance themes have emerged

This overview of governance suggests some growth of policy thinking, if patchily, sometimes crabbily and so far on a limited scale compared with the urgency the evidence suggests is required. We conclude this chapter by summarising some fault lines in the discourse.

### Multi-criteria versus single-issue approach

Some academics have argued that the complexity can be best addressed by focusing on the healthiness of diet: if the public ate healthily, the environmental footprint of diet comes down from the excess exhibited in the West. This is a good, clear message to policy makers but it does not help for developing countries. It also downgrades other factors shaping how consumers eat. It assumes health is the key appeal to consumers; it may be what consumers say they are concerned about but is not what they do. We conclude the case for multi-criteria approaches remains strong.

### Deep versus 'lite' = gradualism versus systems change

A big policy challenge is whether the transition to sustainable diets can be managed quietly and below the radar – if so by whom? – or whether it requires overt systems change. Business-as-usual implies soft change, slowly. Systems change requires preparation and planning for big changes ahead, even if they need to be introduced carefully. Many scientists have concluded that only big changes will go a significant way towards addressing food's environmental crisis.

### Cutting waste is a must

A matter everyone agrees on, whether in developed or developing food economies, is that waste is the enemy of sustainability. Food waste taps into deep moral values. Most religions have warned for centuries against it. The UN encourages young people worldwide to prevent waste through the Think-Eat-Save Campaign.[291] The EU's Food Use for Social Innovation by Optimising Waste Prevention Strategies (FUSIONS) project advises 13 EU member states.[292] Social scientists stress how rich societies waste post-purchase food partly because it is cheap but warn against blaming the consumer for what is structural waste due to overproduction and overselling.[293, 294] Some food waste is inevitable. Even consumers in very poor societies waste some food, that is if bones and peelings are waste. What matters is how this is used: is it recycled, turned into compost and back into the soil or just discarded? Technologists remind us that any waste can always be used beneficially by creating biofuels and/or compost to return to the soil.[61] The income gradient in food waste is a point of both delicacy and importance. Low-income societies waste far less than rich society consumers.

### Power and (im)balance in governance

The meaning of governance and the distribution of power that does or could affect a transition to sustainable diets requires us to consider a number of variables: the different sectional interests across the food system (from farm to consumption), the institutional location of power (from local to global), the role of different sciences and their input to dietary governance (from social to natural science, from public health nutrition to political science) and the different 'channels' through which power is exerted (from financial to information, from regulatory to cultural power).

Food has always been a mechanism for power. It offers opportunities to control people, land, nations and cities. One of the oldest uses of food as a weapon has been deliberate starvation – placing cities under siege. Control food supply and, with time, one can control the people. The same is true of water, the effects of which are felt even faster. Such naked power still happens in modern warfare, as the sieges in the Syrian War (2012ff.) showed,[295] and Collingham documented in her study of the Second World War[195] and Mukerjee for India under the British.[296]

It is not just the actual food that can be the medium of control. Softer and more diffuse forms of control come with the filtering of knowledge flows, marketing, advertising, cultural messaging and public relations. Armies of lobbyists surround power bases such as capital cities and particularly where there are international networks – Washington, DC, Brussels, Beijing, post-USSR Moscow. This soft power can become very important indeed if a company's products are at risk or if there is a regulatory change being mooted to which a sectional interest objects. It was manifest in the USA throughout 2015 when powerful meat lobbies stifled proposals to alter the US government's Dietary Guidelines to include an environmental dimension.

### It all depends on what is meant by sustainability and resilience

The word 'sustainability' and its derivatives have become ubiquitous. Part of its attraction (to some) is its vagueness, but surely governance (like science) needs some precision. Clarity is needed on what it is that we want to 'sustain'. Financiers use the word to mean retaining capital. The Dow Jones Sustainability Index was created in 1999 to begin to audit company impact on the environment. Yet, from Barbara Ward to Gro-Harlan Brundtland, the term 'sustainability' has been used to indicate a challenge to the belief that markets are the answer to everything in governance. Reports from the 1980 Brandt and 1987 Brundtland Commissions both stressed the need for political solutions to unequal use of resources.[297, 298] They were responding to an era of hard liberation struggles in the developing world. In the twenty-first century the pursuit of sustainability became fragmented, with some seeing 'sustainability' as about the environment and others going much broader to include health, equality, employment and food culture, and some seeing it as a radical transformation of the political economy,[299] and others seeing it as a softening, even civilising of capitalism or an appeal to responsible consumerism. We are probably stuck with this fluidity in sustainability. It provides a centre of gravity, a fulcrum, a meeting point for very diverse actions. When policy makers (such as a city food council) are considering sustainability, they will apply a different frame of reference to that taken by a food company perhaps, but also perhaps not.

The word 'resilience' has begun to be used as a substitute in order to provide some desired measurability. Resilience thinking centres on the capacity of a system to bounce back after or from stress, shock and destabilisation. Resilience thinking in the modern sense was first outlined by Holling in 1973,[300] and was taken up by climate change and ecosystems scientists such as Folke.[301] It has been widely used by the military, leading to its take-up by business, which sees itself as responding to risk – not least since risks hit even well-run companies. If resilience is translated as the capacity to respond to and overcome risk, companies will engage more easily. This is also how the notion of tipping points has come into policy discourse.[137] It implies ameliorative action is possible. The data on dietary impacts, however, suggest that they have already transitioned beyond what ought to be tipping points. They have been normalised. The tipping points may have been deferred. If they do occur as the metaphor and modelling imply, will the tipping be too late?[302]

## The importance of systems thinking

A constant theme in sustainable diet governance is how to address complexity. One response from within academia is to engage with systems thinking.[263] This means putting actions and reactions into wider context, to look for interactions, feedback loops and how these operate (if they do) as a system. This is not new and was fashionable in the 1960s, helped by warfare planning work in the USA and also computerisation. But, intellectually, it emerged from earlier thinking, such as by Ludwig von Bertalanffy,[303, 304] also trying to engage with the complexity of interdisciplinary research. More recently, Midgley and others have suggested that systems thinking is essential if humanity is to address twenty-first-century problems because its challenges require thinking that accepts interconnectedness, multiple perspectives, the difficulty of boundaries, the existence of 'wicked' (imponderable) problems and the difficulty of looking to science to resolve value judgements.[305, 306] We noted earlier the importance of the notion of boundaries in the work by Steffen, Rockström and colleagues on planetary boundaries.[307, 308] This conceptualises the planet's ecosystems as a self-regulating system, now destabilised by human intervention in the last two centuries. Scheffer, too, has argued that Planet Earth is experiencing a series of crucial transitions, with thresholds being transcended. Interdisciplinary thinking and policy frameworks are required to protect what he called the 'Social-Eco-Earth-System'.[309, 310]

One thing all agree on is huge shifts are occurring in climate, biological evolution, oceans, in ecosystems and social systems, all the unintended consequences of a pursuit of economic growth. Different paradigms and visions are invoked in the name of sustainable diets, each appealing to policy makers with different policy packages. Lamine and colleagues posit two competing paradigms,[311] while Lang and Heasman see a tension between life sciences and ecologically integrating worldviews.[18] Systems thinking may attempt to stand away from value judgements and the language may be 'cool' and 'flat' but, for policy makers, the challenges still boil down to the need to map systemic options and make choices.

### Skilling consumers: information is not enough

Policy makers have been attracted to 'nudge' and 'below the radar' approaches to dietary change because these seem less draconian than the harder measures such as fiscal or regulatory change. Approaches trying quietly to alter the conditions in which food choices are made, by definition, do not engage the consumer. Yet there is a large body of knowledge that points out that consumers bring very complex understandings of food to their food choices. Some are innate – taste reflexes, for instance – but many are learned.[79, 312] We humans also use food to communicate and send signals of identity, status and aspiration.[313]

There is also a body of literature pointing out that the nutrition transition is accompanied by a skills transition, subtly changing how people eat, what they consider a meal and when to eat.[314-316] This is partly what has accelerated the rise in overweight and obesity. Far from there being a global shortage of food, there is a surplus, even at the global level. In richer societies, as food has become cheaper and the opportunities and signals to eat constantly surround consumers, the environment has become one that reinforces continual snacking, grazing and nibbling. The eating environment has become an obesogenic environment.[89, 317] Deeply embedded norms and habits have been altered, not least by a barrage of marketing. Even supposedly strong food cultures such as the French exhibit these tendencies.[314]

What skills are needed to enable people to eat sustainably? Some argue that beneficial outcomes will follow if people simply eat healthily. The CSIRO, an Australian government–industry research organisation, has stated that, if Australians ate according to their National Dietary Guidelines, the reduction in the over-consumption of calories plus eating whole foods could cut the greenhouse gas contribution of the average diet by 25%. It calculated that 'junk food' accounted for up to 27% of the 14.5 kilograms of diet-related GHGEs produced by the average Australian each day.[318]

Within the organised consumer movement, a key demand is for more and better information. Ever since President Jack Kennedy's 1962 speech on consumer rights, it's been central to the consumer movement's case.[319] In neoliberal thinking, this has become 'put it on the label', yet decades of consumer research has also shown that what is not on the label also matters – issues such as the processing, the hidden additives, the residues, the hidden labour, etc. Indeed, food labelling can too easily become the governance battleground itself with forces arguing over whether it is necessary to inform consumers. It took nearly two decades, for instance, to get the European Union to agree to make quantitative ingredients declaration (QUID) labelling mandatory. This puts ingredients listed by the amount used onto the label. There has been decades of resistance to labelling the level of pesticide residues, for example. If an agrichemical is safe to use and residues are monitored, there's no need, argue the agrichemical industry.

In principle, it could be argued that good food does not need labelling. It can also be argued that sustainable diets are one issue in food policy where labelling and information transfer really might now be helpful. The FCRN study concluded not, and suggested that diverse and tougher multiple interventions are needed.[133] Certainly, there is nervousness within the food industries about ever more labelling and information, unless under its control, such as via in-store information or corporate websites. Indeed, a full label is almost inconceivable; the sheer weight of information would lead to vast labels and information overload. But there are other ways of making information available – on screen/on demand, phone apps, in store, for example. More and more producers and sellers wish either to 'engage' with their customers or to be seen to do so. Some of this is PR and 'greenwash'. Some is genuine. What really matters, if this is a future policy direction on sustainable diet information, is who sets controls for how such information is given, and what standards are applied.

### The bottom line: sustainable diets mean eating differently

This, we think, is the simple truth: sustainable diets mean eating differently, which means a different food supply chain. This may take different forms in different parts of the world – and cost systems – but broadly implies that consumers in high-income developed countries will on the whole eat less but better, while in very low-income developing countries they will eat more but better, while in middle-income countries they broadly will need to eat just differently. This is the contract and converge policy position. It implies a shift from seeing humans as consumers to seeing them as citizens. It redefines what a good consumer is and suggests some tension between ameliorating conventional food systems or whether 'alternative' ones should be expanded.[320] Meanwhile, there is a broad agreement on the need to eat so as to balance intake and output of energy, to eat mostly plant-based diets, to consume little meat (and to eat the whole animal), to avoid waste of food, to eat appropriately for health, environment and culture, and to place food (whether plants, animals or seafood) back into its ecological role.

### Conclusion: achieving action through the SDG$^2$ strategy

This chapter has considered how governance matters for sustainable diets. A process of what might be called 'democratic experimentation' is emerging at different levels around the world. This illustrates the state of local and national political engagement on food and sustainability. At the same time, there is commercial engagement. Food companies are increasingly concerned, some out of self-interest, others to retain consumer loyalty, others for the long-term.

Some strong civil society leadership has also emerged. These all offer hope as well as opportunities to test what works. Indeed, an element of pragmatism is essential in this area. But mass consumer behaviour change to integrate diet's components explored in this book is not yet happening. This is the hard truth.

How can policy specialists, analysts and governance processes give an effective lead on the transition? The niggling worry for governance structures is that, unless there is change, unsustainable diets and food systems will continue to make more catastrophic change more likely via wars, accelerating climate change, ecosystems damage, volatility of food supply or other systemic pressures. Let us hope such shifts are held off. Planned, progressive change is more orderly. It is above the radar, not below. Where might this come from for sustainable diets?

Politicians, the default leaders even in modern governance, are reluctant to mess with their voters' food. Cynics say they are usually voted out before anything serious can be undertaken, but that is not wholly fair or true. Experience suggests that a combination of public pressure, persistent scientific data and good organisation can generate the conditions for progressive policy change. It may take time, it may feel too late, but, pending crises, what is the alternative? In 2015 the world's political elite did agree serious intergovernmental commitments with the Sustainable Development Goals and the Paris Climate Change Accord. These provide the beginnings of a rational framework for change, which we call the SDG$^2$ virtuous circle strategy (see Figure 8.2).

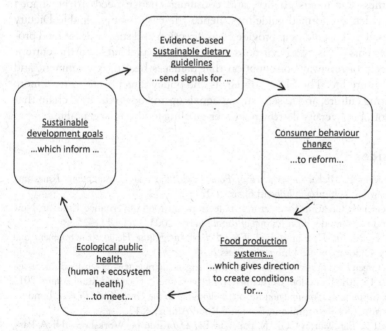

*Figure 8.2* The SDG$^2$ virtuous circle strategy

Source: the authors.

Figure 8.2 presents the process of change as a stylised cycle. In reality, change can be messier. It could be argued, too, that this gives too much emphasis to the creation of formal guidelines when we have just shown that these have proven hard to achieve. Might not 'softer' guidance rather than 'harder' guidelines be the way forward? This is the route Germany and Sweden have taken, the latter under duress when its guidelines were deemed unacceptable by the EU. It did not give up, however. So soft guidance might indeed be the pragmatic first step; but to achieve systemic change there will surely need to be formal, institutionally backed guidelines to translate into standards. An important international review was conducted for FAO in 2016, which showed the growth of interest in this approach.[321] The transition from informal to formal guidelines is gathering interest but there is, as yet, no mass rush by governments, which suggests that the scientists and civil society organisations have much work to do to win more support. One particularly hopeful direction is the development of city/town level food activity all over the world. FAO, together with RUAF and the City Region Food System Alliance, is taking a useful lead here.[322] This has potential to combine the cultural identity element of sustainable diets with the environmental, health and jobs case for change, so important to win local political support.

The SDG[2] strategy is straightforward: to aim for Sustainable Dietary Guidelines to meet the Sustainable Development Goals. The Sustainable Development Goals cannot be met unless the food system changes. The food system cannot change unless consumers change, and consumer change needs to be shaped by clear evidence-informed guidelines, hence the case for Sustainable Dietary Guidelines. These would help provide clear direction and standards for food production systems. This SDG[2] virtuous circle is surely preferable to the current vicious circle of runaway consumption that damages health, environment and quality of future life. The SDG[2] strategy is one policy direction to foster a more benign eating culture, and to send strong signals up and down the food chain that high-carbon, biodiversity destroying, water-guzzling food is unacceptable.

## References

1   Oosterveer P. *Global Governance of Food Production and Consumption: Issues and Challenges*. Cheltenham: Edward Elgar, 2007
2   Le Heron R. Creating food futures: reflections on food governance issues in New Zealand's agri-food sector. *Journal of Rural Studies*, 2003; 19(1): 111–25
3   Lang T, Barling D, Caraher M. *Food Policy: Integrating Health, Environment and Society*. Oxford: Oxford University Press 2009
4   Defra. *Green Food Project*. Available at: http://engage.defra.gov.uk/green-food/ (accessed August 15, 2013). London: Department for Environment, Food and Rural Affairs, 2012
5   Defra. *Sustainable Consumption Report: Follow-Up to the Green Food Project*. London: Department for Environment, Food and Rural Affairs, 2013
6   Arnaud E. *Big Data in CGIAR*, paper to Big Data Europe Workshop. INRA Pars, 22 September. Available at: http://de.slideshare.net/BigData_Europe/big-data-in-cgiar-53151807 (accessed January 6, 2016). Paris: CGIAR, 2015

7 Ruppert E, Harvey P, Lury C, et al. Socialising Big Data: From Concept to Practice. CRESC Working Paper Series. Manchester: CRESC, The University of Manchester and the Open University, 2015

8 Trentmann F. The Making of the Consumer: Knowledge, Power and Identity in the Modern World. New York: Berg, 2005

9 Trentmann F. Empire of Things: How We Became a World of Consumers, Fifteenth Century to the Twenty-First. London: Allen Lane/Penguin, 2016

10 Marsden TK. From post-productionism to reflexive governance: contested transitions in securing more sustainable food futures. Journal of Rural Studies, 2013; 29(2): 123–34

11 Held D, Koenig-Archibugi M. Global Governance and Public Accountability. Oxford: Blackwell, 2005

12 Cockett R. Thinking the Unthinkable: Think-Tanks and the Economic Counter-Revolution, 1931–1983. London: HarperCollins, 1994

13 Hayek F. The Constitution of Liberty. London: Routledge, 1960

14 Hayek FA. The Road to Serfdom. Chicago, IL: University Chicago Press, 1994

15 Friedman M. Capitalism and Freedom. Chicago, IL: University of Chicago Press, 1962

16 Friedman M, Friedman RD. Free to Choose: A Personal Statement (1st Ed.). New York: Harcourt Brace Jovanovich, 1980

17 Gabriel Y, Lang T. The Unmanageable Consumer (3rd Ed.). London: Sage, 2015

18 Lang T, Heasman M. Food Wars: The Global Battle for Mouths, Minds and Markets (2nd Ed.). Abingdon: Routledge Earthscan, 2015

19 Brandt K. The Reconstruction of World Agriculture. London: George Allen & Unwin, 1945

20 Dunman J. Agriculture: Capitalist and Socialist. London: Lawrence & Wishart, 1975

21 Gray J. Beyond the New Right: Markets, Government and the Common Environment. London; New York: Routledge, 1993

22 Mazower M. Governing the World: The History of an Idea. London: Allen Lane, 2012

23 Hager C. Revisiting the ungovernability debate: regional governance and sprawl in the USA and UK. International Journal of Urban and Regional Research, 2012; 36(4): 817–30

24 Hampden-Turner C, Trompenaars A. The Seven Cultures of Capitalism: Value Systems for Creating Wealth in the United States, Japan, Germany, France, Britain, Sweden, and the Netherlands (1st Ed.). New York: Currency/Doubleday, 1993

25 Gereffi G. Global value chains in a post-Washington Consensus world. Review of International Political Economy, 2014; 21(1): 9–37, doi: 10.1080/09692290.2012.756414

26 Williamson J. A Short History of the Washington Consensus. From the Washington Consensus Towards a New Global Governance (hosted by Fundación CIDOB). Barcelona: Institute for International Economics, 2004

27 Bello W, Cunningham S, Rau B. Dark Victory: The United States, Structural Adjustment and Global Poverty. London: Pluto Press with Food First and the Transnational Institute, 1994

28 Khor M. Rethinking Globalization: Critical Issues and Policy Choices. London: Zed Books, 2001

29 Amanor KS. Global food chains, African smallholders and World Bank governance. Journal of Agrarian Change, 2009; 9(2): 247–62, doi: 10.1111/j.1471-0366.2009.00204.x

30 Bello WF. The Food Wars. London: Verso, 2009

31  Jawara F, Kwa A. *Behind the Scenes at the WTO: The Real World of International Trade Negotiations*. London; Bangkok: Zed Books, 2003

32  OECD. *Agricultural Monitoring and Evaluation 2015*. Paris: Organisation for Economic Cooperation and Development, 2015: 35

33  OECD. *Agricultural Policy Monitoring and Evaluation 2016*. Paris: Organisation for Economic Cooperation and Development, 2016

34  Garnett T, Strong M. *The Principles of Healthy and Sustainable Eating Patterns*. Swindon: Global Food Security programme (BBSRC *et al.*), 2015

35  Macdiarmid JI, Douglas F, Campbell J. Eating like there's no tomorrow: public awareness of the environmental impact of food and reluctance to eat less meat as part of a sustainable diet. *Appetite*, 2015; 96: 487–93, doi: 10.1016/j.appet.2015.10.011

36  Which? *Making Sustainable Food Choices Easier: A Consumer-Focussed Approach to Food Labels*. London: Which?, 2010

37  Which? *The Future of Food: Giving Consumers a Say*. London: Which?, 2013

38  Which?, Government Office for Science, TNS BMRB. *Food System Challenges: Public Dialogue on Food System Challenges and Possible Solutions*. London: Which? and Government Office for Science, 2015

39  Fuchs D, Kalfagianni A. The causes and consequences of private food governance. *Business and Politics*, 2010; 12(3)

40  Avery N, Drake M, Lang T. *Cracking the Codex: a Report on the Codex Alimentarius Commission*. London: National Food Alliance, 1993

41  GLOBALG.A.P. *What Is GLOBALG.A.P.?* Available at: www.globalgap.org/ (accessed July 7, 2014). Cologne, Germany: GLOBALG.A.P., 2014

42  Barling D. Food supply chain governance and public health externalities: upstream policy interventions and the UK state. *Journal of Agricultural and Environmental Ethics*, 2007; 20(3): 285–300

43  FDF. *Guideline Daily Amounts*. Available at: www.fdf.org.uk/publicgeneral/gdas_science_Jul09.pdf (accessed June 24, 2016). London: Food and Drink Federation, 2009

44  Kaan C, Liese A. Public private partnerships in global food governance: business engagement and legitimacy in the global fight against hunger and malnutrition. *Agriculture and Human Values*, 2011; 28(3): 385–99

45  Marsden TK. *The New Regulation and Governance of Food: Beyond the Food Crisis?* London: Routledge, 2010

46  Panjwani C, Caraher M. The public health responsibility deal: brokering a deal for public health, but on whose terms? *Health Policy*, 2014; 114(2–3): 163–73, doi: 10.1016/j.healthpol.2013.11.002

47  Marine Stewardship Council. *What Is the Marine Stewardship Council?* Available at: www.msc.org/ (accessed December 2, 2016). London: Marine Stewardship Council

48  Smithsonian Migratory Bird Center. *Bird Friendly Coffee*. Available at: http:// nationalzoo.si.edu/scbi/migratorybirds/coffee/ (accessed July 13, 2016). Washington, DC: Smithsonian Museum

49  Fairtrade International. *About Fairtrade Standards*. Available at: www.fairtrade.net/ standards.html (accessed July 13, 2016). Bonn: Fairtrade International, 2016

50  ETI. *Ethical Trade Initiative: About Us*. Available at: www.ethicaltrade.org/ (accessed August 30, 2015). London: Ethical Trade Initiative, 2015

51  Morgan K, Marsden T, Murdoch J. *Worlds of Food: Place, Power and Provenance in the Food Chain*. Oxford: Oxford University Press, 2006

52  Lawrence F. *Not on the Label*. London: Penguin, 2004

53 Nestle M. *Food Politics: How the Food Industry Influences Nutrition and Health*. Berkeley, CA: University of California Press, 2002

54 Nestle M. *Safe Food: Bacteria, Biotechnology and Bioterrorism*. Berkeley, CA: University of California Press, 2003

55 Elliott C. *Elliott Review into the Integrity and Assurance of Food Supply Networks. Final Report – A Food Crime Prevention Framework*. Available at: www.gov.uk/government/ policy-advisory-groups/review-into-the-integrity-and-assurance-of-food-supply-networks (accessed July 3, 2016 ). London: HM Government, 2014

56 BBC News. *Timeline: China Milk Scandal*. Available at: http://news.bbc.co.uk/1/ hi/7720404.stm (accessed June 8, 2016). London: BBC, 2010

57 Ruijia Yang R, Huang W, Zhang L, et al. Milk adulteration with melamine in China: crisis and response. *Quality Assurance and Safety of Crops & Foods*, 2009; 1(2): 111–16, doi: 10.1111/j.1757-837X.2009.00018.x

58 Merrigan K, Griffin T, Wilde P, et al. Designing a sustainable diet. *Science*, 2015; 350(6257): 165–6, doi: 10.1126/science.aab2031

59 Salter AM. Improving the sustainability of global meat and milk production. *Proceedings of the Nutrition Society*, 2015, doi: 10.1017/S0029665116000276

60 Monteiro CA, Cannon G, Moubarac J-CT. The food system: product reformulation will not improve public health. *World Nutrition*, 2014; 5(2): 140–68

61 Institute of Mechanical Engineers. *Global Food: Waste Not Want Not*. London: Institute of Mechanical Engineers, 2013

62 Gunn M, Mont O. Choice editing as a retailers' tool for sustainable consumption. *International Journal of Retail & Distribution Management*, 2014; 42(6): 464–81, doi: doi:10.1108/IJRDM-12-2012-0110

63 National Consumer Council, Sustainable Development Commission. *Looking Back Looking Forward: Lessons in Choice Editing for Sustainability: 19 Case Studies into Drivers and Barriers to Mainstreaming More Sustainable Products*. London: Sustainable Development Commission, 2006

64 Carlsson-Kanyama A, Ekström MP, Shanahan H. Food and life cycle energy inputs: consequences of diet and ways to increase efficiency. *Ecological Economics*, 2003; 44(2–3): 293–307

65 van Dooren C, Marinussen M, Blonk H, et al. Exploring dietary guidelines based on ecological and nutritional values: a comparison of six dietary patterns. *Food Policy*, 2014; 44: 36–46

66 Wickramasinghe KK, Rayner M, Goldacre M, et al. Contribution of healthy and unhealthy primary school meals to greenhouse gas emissions in England: linking nutritional data and greenhouse gas emission data of diets. *European Journal of Clinical Nutrition*, 2016; 70(10): 1162–7, doi: 10.1038/ejcn.2016.101

67 van Dooren C, Kramer G. *Food Patterns and Dietary Recommendations in Spain, France and Sweden: Healthy People, Healthy Planet*. Godalming: WWF-UK, 2012

68 Carlsson-Kanyama A, Gonzalez AD. Potential contributions of food consumption patterns to climate change. *The American Journal of Clinical Nutrition*, 2009; 89(Supplement): 1S–6S

69 Smith P, Haberl H, Popp A, et al. How much land-based greenhouse gas mitigation can be achieved without compromising food security and environmental goals? *Global Change Biology*, 2013; 19(8): 2285–302, doi: 10.1111/gcb.12160

70 Blake L, Zero Carbon Britain. *People, Plate and Planet: The Impact of Dietary Choices on Health, Greenhouse Gas Emissions and Land Use*. Machynlleth: Centre for Alternative Technology, 2014

71  Lang T. *Re-fashioning Food Systems with Sustainable Diet Guidelines: The SDG² Strategy.* London: Friends of the Earth (England and N. Ireland), 2016

72  McDonald's. *McDonald's to Fully Transition to Cage-free Eggs for all Restaurants in the U.S. and Canada.* Available at: http://news.mcdonalds.com/ (accessed 10 July, 2016). Oak Brook, IL: McDonald's Newsroom, 2015

73  Compassion in World Farming. Personal communication to T Lang, July. Godalming: CIWF, 2016

74  Tareke E, Rydberg P, Karlsson P, *et al.* Analysis of acrylamide, a carcinogen formed in heated foodstuffs. *Journal of Agricultural and Food Chemistry,* 2002; 50(17): 4998–5006, doi: 10.1021/jf020302f

75  Pollan M. *Food Rules: An Eater's Manual.* London: Penguin, 2010

76  Pollan M. *In Defence of Food: The Myth of Nutrition and the Pleasures of Eating.* London: Allen Lane, 2008

77  Ministry of Health (Brazil). *Dietary Guidelines for the Brazilian Population.* Available at: http://189.28.128.100/dab/docs/portaldab/publicacoes/guia_alimentar_populacao_ingles.pdf (accessed November 9, 2014). Brasília: Ministry of Health, 2014: 80

78  Livsmedelsverket, National Food Administration. *Find Your Way to Eat Greener, Not Too Much and Be Active.* Stockholm: Livsmedelsverket/National Food Administration, 2015: 26

79  Warde A. *The Practice of Eating.* Cambridge: Polity Press, 2016

80  G8. 'L'Aquila' *Joint Statement on Global Food Security, L'Aquila Food Security Initiative (AFSI),* 10 July. Available at: www.g8italia2009.it/static/G8_Allegato/LAquila_Joint_Statement_on_Global_Food_Security%5B1%5D,0.pdf (accessed July 15, 2016). Rome: G8 Leaders, 2009

81  G8. *Final Communique of G8 Loch Erne.* Available at: www.gov.uk/government/uploads/system/uploads/attachment_data/file/207583/Lough_Erne_2013_G8_Leaders_Communique__2_.pdf (accessed July 15, 2016). London: HM Government, 2013

82  Global Commission on Economy and Climate. *Final Report: Strategies to Achieve Economic and Environmental Gains by Reducing Food Waste,* report by WRAP for the Global Commission (New Climate Economy). Banbury: WRAP and Global Commission on Economy and Climate, 2015

83  FAO. *Declaration from the World Summit on Food Security.* Available at: www.fao.org/fileadmin/templates/wsfs/Summit/Docs/Final_Declaration/WSFS09_Declaration.pdf (accessed July 15, 2016). Rome: Food and Agriculture Organization, 2009

84  IPES-Food. *From Uniformity to Diversity: A Paradigm Shift from Industrial Agriculture to Diversified Agroecological Systems.* Brussels: International Panel of Experts on Sustainable Food (IPES-Food), 2016: 96

85  Gerber PJ, Steinfeld H, Henderson B, *et al. Tackling Climate Change Through Livestock: A Global Assessment of Emissions and Mitigation Opportunities.* Rome: Food and Agriculture Organization of the United Nations, 2013

86  Godfray HCJ, Garnett T. Food security and sustainable intensification. *Philosophical Transactions of the Royal Society B,* 2014; 369, doi: 10.1098/rstb.2012.0273

87  Lampkin NH, Pearce BD, Leake AR, *et al. The Role of Agroecology in Sustainable Intensification.* Report for the Land Use Policy Group (Natural England, Natural Resources Wales, Scottish Natural Heritage, Scottish Environmental Protection Agency, Northern Ireland Environment Agency, Environment Agency). Hamstead Marshall, Newbury: Organic Research Centre and Game & Wildlife Conservation Trust, 2015

88  Braithwaite T. Lunch with the FT: Rob Rhinehart. His 'future food' began as a life-hack for techies. Now it's a $100m-plus start-up. Over double desserts in LA, he says our eating habits are stuck in the industrial revolution. *Financial Times*, July 23, 2016. Available at: http://on.ft.com/2aiH5yY (accessed July 23, 2016)

89  Egger G, Swinburn B. An 'ecological' approach to the obesity pandemic. *British Medical Journal*, 1997; 315(7106): 477–80

90  Lim GE, Albrecht T, Piske M, *et al.* 14-3-3ζ coordinates adipogenesis of visceral fat. *Nature Communications*, 2015; 6(7671), doi: 10.1038/ncomms8671

91  Shotter J. Nestlé boosts R&D to aid nutrition. *Financial Times*, December 27, 2014: 12

92  Ming T, de Richter R, Liu W, *et al.* Fighting global warming by climate engineering: is the Earth radiation management and the solar radiation management any option for fighting climate change? *Renewable and Sustainable Energy Reviews*, 2014; 31: 792–834

93  Wellesley L, Happer C, Froggatt A. *Changing Climate, Changing Diets: Pathways to Lower Meat Consumption*. London: Chatham House (Royal Institute of International Affairs), 2015: 76

94  National Health and Family Planning Commission of China. *Announcement of Goal to Reduce Meat Consumption by 50%*. Available at: http://mp.weixin.qq.com/s?__biz=MzAxODEwNzYzOA==&mid=2650236377&idx=1&sn=54b06cf4ab6cf2f71a6504c9ca32df59 (accessed July 19, 2016). Beijing: National Health and Family Planning Commission of China, 2016

95  Yang A. China wants to cut its meat consumption in HALF. Available at: http://shanghaiist.com/2016/06/22/china_wants_to_eat_half_the_meat.php (accessed July 19, 2016). *Shanghaiist*, June 22, 2016

96  Jeffries E. Changing course. *Nature Climate Change*, 2015; 5: 405–7

97  Stehfest E, Bouwman L, van Vuuren DP, *et al.* Climate benefits of changing diet. *Climatic Change*, 2009; 95: 83–102, doi: 10.1007/s10584-008-9534-6

98  Smith P. Delivering food security without increasing pressure on land. *Global Food Security* 2013; 2(1): 18–23, doi: 10.1016/j.gfs.2012.11.008

99  Aiking H, De Boer J. Food sustainability: diverging interpretations. *British Food Journal*, 2004; 106(5): 359–65

100  Helms M. Food sustainability, food security and the environment. *British Food Journal*, 2004; 106(5): 380–7, doi: 10.1108/00070700410531606

101  Thaler R, Sunstein C. *Nudge: Improving Decisions about Health, Wealth, and Happiness*. New Haven, CT: Yale University Press, 2008

102  Keats S, Wiggins S. *Future Diets: Implications for Agriculture and Food Prices*. London: Overseas Development Institute, 2014

103  Wiggins S, Keats S, Han E, *et al.* *The Rising Cost of a Healthy Diet*. London: Overseas Development Institute, 2015: 64

104  Brinsden H, Lang T. Reflecting on ICN2: was it a game changer? *Archives of Public Health*, 2015; 73(42), doi: 10.1186/s13690-015-0091-y

105  IFPRI. *Global Nutrition Report 2016*. Washington, DC: International Food Policy Research Institute, 2016

106  Scaling Up Nutrition (SUN). *Scaling Up Nutrition*. Available at: http://scalingupnutrition.org/ (accessed November 11, 2015). Copenhagen: UNOPS, 2013.

107  National Food Administration, Sweden's Environmental Protection Agency. *Environmentally Effective Food Choices*, proposal notified to the EU, 15 May. Stockholm: National Food Administration and Swedish Environmental Protection Agency, 2009

108 German Council for Sustainable Development. *The Sustainable Shopping Basket: A Guide to Better Shopping* (1st Ed.). Berlin: German Council for Sustainable Development, 2003

109 German Council for Sustainable Development. *The Sustainable Shopping Basket: A Guide to Better Shopping* (3rd Ed.). Berlin: German Council for Sustainable Development, 2008

110 German Council for Sustainable Development (RNE). *The Sustainable Shopping Basket: A Guide to Better Shopping.* Available at: www.nachhaltigkeitsrat.de/en/projects/projects-of-the-council/nachhaltiger-warenkorb/ (accessed January 18, 2015). Berlin: Rat für Nachhaltige Entwicklung/German Council for Sustainable Development, 2014: 93

111 Atwater WO. *Foods, Nutritive Value and Cost: US Department of Agriculture, Farmers Bulletin 23.* Washington, DC: US Department of Agriculture, 1894

112 Rowntree BS. *Poverty: A Study of Town Life.* London: Macmillan, 1902

113 Rowntree BS. *How the Labourer Lives.* London: Thomas Nelson & Sons, 1913

114 Astor WA, Rowntree BS. *British Agriculture: A Report of an Inquiry Organised by Viscount Astor and B Seebohm Rowntree* (abridged Ed.). Harmondsworth: Penguin, 1939

115 Beveridge SW. *Food Control.* Oxford: Oxford University Press, 1928

116 Woolton TE. *The Memoirs of the Rt Hon. The Earl of Woolton.* London: Cassell, 1959

117 Davis C, Saltos E. *Dietary Recommendations and How They Have Changed Over Time. America's Eating Habits: Changes and Consequences.* Washington, DC: US Department of Agriculture Economic Research Services, 1999: 33–50

118 Center for Nutrition Policy and Promotion. *A Brief History of USDA Food Guides.* Washington, DC: US Department of Agriculture CNPP, 2011

119 Chiuve SE, Fung TT, Rimm EB, *et al.* Alternative dietary indices both strongly predict risk of chronic disease. *Journal of Nutrition*, 2012; 142(6): 1009–18, doi: 10.3945/jn.111.157222

120 Corvo P. *Food Culture, Consumption and Society.* Basingstoke: Palgrave Macmillan, 2015

121 World Bank. *Global Consumption Database.* Available at: http://datatopics.worldbank.org/consumption/ (accessed July 26, 2015). Washington, DC: World Bank, 2016

122 TEEB. *The Economics of Ecosystems and Biodiversity: Mainstreaming the Economics of Nature: A Synthesis of the Approach, Conclusions and Recommendations of TEEB.* Geneva: UN Environment Programme, 2010

123 TEEB. *The Economics of Ecosystems and Biodiversity (TEEB) for Agriculture and Food: An Interim Report.* Geneva: UN Environment Programme, 2015: 124

124 Imamura F, Micha R, Khatibzadeh S, *et al.* Global burden of diseases: Nutrition and Chronic Diseases Expert Group (NutriCoDE). Dietary quality among men and women in 187 countries in 1990 and 2010: a systematic assessment. *The Lancet Global Health*, 2015; 3(3): e132–42

125 Murray CJL, Lopez AD. *The Global Burden of Disease: A Comprehensive Assessment of Mortality and Disability from Diseases, Injuries and Risk Factors in 1990 and Projected to 2020.* Cambridge, MA: Harvard School of Public Health on behalf of the World Health Organization and the World Bank, 1996

126 Wanless D. *Securing Our Future Health: Taking a Long-Term View.* London: HM Treasury, 2002

127 Wanless D. *Securing Good Health for the Whole Population*. London: HM Treasury, 2004

128 Cabinet Office Strategy Unit. *Food Matters: Towards a Strategy for the 21st Century*. London: Cabinet Office Strategy Unit, 2008

129 Defra. *About Food 2030*. Available at: http://sandbox.defra.gov.uk/food2030/about-food-2030/ (accessed May 5, 2016). London: Department for Environment, Food and Rural Affairs, 2009

130 Defra. *Food 2030 Strategy*. London: Department for Environment, Food and Rural Affairs, 2010: 84

131 Defra. 25-Year Food and Farming Plan (draft March 22, 2016). London: Department of Environment, Food and Rural Affairs, 2016

132 Lang T, Schoen V. *Food, the UK and the EU: Brexit or Bremain?* London: Food Research Collaboration, 2016: 40

133 Garnett T, Mathewson S, Angelides P, *et al. Policies and Actions to Shift Eating Patterns: What Works? A Review of the Evidence of the Effectiveness of Interventions Aimed at Shifting Diets in More Sustainable and Healthy Directions*. Oxford: Food Climate Research Network, University of Oxford, 2015

134 FAO. *The State of World Fisheries and Aquaculture*. Rome: Food and Agriculture Organization, 2014

135 Royal Commission on Environmental Pollution. *Turning the Tide: Addressing the Impact of Fishing on the Marine Environment*, 25th Report. London: Royal Commission on Environmental Pollution, 2004

136 Thurstan RH, Roberts CM. The past and future of fish consumption: can supplies meet healthy eating recommendations? *Marine Pollution Bulletin*, 2014; 89(1–2): 5–11

137 Gladwell M. *The Tipping Point: How Little Things Can Make a Big Difference*. London: Abacus, 2000

138 O'Riordan T, Lenton T (Eds). *Addressing Tipping Points for a Precarious Future*. Oxford: Oxford University Press/British Academy, 2013

139 Butler CD. Sounding the alarm: health in the Anthropocene. *International Journal of Environmental Research and Public Health*, 2016; 13(665), doi: 10.3390/ijerph13070665

140 Rees SM. *Our Final Hour: A Scientist's Warning*. London: Basic Books, 2009

141 de Ruiter H, Macdiarmid JI, Matthews RB, *et al.* Global cropland and greenhouse gas impacts of UK food supply are increasingly located overseas. *Journal of the Royal Society Interface*, 2016; 13(114), doi: 10.1098/rsif.2015.1001

142 Audsley E, Brander M, Chatterton J, *et al. How Low Can We Go? An Assessment of Greenhouse Gas Emissions from the UK Food System and the Scope for Reduction by 2050*. Godalming, Surrey: FCRN and WWF, 2010

143 Barling D, Lang T. Trading on health: cross-continental production and consumption tensions and the governance of international food standards, in: N Fold, B Pritchard (Eds) *Cross-Continental Food Chains*. London: Routledge, 2005: 39–51

144 Loconto A, Dankers C. *Impact of International Voluntary Standards on Smallholder Market Participation in Developing Countries: A Review of the Literature*. Rome: Food and Agriculture Organization, 2014: 104

145 Jones AD, Hoey L, Blesh J, *et al.* A systematic review of the measurement of sustainable diets. *Advances in Nutrition*, 2016; 7: 641–64, doi: 10.3945/an.115.011015

146 IUCN, UNEP, WWF. *Caring for the Earth: A Strategy for Sustainable Living*. Gland, Switzerland: International Union for the Conservation of Nature, the United Nations Environment Program (UNEP) and WWF, 1991

147 Carbon Trust. *The Eatwell Guide: a More Sustainable Diet. Understanding the Environmental Impact of Public Health England's Updated Eatwell Guide Nutritional Guidance*. London: Carbon Trust/Public Health England, 2016

148 Public Health England, Carbon Trust. *Sustainable Diets: Methodology and Results Summary*. London: Public Health England, 2016

149 Leach G. *Energy and Food Production*. Guildford: IPC Science and Technology Press for the International Institute for Environment and Development, 1976

150 ACARD. *The Food Industry and Technology*. London: Cabinet Office, Advisory Committee on Applied Research and Development, 1982

151 Hines C. *Food Co-ops: How to Save Money by Getting Together and Buying in Bulk*. London: Friends of the Earth, 1976

152 Meadows DH, Meadows DL, Randers J, *et al. The Limits to Growth: A Report for the Club of Rome's Project on the Predicament of Mankind*. New York: Universe Books, 1972

153 Jackson T. *Prosperity Without Growth: Economics for a Finite Planet*. London: Earthscan 2009

154 Daly HE. *Steady State Economics*. Boston: Island Press, 1991

155 Daly HE, Cobb JB, Cobb CW. *For the Common Good: Redirecting the Economy Toward Community, the Environment, and a Sustainable Future*. London: Green Print, 1990

156 Jackson T, Webster R. *Limits Revisited: The Limits to Growth Debate Revisited*. London: All Party Parliamentary Group on Limits to Growth, 2016

157 Randers J. *2052: A Report to the Club of Rome Commemorating the 40th Anniversary of The Limits to Growth*. White River Junction, VT: Chelsea Green Publishing, 2012

158 European Commission. *Roadmap to a Resource Efficient Europe*. Communication from the Commission to the European Parliament, the Council, the European Economic and Social Committee and the Committee of the Regions, COM(2011) 571 final. Brussels: European Commission, 2011: 26

159 Ellen Macarthur Foundation, McKinsey. *Towards the Circular Economy*. Cowes, Isle of Wight: Ellen Macarthur Foundation, 2013

160 European Commission. *The Circular Economy: Communication 'Towards a Circular Economy: A Zero Waste Programme for Europe'*. Available at: http://ec.europa.eu/environment/circular-economy/index_en.htm (accessed November 19, 2015). Brussels: European Commission, 2014

161 Innocent. What does sustainable packaging mean to Innocent drinks? *Footprint*, 2013: 10

162 Royal Society. *People and the Planet*. London: Royal Society, 2012

163 Hillman M. *How We Can Save the Planet*. London: Penguin Books, 2004

164 Garnett T, Mathewson S, Angelides P, *et al. Policies and Actions to Shift Eating Patterns: What Works? A Review of the Evidence of the Effectiveness of Interventions Aimed at Shifting Diets in More Sustainable and Healthy Directions*. Oxford and London: Food Climate Research Network, University of Oxford and Chatham House, 2015

165 Colchero MA, Popkin BM, Rivera JA, *et al.* Beverage purchases from stores in Mexico under the excise tax on sugar sweetened beverages: observational study. *BMJ*, 2016; 352: h6704, doi: 10.1136/bmj.h6704

166 UN Framework Convention on Climate Change. *Paris Convention of the Parties (COP21)*. Available at: http://unfccc.int/2860.php (accessed June 21, 2016). Bonn: UNFCCC Secretariat, 2015

167 Bajželj B, Benton TG, Clark M, *et al. Synergies Between Healthy and Sustainable Diets: Brief for Global Sustainable Development Report*. New York: United Nations Sustainable Development Report, 2015

168 Ripple WJ, Smith P, Haberl H, *et al.* Ruminants, climate change and climate policy. *Nature Climate Change*, 2014; 4: 2–5, doi: 10.1038/nclimate2081

169 United Nations. *Sustainable Development Goals*, agreed at the UN Summit, September 27–29. Available at: https://sustainabledevelopment.un.org/post2015/summit (accessed 7 July 7, 2016). New York: United Nations Department of Economic and Social Affairs, Division for Sustainable Development, 2015

170 IPES-Food. *International Panel of Experts on Sustainable Food*. Available at: www.ipes-food.org/ (accessed July 7, 2016). Paris: IPES Food, 2014

171 LIDC. *Global Panel on Agriculture and Food Systems for Nutrition*. Available at: www.lidc.org.uk/globalpanel (accessed May 9, 2015). London: London International Development Centre, 2013

172 FAO. *High Level Panel of Experts on Food Security and Nutrition*. Rome: UN Committee on World Food Security (CFS) and Food and Agriculture Organization, 2010

173 Duncan J. *Global Food Security Governance: Civil Society Engagement in the Reformed Committee on World Food Security*. Abingdon: Routledge, 2015

174 Rockström J, Steffen W, Noone K, *et al.* A safe operating space for humanity. *Nature*, 2009; 461(7263): 472–5

175 USTR. The Trans-Pacific Partnership. Available at: https://ustr.gov/tpp (accessed July 18, 2016). Washington, DC: Office of the United States Trade Representative, 2015

176 TTIP. *The Transatlantic Trade and Investment Partnership*. Available at: http://ec.europa.eu/trade/policy/in-focus/ttip/about-ttip/ (accessed July 21, 2016). Brussels: Commission of the European Communities, 2015

177 Corporate Europe Observatory. *Who Lobbies Most on TTIP?* Available at: http://corporateeurope.org/international-trade/2014/07/who-lobbies-most-ttip (accessed July 3, 2015). Brussels: Corporate Europe Observatory, 2015

178 Hansen-Kuhn K, Suppan S. *Promises and Perils of the TTIP: Negotiating a Transatlantic Agricultural Market*. Minneapolis: Institute for Agriculture and Trade Policy, 2013

179 McKeon N. *The United Nations and Civil Society: Legitimating Global Governance – Whose Voice?* London: Zed Books, 2009

180 National Food Administration, Environment Agency. *Environmentally Effective Food Choices*, proposal notified to the EU. Stockholm: National Food Administration, 2008

181 2015 Dietary Guidelines Advisory Committee. *Scientific Report of the 2015 Dietary Guidelines Advisory Committee (Advisory Report); submitted to the Secretary of Health and Human Services and the Secretary of Agriculture*. Washington, DC: US Department of Agriculture and Deparment of Health and Human Services, 2015: 571

182 Qatar Supreme Council of Health. *Qatar Dietary Guidelines Evidence Base*. Doha: Supreme Council of Health, 2014

183 Qatar Supreme Council of Health. *Diet and Nutrition Profile for Qatar National Dietary Guidelines*. Doha: Supreme Council of Health, 2014

184 Seed B. Sustainability in the Qatar national dietary guidelines, among the first to incorporate sustainability principles. *Public Health Nutrition*, 2014; 18(13): 2303–10, doi: 10.1017/S1368980014002110

185 Health Council of the Netherlands. *Guidelines for a Healthy Diet: The Ecological Perspective*. The Hague: Health Council of the Netherlands, 2011

186 Ministry of Health (Brazil). *Guia Alimentar para a População Brasileira*. Brasília: Ministério da Saúde, 2014

187 Pact MUFP. *Milan Urban Food Policy Pact*, signed by 100 cities October 15, 2015. Milan: Commune di Milano, 2015: 6

188 Declaration IS. *Building a World of Local Action for A Sustainable Urban Future*, declaration signed April 9, 2015. Seoul: ICLEI Local Governments for Sustainability, 2015: 4

189 Calori A, Magarini A. *Food and the Cities: Food Policies for Sustainable Cities*. Milan: Edizioni Ambiente, 2015

190 Sustainable Food Cities. *Sustainable Food Cities Network*. Available at: http://sustainablefoodcities.org/ (accessed July 22, 2016). Bristol, London, Brighton, UK: Soil Association, Food Matters, Sustain, 2014

191 Porter JR, Dyball R, Dumaresq D, *et al.* Feeding capitals: urban food security and self-provisioning in Canberra, Copenhagen and Tokyo. *Global Food Security*, 2014; 3(1): 1–7

192 Barker B. *City Mayors Mayor of the Month: Joko Widodo (Jokowi) Governor of Jakarta*. Available at: www.citymayors.com/mayors/jakarta-widodo.html (accessed December 9, 2015). London, UK and Freiburg, Germany: City Mayors, 2013

193 Balazs B. paper on Hungary, presented to conference: Symposium on Global Sustainability and Local Foods, American University of Rome, October 2, 2015. Rome: American University of Rome and Environmental Social Science Research Group, Budapest, 2015

194 Barnett M. *British Food Policy During the First World War*. Abingdon: Routledge, 2014

195 Collingham L. *Taste of War: World War Two and the Battle for Food*. London: Allen Lane, 2011

196 Smith DF. Nutrition science and the two world wars, in: DF Smith (Ed.) *Nutrition in Britain: Science, Scientists and Politics in the Twentieth Century*. London: Routledge, 1997, 142–65

197 Minns R. *Bombers and Mash: The Domestic Front 1939–1945*. London: Virago, 1980

198 Lappé FM. *Diet for a Small Planet*. New York: Ballantine Books, 1971

199 Smith A, Mackinnon JB. *The 100-Mile Diet: A Year of Local Eating*. New York: Random House, 2007

200 Kinross E, Small K, Small M, *et al. The Fife Diet: About Us*. Available at: www.fifediet.co.uk/about-us/ (accessed July 22, 2016). Burntisland, Fife, Scotland: The Fife Diet, 2012

201 Small M. *The Fife Diet: A Local Experiment*. Available at: http://fifediet.wordpress.com/about/: (accessed July 22, 2016). Fife, Scotland: The Fife Diet, 2007

202 The Food Assembly. *Who We Are*. Available at: https://thefoodassembly.com (accessed May 4, 2016). London: The Food Assembly, 2015

203 O'Connell J. A new way to buy local produce? Food assembly is coming to Britain. *The Guardian*, July 10, 2014. Available at: www.theguardian.com/lifeandstyle/2014/jul/10/new-way-buy-local-produce-food-assembly-coming-britain (accessed July 22, 2016).

204 Greenpeace International. *Eating Up the Amazon*. Amsterdam: Greenpeace International, 2006

205 Friends of the Earth. *Pesticides in Supermarket Food*. Available at: www.foe.co.uk/resource/briefings/pesticide_supermarket_food.pdf (accessed June 9, 2006). London: Friends of the Earth, 2004

206 RSPB WT, Friends of the Earth, Sustain, National Trust, Eating Better, Compassion in World Farming, Food Research Collaboration, Food Ethics Council, Soil Association. *Square Meal: Why We Need a Better Recipe for the Future*. London: Food Research Collaboration, 2014

207 Birdlife. *Agriculture: Food for the Future*. Available at: www.birdlife.org/sites/default/files/attachments/factsheet%20agriculture%20HR%20.pdf (accessed December 2, 2016). Brussels: Birdlife International, 2016

208 Birdlife International. *State of the World's Birds: Seabirds Are in Serious Danger from Fisheries Bycatch*. Available at: www.birdlife.org/datazone/sowb/pressure/PRESS8 (accessed July 17, 2016). Brussels: Birdlife International, 2016

209 National Trust. *Principles of the Food Policy*. Available at: www.nationaltrust.org.uk/documents/download-the-food-policy.pdf (accessed July 17, 2016). Swindon: National Trust, 2016

210 National Trust. *Why We Champion Sustainable Food*. Swindon: National Trust, 2016

211 National Trust. *Appetite for Change*. Swindon: National Trust, 2009: 36

212 Jacobson MF. *Six Arguments for a Greener Diet: How a More Plant-Based Diet Could Save Your Health and the Environment*. Washington, DC: Center for Science in the Public Interest, 2006

213 Meatless Mondays Global and Meat-Free Mondays. Available at: www.meatlessmonday.com/the-global-movement/ (accessed January 21, 2017) and www.meatfreemondays.com/ (accessed April 25, 2016)

214 Growing Communities. *Transforming Food and Farming through Community-Led Trade*. Available at: www.growingcommunities.org/ (accessed May 21, 2016). London: Hackney Growing Communities, 2015

215 McLaren D, Agyeman J. *Sharing Cities: A Case for Truly Smart and Sustainable Cities*. Cambridge, MA: MIT Press, 2015

216 City Growers. *About Us*. Available at: https://citygrowers.wordpress.com/ (accessed May 21, 2016). Boston, MA: City Growers, 2016

217 WWF. *Thirsty Crops: Our Food and Clothes: Eating Up Nature and Wearing Out the Environment?* Zeist (NL): WWF, 2006

218 WWF, Zoological Society of London. *Living Blue Planet Report 2015: Species, Habitats and Human Well-Being*. Gland, Switzerland: WWF and ZSL, 2015

219 WWF-UK. *One Planet Food Strategy 2009–2012*. Godalming, Surrey: WWF UK, 2009

220 Gladek E, Fraser M, Roemers G, et al. *The Global Food System: An Analysis*, Report to WWF. Amsterdam: WWF Netherlands, 2016: 188

221 IBLF. IBLF Global. London: International Business Leaders Forum (IBLF) Global, 2016

222 B20 Coalition. *What Is B20?* Available at: www.b20businesssummit.com/b20/ (accessed July 25, 2016). Berlin/Paris: B20 Business Summit, 2011

223 BIAC. Business and Industry Advisory Committee to the OECD. Available at: http://biac.org/ (accessed July 2, 2016). Paris: BIAC/OECD, 2016

224 SAI. *Sustainable Agriculture Initiative Platform*. Available at: www.saiplatform.org/ (accessed July 25, 2016). Brussels: Sustainable Agriculture Initiative, 2016

225 Dow Jones. *Dow Jones Sustainability Indices*. Available at: www.sustainability-indices.com/index-family-overview/djsi-family-overview/index.jsp (accessed July 17, 2016). New York: Dow Jones, 2016

226 World Business Council for Sustainable Development. *A Vision for Sustainable Consumption*. Available at: www.wbcsdpublications.org/cd_files/datas/capacity_building/consumption/pdf/AVisionForSustainableConsumption.pdf (accessed July 12, 2014). Conches-Geneva: World Business Council for Sustainable Development, 2011

227 World Business Council for Sustainable Development. Food and Land Use. Available at: www.wbcsd.org/Overview/Our-approach/Food-and-land-use (accessed December 2, 2016). Geneva: World Business Council for Sustainable Development, 2016

228 UNFCCC. *Copenhagen Accord*, 15th session of the Conference of the Parties to the UNFCCC and the 5th session of the Conference of the Parties serving as the Meeting of the Parties to the Kyoto Protocol took place in Copenhagen. Bonn: United Nations Framework Convention on Climate Change, 2009

229 World Economic Forum, McKinsey & Co. *Realizing a New Vision for Agriculture: A Roadmap for Stakeholders*. Davos: World Economic Forum, 2010

230 Murphy J, Thomas M. *We Will Live as We Will Eat: Anticipating the Future Power of Sustainability Amid Our Shifting Food Culture*. London: Dissident, 2016

231 Unilever. *Sustainable Living Plan 2010*. Available at: www.sustainable-living.unilever.com/the-plan/ (accessed December 12, 2010). London: Unilever plc, 2010

232 Marks & Spencer plc. *About Plan A: Plan A is Our Five-Year, 100 Point Plan*. Available at: http://plana.marksandspencer.com/about (accessed May 6, 2012). London: Marks & Spencer plc, 2009

233 Marks and Spencer. *About Plan A*. Available at: https://corporate.marksandspencer.com/plan-a/our-stories/about-plan-a (accessed July 17, 2016). London: Marks and Spencer plc, 2016

234 Barilla Center for Food & Nutrition. *Eating Planet: Diet and Sustainability to Build Our Future*. Milan: Edizioni Ambiente, 2016

235 Barilla Center for Food & Nutrition. *The Milan Protocol*. Available at: www.milanprotocol.com/ (accessed July 27, 2016). Parma: Barilla Center for Food & Nutrition, 2014

236 Barilla Center for Food & Nutrition Foundation. *Double Pyramid: Health Food for People, Sustainable Food for the Planet*. Parma: Barilla Center for Food & Nutrition Foundation, 2014

237 Culinary Institute of America, Harvard School of Public Health. *Menus of Change Initiative*. Available at: www.menusofchange.org/ (accessed 9 September 2016). Hyde Park, NY: Culinary Institute of America and Harvard School of Public Health Department of Nutrition, 2013

238 Harvard School of Public Health. *Food Pyramids and Plates: What Should You Really Eat?* Available at: www.hsph.harvard.edu/nutritionsource/pyramid-full-story/ (accessed April 7, 2014). Boston, MA: Harvard University, 2014

239 *Relais et Chateau*, UNESCO. *Le Manifeste: un Monde Meilleur, par la Table et l'Hospitalité*. Paris: Relais et Chateau, 2014

240 Food Ethics Council. *Catering for Sustainability: Making the Case for Sustainable Diets in Foodservice*. London: Food Ethics Council, WWF-UK, Sodexho, 2016

241 Watson G. Personal communication to T Lang, March 18 and *Riverford Newsletter 176*, February 1. Buckfastleigh: Riverford, 2016

242 Riverford. *How Much Meat London debate?* Available at: https://www.riverford.co.uk/blog/2016/03/25/guys-newsletter-how-much-meat/ (accessed December 2, 2016). Buckfastleigh: Riverford, 2016

243 Iejlersen S. Talk on Aarstiderne to EAT Forum, June 14. Available at: www.aarstiderne.com/ (accessed December 5, 2016). Stockholm: personal communication, 2016

244 Hammond RJ. *Food: The Growth of Policy*. London: HMSO/Longmans, Green and Co., 1951

245 Inter-departmental Committee on Physical Deterioration (chaired by Sir Almeric W Fitzroy). *Report of the Inter-Departmental Committee on Physical Deterioration* (vol. 1, Cd.2175). London: HMSO, 1904: v + 137

246 Ehrlich PR, Ehrhich AH. The population bomb revisited. *The Electronic Journal of Sustainable Development*, 2009; 1(3): 63–71

247 Ehrlich PR. *The Population Bomb*. New York: Ballantine Books, 1968

248 Eide A, Eide WB, Goonatilake S, et al. (Eds). *Food as a Human Right*. Tokyo: United Nations University, 1984

249 Gussow JD, Clancy KL. Dietary guidelines for sustainability. *Journal of Nutrition Education*, 1986; 18(1): 1–5

250 Herrin M, Gussow JD. Designing a sustainable regional diet. *Journal of Nutrition Education*, 1989; 21(6): 270–5

251 WHO. *The Ottawa Charter for Health Promotion*, First International Conference on Health Promotion, Ottawa, November 21. Geneva: World Health Organization, 1986

252 Keys A (Ed.). Coronary heart disease in seven countries. *Circulation*, 1970; 41 (supp. 1): 1–211

253 COMA. *Diet and Coronary Heart Disease*, Report of the Advisory Panel of the Committee on Medical Aspects of Food Policy (COMA). London: Department of Health and Social Security, 1974

254 Gussow JD. Mediterranean diets: are they environmentally responsible? *American Journal of Clinical Nutrition*, 1995; 61(6 Suppl): 1383S–9S

255 Popkin BM. The nutrition transition in low-income countries: an emerging crisis. *Nutrition Reviews*, 1994; 52: 285–98

256 Popkin BM. Reducing meat consumption has multiple benefits for the world's health. *Archives of International Medicine*, 2009; 169(6): 543–5

257 Steinfeld H, Gerber P, Wassenaar T, et al. *Livestock's Long Shadow: Environmental Issues and Options*. Rome: Food and Agriculture Organization, 2006

258 WHO. *Obesity: Preventing and Managing the Global Epidemic*, Report of a WHO Consultation, WHO Technical Series 894. Geneva: World Health Organization, 2000

259 WHO. *Global Strategy on Diet, Physical Activity and Health*, 57th World Health Assembly, WHA 57.17, agenda item 12.6. Geneva: World Health Assembly, 2004

260 Kolbert E. *The Sixth Extinction: An Unnatural History*. New York: Henry Holt, 2015

261 Hallström E, Carlsson-Kanyama A, Börjesson P. Environmental impact of dietary change: a systematic review. *Journal of Cleaner Production*, 2015; 91(0): 1–11

262 Bresalier M, Cassidy A, Woods A. One health in history, in: J Zinsstag, E Schelling, D Waltner-Toews, et al. (Eds) *One Health: the Theory and Practice of Integrated Health Approaches*. Wallingford: CABI International, 2015: Ch. 1

263 Wallace RG, Bergmanm L, Kock R, et al. The dawn of Structural One Health: a new science tracking disease emergence along circuits of capital. *Social Science and Medicine*, 2015; 129: 68–77, doi: 10.1016/j.socscimed.2014.09.047

264 Zinsstag J, Schelling E, Waltner-Toews D, et al. (Eds). *One Health: the Theory and Practice of Integrated Health Approaches*. Wallingford: CABI Publishing, 2015

265 CBC, UNEP, WHO. *Connecting Global Priorities: Biodiversity and Human Health, a State of Knowledge Review*. Nairobi and Geneva: UNEP, Convention on Biological Diversity and World Health Organization, 2015

266 Rayner G, Lang T. *Ecological Public Health: Reshaping the Conditions for Good Health*. Abingdon: Routledge/Earthscan, 2012: 409

267 Rayner G, Lang T. Ecological public health: leaders, movements and ideas to shift the boundaries between the normal and the desirable, in: CD Butler, J Dixon, AG Capon (Eds) *Health of People, Places and Planet: Reflections Based on Tony McMichael's Four Decades of Contribution to Epidemiological Understanding.* Canberra: Australian National University Press, 2015: 617–41

268 Still J. Top 10 sustainable food apps. Available at: www.theguardian.com/sustainable-business/sustainable-food-apps-smartphone-menu (accessed December 5, 2016). *The Guardian,* June 9, 2014

269 CAT. Laura's Larder 'app'. Available at: http://blog.cat.org.uk/2014/07/18/want-to-eat-a-healthy-and-sustainable-diet-ask-laura/ (accessed August 10, 2016). Macchynlyth: Centre for Alternative Technology, 2014

270 Big Data Europe. *Big Data for Food, Agriculture and Forestry: Opportunities and Challenges,* Big Data Europe workshop, Paris, September 22. Sankt Augustin, Germany: Big Data Europe, 2015

271 Manyika J, Chui M, Brown B, *et al. Big Data: The Next Frontier for Innovation, Competition, and Productivity.* San Francisco and London: McKinsey Global Institute, 2011

272 Anderson K. Duality in climate science. *Nature Geoscience,* 2015; 8: 898–900, doi: 10.1038/ngeo2559

273 Bajzelj B, Richards KS, Allwood JM, *et al.* Importance of food-demand management for climate mitigation. *Nature Climate Change,* 2014; 4: 924–9, doi: 10.1038/nclimate2353

274 Carlsson-Kanyama A. Climate change and dietary choices: how can emissions of greenhouse gases from food consumption be reduced? *Food Policy,* 1998; 23(3/4): 277–93

275 Garnett T. *Cooking Up a Storm: Food, Greenhouse Gas Emissions and Our Changing Climate.* Guildford: Food and Climate Research Network University of Surrey, 2008

276 Garnett T. Where are the best opportunities for reducing greenhouse gas emissions in the food system (including the food chain)? *Food Policy,* 2011; 36: S23–S32

277 Garnett T. Food sustainability: problems, perspectives and solutions. *Proceedings of the Nutrition Society,* 2013; 72 (1): 29–39

278 Garnett T. *What Is a Sustainable Diet? A Discussion Paper.* Oxford: Food and Climate Research Network, Oxford Martin School, University of Oxford, 2014: 31

279 Cabinet Office Behavioural Insights Team. *Applying Behavioural Insight to Health.* London: Cabinet Office, 2010

280 Rayner G, Lang T. Is nudge an effective public health strategy to tackle obesity? No. BMJ, 2011; 342: d2177, doi: 10.1136/bmj.d2177

281 Wise J. Nudge or fudge? Doctors debate best approach to improve public health. BMJ (Clinical Research Ed.), 2011; 342, doi: 10.1136/bmj.d580

282 Reisch L, Eberle U, Lorek S. Sustainable food consumption: an overview of contemporary issues and policies. *Sustainability: Science, Practice, & Policy,* 2013; 9(2): 7–25

283 Reisch LA, Lorek S, Bietz S. *Policy Instruments for Sustainable Food Consumption. Paper 2 for CORPUS (Enhancing the Connectivity between Research and Policy-Making in Sustainable Consumption),* European Commission FP 7 Project No. 244103, January. Available at: http://cri.dk/publications/corpus-enhancing-connectivity-between-research-and-policymaking-in-sustainable (accessed December 2, 2016). CORPUS/SCP, 2011

284 OPUS. *Developing the New Nordic Diet*. Available at: http://foodoflife.ku.dk/opus/english/wp/nordic_diet/ (accessed December 5, 2015). Copenhagen: University of Copenhagen Research Center OPUS, 2009

285 Barsac Declaration Group. *The Barsac Declaration: Environmental Sustainability and the Demitarian Diet*. Available at: www.nine-esf.org/sites/nine-esf.org/files/Barsac%20Declaration%20V5.pdf (accessed December 5, 2015). Barsac, France: European Science Foundation Nitrogen in Europe (NinE) Research Networking Programme, Biodiversity in European Grasslands: Impacts of Nitrogen Deposition (BEGIN) Research Programme of the European Science Foundation, Task Force on Reactive Nitrogen (TFRN) of the UNECE Convention on Long-Range Transboundary Air Pollution, International Nitrogen Initiative (INI), COST Action 729 on Assessing and Managing Nitrogen in the Atmosphere Biosphere System in Europe, and NitroEurope Integrated Project, 2009

286 Sutton MA, Howard CM, Erisman JW, *et al. The European Nitrogen Assessment Sources, Effects and Policy Perspectives*. Cambridge: Cambridge University Press, 2011

287 Harvard TH Chan School of Public Health. *5 Tips for Sustainable Eating*. Available at: www.hsph.harvard.edu/nutritionsource/2015/06/17/5-tips-for-sustainable-eating/ (accessed July 25, 2016). Boston, MA: Harvard University TH Chan School of Public Health Nutrition Source, 2016

288 Harvard TH Chan School of Public Health. *Nutrition Source: Sustainability: What Can I Do About Sustainability?* Boston, MA: Harvard TH Chan School of Public Health Nutrition Source, 2016

289 Lang T, Heasman M. *Food Wars: The Global Battle for Mouths, Minds and Markets*. London: Earthscan, 2004

290 Garnett T. *Changing What We Eat: A Call for Research and Action on Widespread Adoption of Sustainable Healthy Eating*. Oxford: Food Climate Research Network, University of Oxford, 2014: 27

291 UNEP, FAO, Messe Düsseldorf. *ThinkEatSave: Campaign in Support of the UN Secretary-General's Zero Hunger Challenge*. Available at: www.thinkeatsave.org/ (accessed August 11, 2016). Nairobi, Rome and Düsseldorf: United Nations Environment Programme and UN Food and Agriculture Organization, 2016

292 EU Fusions. *Fusions Programme to Reduce Food Waste in the European Union*. Available at: www.eu-fusions.org/ (accessed July 25, 2016). Wageningen: WUR, 2014

293 Evans D. Blaming the consumer – once again: the social and material contexts of everyday food waste practices in some English households. *Critical Public Health*, 2011; 21(4): 429–40

294 Evans D. Beyond the throwaway society: ordinary domestic practice and a socio-logical approach to household food waste. *Sociology*, 2011; 46(1): 41–56, doi: 10.1177/0038038511416150

295 Naylor H. Death by siege in Syria's civil war: hundreds of thousands at risk. *Washington Post*, January 23, 2016. Available at: www.washingtonpost.com/world/middle_east/death-by-siege-in-syrias-civil-war-we-have-no-food/2016/01/21/0bb14f4c-bbd7-11e5-85cd-5ad59bc19432_story.html (accessed 16 March 2016).

296 Mukerjee M. *Churchill's Secret War: The British Empire and the Ravaging of India During World War II*. New York: Basic Books, 2010

297 Brundtland GH. *Our Common Future*, report of the World Commission on Environment and Development (WCED) chaired by Gro Harlem Brundtland. Oxford: Oxford University Press, 1987

298  Brandt W. *North-South: A Programme for Survival.* London: Pan Books, 1980

299  Ranganathan J, Vennard D, Waite R, *et al. Shifting Diets for a Sustainable Food Future: Creating a Sustainable Food Future, Installment Eleven.* Washington, DC: World Resources Institute, 2016

300  Holling CS. Resilience and stability of ecological systems. *Annual Review of Ecology and Systematics,* 1973; 4: 1–23

301  Folke C, Carpenter SR, Walker B, *et al.* Resilience thinking: integrating resilience, adaptability and transformability. *Ecology and Society,* 2010; 15(4): 20

302  Lang T, John I. Food security twists and turns: why food systems need complex governance, in: T O'Riordan, T Lenton (Eds) *Addressing Tipping Points for a Precarious Future.* Oxford: Oxford University Presss and The British Academy, 2013: 81–103

303  Bertalanffy Lv. *Das biologische Weltbild.* Bern: A. Francke, 1949

304  Bertalanffy Lv. *General System Theory: Foundations, Development, Applications.* New York: Braziller, 1968

305  Midgley G. *Systemic Intervention: Philosophy, Methodology, and Practice.* New York: Kluwer, 2000

306  Midgley G. Systems thinking for the 21st Century, in: G Ragsdell, J Wilby (Eds) *Understanding Complexity.* Dordrecht: Springer, 2001: 249–56

307  Rockström J, Steffen W, Noone K, *et al.* Planetary boundaries: exploring the safe operating space for humanity. *Ecology and Society,* 2009; 14(2): 32

308  Steffen W, Richardson K, Rockström J, *et al.* Planetary boundaries: guiding human development on a changing planet. Available at: http://science.sciencemag.org/content/early/2015/01/14/science.1259855 (accessed June 22, 2016). *Science,* Jan 15, 2015, doi: 10.1126/science.1259855

309  Scheffer M. *Critical Transitions in Nature and Society.* Princeton; Oxford: Princeton University Press, 2009

310  Scheffer M, Bascompte J, Brock WA, *et al.* Early-warning signals for critical transitions. *Nature,* 2009; 461(7260): 53–9

311  Lamine C, Renting H, Rossi A, *et al.* Agri-food systems and territorial development: innovations, new dynamics and changing governance mechanisms, in: I Darnhofer, D Gibbon, B Dedieu (Eds). *Farming Systems Research into the 21st Century: The New Dynamic.* Dordrecht: Springer Science+Business Media, 2012: 229–56

312  Wilson B. *First Bite: How We Learn to Eat.* London: Fourth Estate, 2015

313  Douglas M. Deciphering a meal. *Daedalus,* 1972; 101: 61–82

314  Gatley A, Caraher M, Lang T. A qualitative, cross cultural examination of attitudes and behaviour in relation to cooking habits in France and Britain. *Appetite,* 2014; 75: 71–81, doi: 10.1016/j.appet.2013.12.014

315  Lang T, Caraher M. Is there a culinary skills transition? Data and debate from the UK about changes in cooking culture. *Journal of the Home Economics Institute of Australia,* 2001; 8(2): 2–14

316  Short F. *Kitchen Secrets: The Meaning of Cooking in Everyday Life.* Oxford: Berg, 2006

317  Foresight. *Tackling Obesities: Future Choices.* London: Government Office of Science, 2007

318  Anon. CSIRO to examine environmental impact of poor eating. Available at: https://foodmag.com.au/csiro-to-examine-environmental-impact-of-poor-eating/?utm_content=buffer85932&utm_medium=social&utm_source=twitter.com&utm_campaign=buffer (accessed August 10, 2016). *Food and Beverage Industry News (Australia),* May 10, 2016

319 Kennedy JF. *Special Message on Protecting the Consumer Interest*, Statement read to Congress by President John F Kennedy, Thursday, 15 March. Washington, DC: Presidential Papers, President's Office Files, Speech Files, 1962

320 Goodman D, Goodman M. Alternative food networks, in: R Kitchin and N Thrift (Eds). *International Encyclopedia of Human Geography*. Oxford: Elsevier, 2008

321 Gonzalez Fischer C, Garnett T. *Plates, Pyramids, Planet: Developments in National Healthy and Sustainable Dietary Guidelines: A State of Play Assessment*. Rome and Oxford: Food and Agriculture Organization and Food & Climate Research Network, 2016: 80

322 FAO, RUAF, City Region Food System Alliance. *Food for Cities Programme: Building Sustainable and Resilient City Region Food Systems*. Available at: www.fao.org/in-action/food-for-cities-programme/en/ (accessed October 10, 2016). Rome: Food and Agriculture Organization, 2016

# Chapter 9

# Conclusions
## Why sustainable diets matter now

## Contents

## Core arguments

The problem of sustainable diets will not go away. The issue is complex but that is not an excuse to duck it. Updating what is considered a good diet is almost inevitable. The evidence of the Western diet's damage is too strong. The world cannot afford for high carbon, high water, excess nutrient, wasteful, health-damaging diets to be the 'role model' for what is considered progress. Nor is the West's dietary impact a good role model for the developing world. We see strong arguments for setting new sustainable dietary guidelines as the new level playing field for the food system. Battles over this have already begun and are likely to continue. Uncertainties in the food system will exacerbate this. Much depends on whether the notion of sustainable diet adopted is 'lite' or 'deep', introduced firmly by consensus or suddenly in a crisis. Some argue that consumer choice will be the deciding factor. The battle for consumers' hearts and minds is already underway. We see a crucial role for interdisciplinary collaboration in that process. Food and dietary sustainability are not the intellectual property of any one discipline. Collaboration is required between the natural and social sciences, arts and culture, policy makers and providers. We find it hopeful that many organisations, people, professions, movements and some commercial companies are engaging with the transition to sustainable diets. The challenge remains awesome.

## A focus on consumption

Food and diets have become problems in the twenty-first century. This might sound strange. Surely they are not of the magnitude they were in much of the nineteenth or twentieth centuries? Nor surely in such stress as when raddled by wars and insufficiency in the pre-industrial era? Yes, they are; and greater. And they are human-made problems, often the result of deliberate political acts; sometimes the unintended consequences; some a mixture.[1-8] It is also true, however, that an optimistic picture of twentieth-century progress can be painted: more food, more people fed, greater scientific understanding. Output rose. Knowledge of food and diet's potential to cause harm and to prevent harm has grown. These are great successes. Yet the harsh truth remains that food systems now pose one of the biggest challenges facing humanity in the twenty-first century.[9, 10] The gaps between evidence, policy and behaviour are great and widening, despite the many grand reports and international conventions referred to in this book.

So enormous is the challenge of tackling the six issues in Chapters 3–8 that one could conclude they are collectively beyond control. Daunting, yes, but face them we must. A motivation for this book was to encourage coordinated action and policy engagement. The old reflex on raising food production. This is the policy comfort zone. Food problems? Just produce more and let markets sort it all out. The banking crisis of 2007–8 and ensuing Great Recession rekindled a neo-Malthusian fear that there will not be enough food to feed the 9 or 10 billion people anticipated to be on the planet by 2050 or 2100; that a 'perfect storm' is on its way; that technologists must be given more freedom to alter the biosphere (not just genes). The core thread running through those analyses is that humanity must above all increase food output. 'More from less' has been the cry in the name of sustainable intensification.[11-14] In fact, sustainable intensification can be taken in different directions.[13] It can mean more people fed per hectare or more output as measured by profit and turnover; a more plant-based diet or more resources going into feeding inefficient meat-oriented diets; pushing nature further off the field or bringing biodiversity into the field.

Our argument is that more attention needs to be given to consumption in this overall problem of the unsustainability of the food system. A predominantly productionist focus tends to ignore the crucial dynamics driven by consumption. It has also ignored the complexity of social change. Simply on the grounds that the world is urbanised, with town-dwellers fed by others, it makes sense to consider what responsible consumption looks like. We need to debate once more what a good diet is. That is why the notion of sustainable diets is so important. Not only does it reconnect production with consumption but it also suggests that consumption, just as much as production, needs to be recalibrated to deliver a clearer approach to whatever is meant by 'sustainability'.

For some, sustainability is just a shorthand for the environment alone. But that turns the clock back to pre-Brundtland, ignoring society and economy in her terms. The environment inevitably connects with other dimensions of existence. That is why this book used the six-heading approach to sustainable food systems proposed by the UK's Sustainable Development Commission: quality, social values, environment, economy, health and governance.[15] These bring some order, clarity and focus, without downplaying the complexity and connections. Environment is shaped by society. Notions of quality are altered by economic status. Gender issues appear almost everywhere, as do inequalities. Far from being separate, the six headings show the need for policy to 'cross-pollinate', even though in reality policy makers focus on issue by issue. Figure 9.1 schematically represents the six discrete but overlapping issues. This provides a useful heuristic, a working model with which to explore and order the complexity of factors that nestle under the deceptively simple term 'sustainable diet'.

The question at the heart of this book remains at the end as it was at the start: what is a good diet for the twenty-first century?[16, 17] This question runs throughout the vast edifice of science and policy papers, books and reports that we have reviewed. They reinforce why and how sustainable diets remain one of

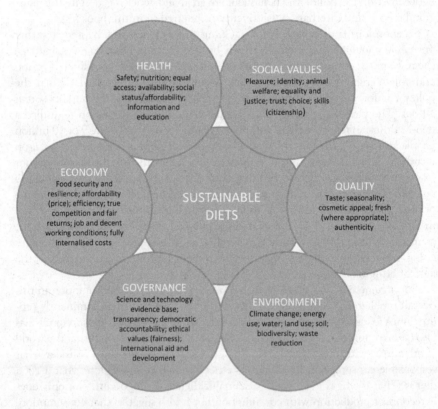

*Figure 9.1* The key features and determinants of a sustainable diet

Source: the authors.

society's great challenges. The twentieth-century success of producing and being able to consume more food than ever before has come at a cost for public health in terms of the rise in obesity and non-communicable diseases, for the environment in terms of loss of biodiversity and loss or pollution of other natural resources such as water and land with associated social injustices, and challenges for economics and food policy. The twentieth-century food fest looks ragged.

The sustainable diet challenge was identified in academic terms in the 1980s by Joan Dye Gussow and Kate Clancy in papers outlining the need for dietary guidelines to consider diets not only for public health but also for preserving natural resources. Although policy makers and industry have been grappling with aspects of sustainable diets since the early 2000s, and academics for longer, not enough has emerged to shift mass consumption into a sustainable diet transition. Chapter 8 outlined important opening forays such as the guidelines from Brazil's Department of Health and Sweden's National Food Administration or WWF's Livewell and Barilla's Double Pyramid. Many such pioneers have offered early warnings and signposts but the world has not yet realised the great Transition itself.

The UN Sustainable Development Goals provide an overdue intergovernmental framework, but more detail and coordination is needed at national, city and local levels. This is where sustainable dietary guidelines would be so useful to help the public engage with the great Transition. Such guidelines can translate the SDG aspirations into dietary terms. Without changing food consumption, the UN's SDGs will not be fully delivered. That is why we propose the $SDG^2$ strategy.

## The problem is real (not a conspiracy to undermine rights or choice)

Why is the transition to sustainable diets not happening if the evidence for change is overwhelming? We have pointed to sources of resistance. Sustainable diets can be dismissed as restrictive, controlling, rolling back the joys of untrammelled choice, implying the unwelcome charms of a nanny corporation or state. It can also always be parked with the call for more research (if in doubt, always call for more research). In our view, such views are understandable but self-defeating. They are rationalisations of the status quo, yet the status quo is already causing us humans damage, let alone the ecosystems on which we depend. Enough is known to act. Our view is that the appeal for sustainable diets probably ultimately comes down to self-interest. The Benthamite case of good governance being the pursuit of 'the greatest happiness of the greatest number' can be updated. Modern ecological public health thinking offers a more sophisticated moral compass than simply the polarity of pain versus pleasure. In this post-Darwinian world, ecological thinking based on myriad interactions is essential. It is in people's own interests to ensure their grandchildren eat, that the climate does not displace hundreds of millions of people, that soil is nurtured to be in a fit state to maintain life, that desertification is kept at bay, that humans don't raise life-giving grains only to feed nearly half to animals in conditions where they become vectors of human ill-health, and so on. This is more than pleasure versus pain. It is why we have located sustainable diets as part of the pursuit of One Health,[18-20] and Ecological Public Health.[21, 22] Sustainable diets are a vehicle for planetary and social justice.

The problem of how to effect the transition is a real one for society and politics. Despite the twentieth-century food system's successes, we now know it is a fantasy that consumers can eat what they like *ad libitum* (unchecked) while maintaining health and preserving natural resources. It is abundantly clear how the modern food system has an impact on health, the environment, social justice, food quality and financial costs. It is time to face facts.

To recap, worldwide, obesity has nearly doubled since 1980. Globally, there are now more than two and a half times more obese and overweight people than there are undernourished people. In 2014, more than 2.1 billion people – nearly 30% of the global population – were overweight or obese.[23] There is a global trend towards over-consumption of energy (calories) even though many people remain hungry. While availability of calories per person may be peaking in developed countries, it is rising across the developing world, particularly in emerging economies like Brazil and China – hence the urgency and rationality of those governments for recalibrating dietary advice to lower meat consumption and to simplify intake.[24-26] Once considered a high-income country problem, the number of obese or overweight people is now increasing in low- and middle-income countries, especially in urban areas. Obesity harms human health and contributes to rising healthcare costs and lost productivity. The healthcare and economic costs are linked and enormous. In 2012, the global economic cost of obesity was estimated to be around $2 trillion, roughly equivalent to the global cost of smoking or armed conflict. Non-communicable diseases (NCDs) kill more than 38 million people each year, among which three quarters – 28 million – occur in low- and middle-income countries.[27]

Alongside the problems related to over-consumption of energy, undernutrition remains significant. While the modern food system generates enough food energy for the global population of over 7 billion, it does not deliver adequate and affordable nutrition for all. In 2014, 795 million people (11% of the world's population) remained undernourished due to the inability to obtain sufficient food to meet their dietary energy requirements, and about 2 billion people or 30% of the world's population are affected by deficiencies of micronutrients, in particular that of vitamin A, iron and iodine.[28] More than half the global population is inadequately or inappropriately nourished, once the combined burdens of hunger, micronutrient deficiencies and obesity are taken into account.

In addition to these well-recognised problems of public health, the food system today is also destroying the environment upon which future food production depends. It contributes to some 20–30% of anthropogenic greenhouse gas emissions, and is the leading cause of deforestation, land use and biodiversity loss. It accounts for 70% of all human water use and is a major source of water pollution. Unsustainable fishing practices deplete the seas of stocks of species we consume and also cause wider disruption to the marine environment. At the same time, the impacts of climatic and environmental change are starting to make food production more difficult and unpredictable in many regions of the world. North America and Europe consume biological resources as though they inhabit multiple planets; the USA consuming as though it inhabits five planets, Europe three.[29] The modern food system represents a major force driving the environment beyond the planet's boundaries.[30] Although the whole food system from farming through to transport, processing and manufacture, retailing, cooking and waste disposal contribute to these problems, it is at the agricultural stage where the greatest impacts tend to occur. Both crop and livestock production generate environmental costs and during recent years the focus of attention has fallen particularly on the latter. The rearing of livestock for meat, eggs and milk generates some 14.5% of total global GHG emissions and uses 70% of agricultural land, including a third of arable land needed also for crop production. Grazing livestock and less directly the production of feed crops are together the main agricultural drivers of deforestation, biodiversity loss and land degradation.

On top of these health and environmental problems, the modern food system is also a source of considerable social injustice – both globally and within countries and localities. Despite overall advances in access to affordable food in many countries, low-income households have been left behind. While most people in high-income countries such as the USA, Canada and the UK are spending less than ever on food as a proportion of their household budget, some low-income families may be spending a third or more of their budget on food. Although food prices fell consistently from the 1970s, a rise in prices since 2006 has combined with rising housing and energy prices to push many low-income households closer to crisis. The cost of healthy foods in particular has risen more than less healthy options. A squeeze in incomes and rising costs of living means those on low incomes trade down towards less nutritious diets high in fat, sugar and salt. Food banks have become institutionalised in wealthy countries, replacing social welfare.[31-33] The proliferation of supermarkets has meant most people in rich countries have more access to nutritious food, but many low income areas suffer from relatively restricted access to nutritious, affordable food. Obesity also differs by socio-economic status. In rich countries, women with more education and a higher income are less likely to become obese, while in the poorest countries the opposite is the case with richer women at the highest risk of obesity. Although obesity in poorer countries is no longer solely a condition of wealthy people, the burden of overweight remains concentrated among wealthier people in low- and middle-income countries.

Although food production and distribution contribute huge economic value both at national and international level, the distribution of that value is not even. Many of the world's 1.3 billion smallholders and landless agricultural workers live on or below the poverty line. In rich countries such as the UK and USA, the farmer and primary producers' share of the consumer spend on food is small – 10% or less. Throughout much of the food system, wages are low and work insecure with much of the labour involved in bringing food to our plates now employed off the land in urban areas. Working conditions can be poor worldwide, both on and off the land, involving a surprising and shocking state of slavery in some parts of the global food system. All of this helps to keep the price of food commodities down, suiting processors off the land, yet workers throughout the food system struggle with the costs of living. The flow of power and profits is off the land and down extended supply chains, with ever more economic actors taking a cut and vying for influence.[34, 35]

The price of food fails to convey the true costs of production in terms of returns to primary producers and labourers' wages while maintaining high profits elsewhere in the food system. Food makes a lot of money for some. The price of food also fails to convey the costs of production in terms of the environment as well as the costs of consumption in terms of public health, and the costs of both production and the burden of waste. Although these costs remain largely hidden from the shopping basket, they must be paid for somewhere, such as, for example, in healthcare costs and food subsidies. Information about diet and health has become more widely available since the 1980s, but the impact of what we eat on the environment and issues of social justice is regrettably patchy. Some consumers have a desire to do the right thing, as evidenced, for example, by the growth of fair trade produce but, for the most part, consumers remain in the dark on food's impacts through no fault of their own.

Given the huge hidden health and environmental costs embedded in the food system, consumers are living on borrowed time. Without action, all these problems are set to become acute. As the global population increases, urbanises and becomes wealthier, people are demanding more energy-rich and resource-intensive foods, including animal foods, potentially increasing energy intake and the risk of obesity and non-communicable diseases (NCDs), as well as further damaging the environment and challenging access to healthy, affordable food for poor people, including the world's smallholders, many of whom are at risk of losing their land and livelihoods. At the same time, technological advances, business and economic changes and government policies are transforming the entire food system from farm to fork. Multinational businesses are increasingly influencing what is grown, how far it travels, what food products are available and hence what people eat, leading to some convergence in diets and certainly to an explosion of processed foods. Although this dietary shift brings health and welfare gains for some people, the sheer scale of these trends could well make it harder for the world to achieve several of the United Nations Sustainable Development Goals, including those on hunger, healthy lives, water management, climate change and terrestrial ecosystems.

## Need for change

The current food system from farm to fork needs to change. That is well recognised, and over time, the detail and case expands. But there is less agreement on exactly what should be done. Our suggestion is to build what we have called an SDG[2] strategy. Might improving the environmental efficiency of production generate more food with less impact? Using inputs more effectively and managing resources, the so-called 'sustainable intensification' approach, would help, but it will not be sufficient. Dietary patterns need to change too. Only when we know what such a diet looks like can production-side approaches be shifted to produce the healthy, low environmental impact food needed and can the whole food system shift in a more sustainable direction.

If sustainable diet became the goal, this would set new indicators for production. The IPCC *Fifth Assessment Report* has already highlighted the potential of demand-side changes to reduce GHG emissions from the food system, while other academics have also shown the mutual benefit that widespread adoption of healthy and sustainable dietary patterns could play in aligning health and environmental goals.[36] Instead of aiming for tonnage yield per hectare, more subtle indicators are needed such as nutrients per hectare or people fed per hectare. These reconnect the land to consumers; they align sustainable consumption to production. Output *per se* does not. The power imbalances and price signals currently distort the food system. The real goals for a better food system ought to be sustainable diets, not just fairer terms of trade. The land ought to grow more food direct for human consumption. There needs to be a reinjection of dignity in land work, and better working conditions and living wages. A sustainable diet also requires improved transport, storage and market infrastructure. Loss and waste of food throughout the food system need to be reduced, not only because this undermines food security but also because it reflects a waste of land, water and other inputs as well as unnecessary emissions and pollutants. This is a big agenda.

## What action is needed, and by whom?

Although there are good pointers, policy responses have so far been too timid at the national level. We see more vibrancy at the city region level of governance. Academics and scientists must continue to study the complexity and clarify the evidence but must engage. They can help the strong, articulate, well-informed and 'noisy' civil society pressure alongside those inside commerce who see the logic and advantage of better diet. This coalition faces resistance, of course; people lobbying and deploying delaying tactics, calling for more evidence. It was ever thus. Proponents of sustainable diets will expect that. We remain convinced, however, by the notion of sustainable diet as something around which disparate interests could agree. This is a term and goal that binds otherwise fragmented single issues. The complexity, in fact, provides unity and strength.

This is ultimately an issue that requires a policy actor to 'chair' and facilitate the Transition. Markets are too anarchic. Only democratically accountable governments ultimately have that remit and responsibility to institute new frameworks. Then let markets work. To achieve framework change sometimes means knocking heads together (politely but firmly). Sometimes, it is simply a matter of shepherding interests to go in the same direction. And it always means taking the long view. Governments (from local to global) need to demonstrate commitment to what is, at heart, a more socially just dietary future everywhere. This is an issue which can reconnect elected politicians and the machinery of government to the interests of the people.

Sustainable dietary guidelines are an essential component of a coherent twenty-first-century food policy. They provide an essential first policy step, a clear steer on how people should and could be eating at the population level. While taxes and incentives on ingredients and macronutrients could contribute to improved diets, as could developing of food policy to nourish people by, for example, paying producers to produce fruit and vegetables and grain for direct human consumption, we think that sustainable dietary guidelines should be developed as a first step. Whether one considers a hungry or obese population, it makes sense.

The academic case for sustainable diets made in this book is interdisciplinary. No one discipline holds all the answers. Sustainable diets do pose a particular challenge for nutrition scientists in particular that they cannot avoid. The focus and excitement of dietetics and nutrition in recent decades has been on the life sciences where there has been an explosion of scientific understanding since the mapping of the genome. But the social and environmental traditions of nutrition also need to come back into play. Behavioural changes to improve diet are not reducible to genomics or nutrients. Dietitians and nutritionists provide information on food and diet to individuals, communities, governments, NGOs and industry. Their potential influence as actors for the sustainable diet transition is considerable. We note there is 'professional' argument that dietetics and nutrition should not engage with wider environmental or socio-economic issues in the food system, arguing that these are beyond the various nutrition professions' remit or competence. We believe that as key advisers on food, who engage with and work in the food system, the professions cannot bury their heads in the sand over sustainable diets. The issues raised in this book alter the focus of nutrition sciences and what the professions can do.

We see this as a wonderful opportunity for interprofessional collaboration and learning. Nutrition, public health, medicine, geography and engineering have all much to say, and published reports and opinions, which show the need for effective multidisciplinary response and less working in silos. While guidelines for the public need to be simple, the complexities of sustainable diets must continue to be studied by scientists and academics. We welcome the emergence of multi-criteria, multi-factor research into sustainable diets, particularly the welcome bridge between health and environmental scientists. We note the problem of trade-offs, but caution against accepting they are inevitable too much in advance. One should aim for improvements across all fronts. It would be absurd to trade-off poor wages for low carbon, for example!

One issue which warrants clarification is the quantity of meat consistent with health, the environment, animal welfare, incomes and labour conditions. Several governments have recommended meat intakes for health, but not enough note has been taken of the environment, including land and water use, biodiversity and animal welfare. This is almost certainly a matter not just of quantity but of the mode of production. Similar questions arise for seafood; can sufficient fish be sourced sustainably, to allow equitable access for all and fairness for those whose livelihoods depend on catching it? Is this a matter of line-caught versus giant 'factory' trawler-caught methods? Alternative sources of omega-3 fatty acids also need more study to reduce risks to fish numbers and species. Similarly, for milk and dairy, not enough is known about the amounts commensurate with health, the environment and animal welfare and what alternative plant-based foods might be suitable sources of the nutrients contained in milk. Also, is, for example, all packaging bad? Packaging can help hygiene. So what is good packaging for sustainable diets?

Academics must help develop better metrics for sustainable diets. We are wary of seeking a single measurement of sustainable diet and think that multiple indicators are almost certainly appropriate. A multi-criteria approach has to be interdisciplinary and must draw across the sciences and humanities for expertise. All of this must be fed into standards for industry.

Commercial interests are divided on sustainable diets. As we have shown (in Chapters 7 and 8), there are strong lobbies against, notably from the meat and dairy sectors, but there is a really encouraging recognition in some quarters of industry that change is inevitable. The Institute of Grocery Distribution (IGD), a UK industry think-tank, highlighted the importance of sustainable diets in 2013, citing its survey that shows consumers expect industry to take the lead.[37] The Barilla Center for Food and Nutrition, created by the Italian food manufacturing company Barilla, has developed and promoted its Double Pyramid dietary guidance model to show how food choice impacts health and the environment. The multinational Unilever developed its *Sustainable Living Plan* in 2010. Also, in an unusual move, Mars recommended in 2016 that some of its processed food products should be consumed only once a week due to their fat, sugar and salt content, and the company said it will distinguish between occasional and everyday foods on its packs and website.[38] These moves would have been unthinkable two decades ago. Sceptics might see these actions as brand protection, 'green/health-wash' or pre-empting legal attack. We see them also as signs companies read the writing on the wall.

Consumers, too, will need to change. Sustainable diet guidelines should help them, but putting the onus on consumers alone is unrealistic. A sizeable section of the consuming public is simply not interested; others are in the dark or in denial; but others are waiting for someone else to do something or take a lead.[39] The plethora of nutrition and healthy eating information over the years has helped to make consumers sceptical, making them continue to eat as they like with food choice largely governed by price and taste. Dietary behaviour change for progressive ends is often said to be difficult to achieve, yet diets have changed considerably in Western countries since the 1960s and they are changing now in emerging economies. To date, efforts to encourage more sustainable eating have largely focused on consumer education, branding, some labelling and suggestions of abstinence such as vegetarianism and 'meat-free days', but with limited success.

They have tended to be small scale or to use the softer end of change agents.[40] Consumers purchase food typically on price, taste and habit rather than sustainability.[41] A World Resources Institute report has suggested that strategies to address these food purchasing decisions are needed and has proposed a framework in the form of a 'Shift Wheel', which involves four mechanisms for addressing dietary change behaviour: minimising disruption to change by developing sustainable dietary choices with appealing taste and packaging; selling a compelling benefit such as health or affordability; maximising awareness of sustainable food choices by, for example, advertising and retail placement; and evolving social norms by providing information and making sustainable dietary choices socially desirable.[41]

Initiatives like this make a positive contribution and they are trying to fill policy space in which it would be more efficient and effective to have simply one

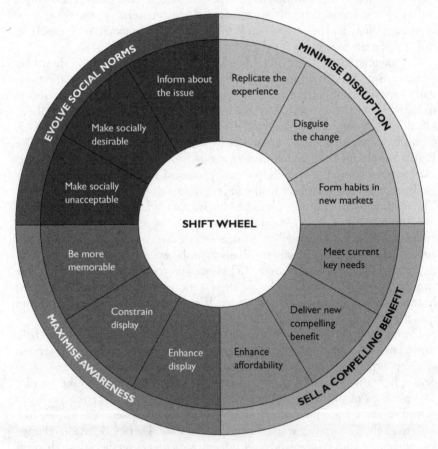

*Figure 9.2* The WRI Shift Wheel: changing consumer purchasing

Source: WRI, 2016.[41]

set of guidance for each regulatory regime, as appropriate. If city regions want to produce these and can use them effectively, then great. If it can be done nationally or, as the Nordic Council is beginning to, at the international level, even better. The goal is to provide the public with new, simple, appropriate 'rules' for everyday eating – in short, sustainable dietary guidelines. What is needed is effort to pull all the experimentation and forays in the same direction and under one common umbrella.

## The core messages of a sustainable diet

A sustainable diet is simply a good diet for human and ecosystem health. But what would a sustainable diet look like? Would it be different in different parts of the world? Are there principles that can then be drilled down into culturally appropriate foods and diets for different populations? The broad characteristics of a diet consistent with public health and of low environmental impact are already clear. They have been summarised by the Food Climate Research Network, University of Oxford.[40, 42] It is a diet that:

- provides diversity – with a wide variety of foods eaten;
- achieves balance between energy intake and energy needs;
- is based around minimally processed tubers and whole grains, legumes; fruits and vegetables, particularly those that are field grown, robust (less prone to spoilage) and less requiring of rapid and more energy-intensive transport modes;
- includes meat, if eaten in moderate amounts and all animal parts consumed;
- includes dairy products or alternatives (for example, fortified milk substitutes and other foods rich in calcium and micronutrients) consumed in moderation;
- includes unsalted seeds and nuts;
- includes small quantities of fish and aquatic products sourced from certified fisheries;
- includes very limited consumption of foods high in fat, sugar or salt and low in micronutrients (for example, crisps, confectionery, sugary drinks);
- includes oils and fats with a beneficial omega 3:6 ratio such as rapeseed and olive oil;
- includes tap water in preference to other beverages, particularly soft drinks.

These broad principles can be used as a basis for developing sustainable dietary guidelines for the public and that, very importantly, could also help to inform policy and create more agreement on ways to shift the whole food system in a more sustainable direction. While broad principles can be the basis for sustainable dietary guidelines in every country, detail can and should be adjusted according to local cultural preferences.

Many high-income countries have healthy eating food-based dietary guidelines, although there is a dearth of them in most low-income countries. Existing food-based dietary guidelines offer a starting point for developing sustainable dietary guidelines that align public health and environmental goals and social justice. Moreover, even where sustainability is not mentioned in dietary guidelines, much of the advice offered in food-based dietary guidelines such as, for example, to increase consumption of fruits, vegetables and whole grains, to limit red and processed meat consumption and to maintain energy balance, is also likely to reduce environmental impacts, if those are already high in mainstream dietary patterns. The first 2009 Swedish guidelines are a role model.

## The last word on sustainable dietary guidelines

As we summarised in Chapter 8, clear policy direction is emerging from science but it is not, as yet, adopted or pursued by governments, leaving industry and consumers rudderless. A largely plant-based diet has advantages for health and the environment. Most scientific reviews point to the high environmental impact of meat and dairy, and recommend reducing intake or eating meat in moderation, but the advice is not quantified and, where maximum amounts are given, they are similar to those given in healthy eating guidelines. Further research is needed to quantify a level of meat consumption consistent with health and the environment. The 2014 Brazilian guidelines are distinct in emphasising the social and economic aspects of sustainable consumption, advising people to avoid ultra-processed food that undermines traditional food cultures and to be wary of advertising, to develop cooking skills and to make food and eating an important part of life. We welcome this focus, noting the second 2015 Swedish guidelines also led on culture. Further research is also needed on the amounts of dairy foods consistent with health and the environment and the role of alternative sources of the key nutrients in these foods. Advice on fish in guidelines with a sustainability dimension is usually similar to healthy eating guidelines, i.e. once or twice a week, which is not sustainable for the entire global population in the context of current fish sourcing practice. Again, more research attention needs to be given to sustainable, including non-fish, sources of omega-3 fatty acids.

Most food-based dietary guidelines, both those incorporating sustainability and those that do not, are led by the Ministry of Health or its equivalent and most of the external experts tend to be from the fields of nutrition and public health. Guidelines should certainly be owned by government but more ministries should be involved in development and more experts from a wider variety of fields such as, for example, agriculture, economics, environmental science, geography and social science, should be involved. This process requires new institutional structures such as standing commissions or expert panels. It should not be left to whim.[42]

Sustainable dietary guidelines should:

- Be established in every country of the world

  - according to the same basic principles, but
  - with differences in detail to reflect the local context and culture.

- Be developed in two stages,

  - first, involving a wide range of independent expertise spanning health, the environment, social science and economics in their development;
  - second, involving consultation with civil society organisations and industry but only after development by independent experts.

- Be owned by government and championed by more than one government department or agency.
- Be disseminated to the public, health professionals, consumer organisations and those working in the food sector. Everyone should know about them.
- Be accompanied by information highlighting the links between food, health, the environment, social justice and economics so that people understand the problems of current dietary patterns and the need for dietary change.
- Recognise current dietary patterns and be realistic in their goals yet ambitious in promoting clear dietary change.
- Include clear guidance on:

  - limiting meat consumption in high-income countries where consumption has plateaued;
  - moderating meat consumption in countries where consumption is increasing;
  - focusing on dietary diversity, including some meat consumption, in low-income countries, while
  - explaining the rationale for health and the environment and
  - how to make dietary changes that are appealing and accessible, taking context into account.

- Highlight the environmental impact of excessive consumption of food energy and food waste.
- Provide guidance on food shopping, encourage some home or community growing, safe and energy efficient food preparation and highlight the importance of food planning and the social and cultural importance of food in lives.
- Be used as the first step to develop and implement food policies, such as public sector procurement, school and hospital meals, industry standards and advertising regulations. Links between food policies and SDGs should be clearly visible.

# References

1  Kent G. *The Political Economy of Hunger: The Silent Holocaust*. New York: Praeger, 1984

2  Russell SA. *Hunger: An Unnatural History*. New York: Basic Books, 2005

3  Conquest R. *The Harvest of Sorrow: Soviet Collectivization and the Terror-Famine*. London: Hutchinson, 1986

4  George S. *How the Other Half Dies: The Real Reasons for World Hunger*. Harmondsworth: Penguin, 1976

5  Haggard S, Noland M. *Famine in North Korea: Markets, Aid, and Reform* (foreword by Amartya Sen). New York: Columbia University Press, 2007

6  Mukerjee M. *Churchill's Secret War: The British Empire and the Ravaging of India During World War II*. New York: Basic Books, 2010

7  Smil V. China's great famine: 40 years later. BMJ, 1999; 319: 1619–21

8  Woodham Smith CBF. *The Great Hunger: Ireland, 1845–9*. London: Hamish Hamilton, 1962

9  UNEP. *Avoiding Future Famines: Strengthening the Ecological Basis of Food Security through Sustainable Food Systems*. Nairobi: United Nations Environment Programme, 2012

10  UNEP, Nellemann C, MacDevette M, et al. *The Environmental Food Crisis: The Environment's Role in Averting Future Food Crises*. A UNEP rapid response assessment. Arendal, Norway: United Nations Environment Programme/GRID-Arendal, 2009

11  Buckwell A, Nordang Uhre A, Williams A, et al. *Sustainable Intensification of European Agriculture*. Brussels: RISE Foundation, 2014

12  Garnett T, Appleby M, Balmford A, et al. Sustainable intensification in agriculture: premises and policies. *Science*, 2013; 341(6141): 33–34

13  Garnett T, Godfray C. *Sustainable Intensification in Agriculture: Navigating a Course Through Competing Food System Priorities*. Oxford: Food Climate Research Network and the Oxford Martin Programme on the Future of Food, University of Oxford, 2012

14  Godfray HCJ, Garnett T. Food security and sustainable intensification. *Philosophical Transactions of the Royal Society B*, 2014; 369: 2012.0273

15  Sustainable Development Commission. *Looking Forward, Looking Back: Sustainability and UK Food Policy 2000–2011*. Available at: www.sd-commission.org.uk/publications.php?id=1187 (accessed July 8, 2016). London: Sustainable Development Commission, 2011

16  Gussow JD. Dietary guidelines for sustainability: twelve years later. *Journal of Nutrition Education*, 1999; 31: 194–200

17  Gussow JD, Clancy KL. Dietary guidelines for sustainability. *Journal of Nutrition Education*, 1986; 18(1): 1–5

18  Bresalier M, Cassidy A, Woods A. One health in history, in: Zinsstag J, Schelling E, Waltner-Toews D, et al. (Eds). *One Health: The Theory and Practice of Integrated Health Approaches*. Wallingford: CABI International, 2015: Chap. 1

19  Wallace RG, Bergmanm L, Kock R, et al. The dawn of Structural One Health: a new science tracking disease emergence along circuits of capital. *Social Science and Medicine*, 2015; 129: 68–77

20  Zinsstag J, Schelling E, Waltner-Toews D, et al. (Eds). *One Health: The Theory and Practice of Integrated Health Approaches*. Wallingford: CABI Publishing, 2015

21 Lang T, Rayner G. Ecological public health: the 21st century big idea? *BMJ*, 2012; 345(e5466)

22 Rayner G, Lang T. *Ecological Public Health: Reshaping the Conditions for Good Health.* Abingdon: Routledge/Earthscan, 2012

23 Dobbs R, Sawers C, Thompson F, *et al. Overcoming Obesity: An Initial Economic Analysis.* Discussion paper. McKinsey Global Institute, 2014

24 National Health and Family Planning Commission of China. Announcement of goal to reduce meat consumption by 50%. Available at: http://mp.weixin.qq.com/s?__biz =MzAxODEwNzYzOA==&mid=2650236377&idx=1&sn=54b06cf4ab6cf2f71a6504 c9ca32df59 (accessed July 19, 2016). Beijing: National Health and Family Planning Commission of China, 2016

25 Ministry of Health (Brazil). *Guia Alimentar para a População Brasileira.* Brasilia: Ministério da Saúde, 2014

26 Ministry of Health (Brazil). *Dietary Guidelines for the Brazilian Population:* Available at: http://189.28.128.100/dab/docs/portaldab/publicacoes/guia_alimentar_populacao_ ingles.pdf (accessed November 9, 2015). Brazilia Ministry of Health, 2014: 80

27 World Health Organization. *Global Status Report on Noncommunicable Diseases 2014.* Geneva: World Health Organization, 2014

28 FAO, IFAD, WFP. *The State of Food Insecurity in the World 2014: Strengthening the Enabling Environment for Food Security and Nutrition.* Rome: FAO, 2014

29 Lang T, Barling D. Nutrition and sustainability: an emerging food policy discourse. *Proceedings of the Nutrition Society*, 2013; 72(01): 1–12

30 Rockström J, Steffen W, Noone K, *et al.* A safe operating space for humanity. *Nature*, 2009; 461(7263): 472–5

31 Garthwaite K. *Hunger Pains: Life Inside Foodbank Britain.* Bristol: Policy Press, 2016

32 Caraher M, Coveney J (Eds). *Food Poverty and Insecurity: International Food Inequalities.* Cham (Switzerland): Springer, 2015

33 Loopstra R, Reeves A, Taylor-Robinson D, *et al.* Austerity, sanctions, and the rise of food banks in the UK. *British Medical Journal*, 2015; 350(1775)

34 Howard PH. *Concentration and Power in the Food System: Who Controls What We Eat?* London: Bloomsbury, 2016

35 Burch D, Lawrence G (Eds). *Supermarkets and Agri-food Supply Chains.* Cheltenham: Edward Elgar, 2007

36 IPCC. *Climate Change 2014: Synthesis Report.* Geneva: Intergovernmental Panel on Climate Change, 2014

37 IGD ShopperVista, Arnold H, Pickard T. *Sustainable Diets: Helping Shoppers.* Letchmore Heath: IGD, 2013

38 BBC News. Dolmio and Uncle Ben's Firm Mars Advises Limit on Products, 15 April. Available at: www.bbc.co.uk/news/uk-36051333 (accessed July 29, 2016). London: British Broadcasting Corporation, 2016

39 Which?, Government Office for Science, TNS BMRB. *Food System Challenges: Public Dialogue on Food System Challenges and Possible Solutions.* London: Which? and Government Office for Science, 2015

40 Gonzalez Fischer C, Garnett T. *Plates, Pyramids, Planet: Developments in National Healthy and Sustainable Dietary Guidelines: A State of Play Assessment.* Rome and Oxford: Food and Agriculture Organization and Food & Climate Research Network, 2016: 80

41  Ranganathan J, Vennard D, Waite R, *et al. Shifting Diets for a Sustainable Food Future: Creating a Sustainable Food Future, Installment Eleven.* Washington, DC: World Resources Institute, 2016

42  Garnett T. *What Is a Sustainable Diet? A Discussion Paper.* Oxford: Food & Climate Research Network, Oxford Martin School, University of Oxford, 2014: 31

# Index

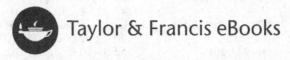

Printed in the United States
by Baker & Taylor Publisher Services

Printed in the United States
by Baker & Taylor Publisher Services